T0331836

Perspectives on Nuclear Medicine for Molecular Diagnosis and Integrated Therapy

Yuji Kuge • Tohru Shiga • Nagara Tamaki
Editors

Perspectives on Nuclear Medicine for Molecular Diagnosis and Integrated Therapy

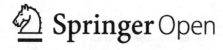

Editors
Yuji Kuge
Central Institute of Isotope Science
Hokkaido University
Department of Integrated Molecular
    Imaging
Graduate School of Medicine
Hokkaido University
Sapporo
Japan

Tohru Shiga
Department of Nuclear Medicine
Graduate School of Medicine
Hokkaido University
Sapporo
Japan

Nagara Tamaki
Department of Nuclear Medicine
Graduate School of Medicine
Hokkaido Univeristy
Sapporo
Japan

ISBN 978-4-431-55892-7   ISBN 978-4-431-55894-1   (eBook)
DOI 10.1007/978-4-431-55894-1

Library of Congress Control Number: 2015959921

Springer Tokyo Heidelberg New York Dordrecht London

Printed on acid-free paper

Springer Japan KK is part of Springer Science+Business Media (www.springer.com)

Preface

Molecular imaging aims to visualize specific molecular and cellular targets that are relevant to tissue characterization. Molecular imaging technologies have rapidly developed worldwide in recent years. Among such developments, nuclear medicine technologies using PET and SPECT have come to play important roles in quantitative analysis of biological processes in vivo and are now widely used in clinical settings. In particular, serial assessments of molecular function are commonly used for monitoring efficacy of various treatments. Prediction of treatment outcome is also an attractive field, in which nuclear medicine technologies may be applied. Indeed, a new era has arrived with the clinical use of nuclear medicine and molecular imaging for personalized medicine. However, in order to further facilitate the use of these technologies for the precise assessment of tissue function and planning of treatment strategies, significant improvement in imaging modalities, selection of optimal imaging biomarkers, and appropriate clinical applications are required.

We conducted international symposia on PET and molecular imaging in 1999, 2003, and 2009 and published the proceedings each time. Rapid progress has been made since then; therefore, we decided to organize another international symposium in order to extend our discussion on the recent progress and future perspectives on nuclear medicine in terms of molecular diagnosis and integrated therapy. Accordingly, we invited our old and new colleagues all over Japan and overseas to this latest international symposium entitled "Perspectives on Nuclear Medicine for Molecular Diagnosis and Integrated Therapy." Over 100 physicians and scientists attended our symposium for two days on July 31 to August 1, 2015. It was a great and unique opportunity to interactively exchange ideas and information among researchers on various related fields.

In order to keep a record of the symposium and share our great experiences with many specialists worldwide who are interested in these research fields, we decided to publish this new volume on the proceedings of the symposium. This volume should be helpful for understanding new advances of nuclear medicine and molecular imaging technologies and their applications to integrated medical therapy and future drug development. We sincerely hope that this volume will benefit researchers in various fields of life sciences, including those working in drug development, molecular imaging, and medical therapy, as well as physicians who utilize diagnostic imaging.

Finally, we would like to express our thanks to Drs. Masako Wada and Eriko Suzuki for their support during the preparation of the manuscripts.

Sapporo, Japan   Yuji Kuge
                                                                                  Tohru Shiga
                                                                             Nagara Tamaki

Contents

Part IV   Neurology

Part V   Oncology

Contributors

Norifumi Abo
Hokkaido University, Sapporo, Japan

M. Roselle Abraham
Johns Hopkins Medical Institute, Baltimore, MD, USA

Hiromichi Akizawa
Showa Pharmaceutical University, Machida, Japan

Yukako Asano
Hitachi, Ltd., Tokyo, Japan

Rob SB Beanlands
University of Ottawa Heart Institute, Ottawa, ON, Canada

Huiting Che
The Second Affiliated Hospital of Zhejiang University, Hangzhou, China

Ling Chen
The Second Affiliated Hospital of Zhejiang University, Hangzhou, China

Robert A. deKemp
University of Ottawa Heart Institute, Ottawa, ON, Canada

Ying Dong
The Second Affiliated Hospital of Zhejiang University, Hangzhou, China

Yutaka Eki
Hitachi General Hospital, Hitachi, Japan

Junichiro Enmi
National Cerebral and Cardiovascular Center Research Institute, Suita, Japan

Fei Feng
Hokkaido University, Sapporo, Japan

Tao Feng
Johns Hopkins Medical Institute, Baltimore, MD, USA

Sagiri Fukura
Hokkaido University, Sapporo, Japan

Hiroko Hanzawa
Hitachi, Ltd., Tokyo, Japan

Rodney J. Hicks
The University of Melbourne, Melbourne, VIC, Australia

Haruhiko Higuchi
Hitachi General Hospital, Hitachi, Japan

Makoto Higuchi
National Institute of Radiological Sciences, Chiba, Japan

Kenji Hirata
Hokkaido University, Sapporo, Japan

Masanori Ichise
National Institute of Radiological Sciences, Chiba, Japan

Kana Ide
Ehime University, Matsuyama, Japan

Satoshi Iguchi
National Cerebral and Cardiovascular Center Research Institute, Suita, Japan

Hidehiro Iida
National Cerebral and Cardiovascular Center Research Institute, Suita, Japan

Takayoshi Ishimori
Kyoto University, Kyoto, Japan

Hayato Ishimura
Ehime University, Matsuyama, Japan

Kiwamu Kamiya
Hokkaido University, Sapporo, Japan

Katsuhiko Kasai
Hokkaido University, Sapporo, Japan

Chietsugu Katoh
Hokkaido University, Sapporo, Japan

Pei Yuin Keng
University of California, Los Angeles, CA, USA

Yasuyuki Kimura
National Institute of Radiological Sciences, Chiba, Japan

Chi-Lun Ko
National Taiwan University Hospital, Taipei, Taiwan

Keiji Kobashi
Hitachi, Ltd., Tokyo, Japan

Kentaro Kobayashi
Hokkaido University, Sapporo, Japan

Naoya Kondo
National Cerebral and Cardiovascular Center Research Institute, Suita, Japan

Kazuhiro Koshino
National Cerebral and Cardiovascular Center Research Institute, Suita, Japan

Naoki Kubo
Hokkaido University, Sapporo, Japan

Yuji Kuge
Hokkaido University, Sapporo, Japan

Norihito Kuno
Hitachi, Ltd., Tokyo, Japan

Osamu Manabe
Hokkaido University, Sapporo, Japan

Naomi Manri
Hitachi, Ltd., Tokyo, Japan

Lidia Matesic
ANSTO Life Sciences, Sydney, NSW, Australia

Masao Miyagawa
Ehime University, Matsuyama, Japan

Teruhito Mochizuki
Ehime University, Matsuyama, Japan

Nobutoku Motomura
Toshiba Medical Systems Co Ltd., Otawara, Japan

Jyoji Nakagawara
National Cerebral and Cardiovascular Center Research Institute, Suita, Japan

Yuji Nakamoto
Kyoto University, Kyoto, Japan

Ken-ichi Nishijima
Hokkaido University, Sapporo, Japan

Masaharu Nishimura
Hokkaido University, Sapporo, Japan

Yoshihiro Nishiyama
Kagawa University, Kagawa, Japan

Yoshiko Nishiyama
Ehime University, Matsuyama, Japan

Hiroshi Ohira
Hokkaido University, Sapporo, Japan

Kazue Ohkura
Health Sciences University of Hokkaido, Sapporo, Japan

Shozo Okamoto
Hokkaido University, Sapporo, Japan

Noriko Oyama-Manabe
Hokkaido University Hospital, Sapporo, Japan

Wensheng Pan
The Second Affiliated Hospital of Zhejiang University, Hangzhou, China

Giancarlo Pascali
ANSTO Life Sciences, Sydney, NSW, Australia

Mamoru Sakakibara
Hokkaido University, Sapporo, Japan

Takeshi Sakamoto
Hitachi, Ltd., Tokyo, Japan

Takahiro Sato
Hokkaido University, Sapporo, Japan

Thomas H. Schindler
Johns Hopkins Medical Institute, Baltimore, MD, USA

Maxim Sergeev
University of California, Los Angeles, CA, USA

Tohru Shiga
Hokkaido University, Sapporo, Japan

Hitoshi Shimada
National Institute of Radiological Sciences, Chiba, Japan

Yoichi Shimizu
Hokkaido University, Sapporo, Japan

Eku Shimosegawa
Osaka University, Suita, Japan

Chiaki Sugano
Hitachinaka General Hospital, Hitachinaka, Japan

Tetsuya Suhara
National Institute of Radiological Sciences, Chiba, Japan

Akihiro Suzuki
Hitachi General Hospital, Hitachi, Japan

Atsuro Suzuki
Hitachi, Ltd., Tokyo, Japan

Wataru Takeuchi
Hitachi, Ltd., Tokyo, Japan

Yasuyuki Taki
Tohoku University, Sendai, Japan

Nagara Tamaki
Hokkaido University, Sapporo, Japan

Rami Tashiro
Ehime University, Matsuyama, Japan

Takashi Temma
National Cerebral and Cardiovascular Center Research Institute,
Suita, Japan

Mei Tian
The Second Affiliated Hospital of Zhejiang University, Hangzhou, China

Kaori Togashi
Kyoto University, Kyoto, Japan

Yuuki Tomiyama
Hokkaido University, Sapporo, Japan

Benjamin M.W. Tsui
Johns Hopkins Medical Institute, Baltimore, MD, USA

Ichizo Tsujino
Hokkaido University, Sapporo, Japan

Hiroyuki Tsutsui
Hokkaido University, Sapporo, Japan

Yuichiro Ueno
Hitachi, Ltd., Tokyo, Japan

Kikuo Umegaki
Hokkaido University, Sapporo, Japan

R. Michael van Dam
University of California, Los Angeles, CA, USA

Jizhe Wang
Johns Hopkins Medical Institute, Baltimore, MD, USA

Shiro Watanabe
Hokkaido University, Sapporo, Japan

Yen-Wen Wu
National Yang-Ming University, Taipei, Taiwan

Jingyan Xu
Johns Hopkins Medical Institute, Baltimore, MD, USA

Shiro Yamada
Hokkaido University, Sapporo, Japan

Yuka Yamamoto
Kagawa University, Kagawa, Japan

Miho Yamauchi
National Cerebral and Cardiovascular Center Research Institute, Suita, Japan

Taiga Yamaya
National Institute of Radiological Sciences, Chiba, Japan

Makoto Yamazaki
National Cerebral and Cardiovascular Center Research Institute, Suita, Japan

Keiichiro Yoshinaga
National Institute of Radiological Sciences, Chiba, Japan

Tsutomu Zeniya
National Cerebral and Cardiovascular Center Research Institute, Suita, Japan

Hong Zhang
The Second Affiliated Hospital of Zhejiang University, Hangzhou, China

Ying Zhang
The Second Affiliated Hospital of Zhejiang University, Hangzhou, China

Songji Zhao
Hokkaido University, Sapporo, Japan

Yan Zhao
Hokkaido University, Sapporo, Japan

Stefan L. Zimmerman
Johns Hopkins Medical Institute, Baltimore, MD, USA

Part I
Instrument and Data Analysis

Chapter 1
Advances in 4D Gated Cardiac PET Imaging for Image Quality Improvement and Cardiac Motion and Contractility Estimation

Benjamin M.W. Tsui, Tao Feng, Jizhe Wang, Jingyan Xu, M. Roselle Abraham, Stefan L. Zimmerman, and Thomas H. Schindler

Abstract Quantitative four-dimensional (4D) image reconstruction methods with respiratory and cardiac motion compensation are an active area of research in ECT imaging, including SPECT and PET. They are the extensions of three-dimensional (3D) statistical image reconstruction methods with iterative algorithms that incorporate accurate models of the imaging process and provide significant improvement in the quality and quantitative accuracy of the reconstructed images as compared to that obtained from conventional analytical image reconstruction methods. The new 4D image reconstruction methods incorporate additional models of the respiratory and cardiac motion of the patient to reduce image blurring due to respiratory motion and image noise of the cardiac-gated frames of the 4D cardiac-gated images. We describe respiratory motion estimation and gating method based on patient PET list-mode data. The estimated respiratory motion is applied to the respiratory gated data to reduce respiratory motion blur. The gated cardiac images derived from the list-model data are used to estimate cardiac motion. They are then used in the cardiac-gated images summing the motion-transformed cardiac-gated images for significant reduction in the gated images noise. Dual respiratory and cardiac motion compensation is achieved by combining the respiratory and cardiac motion compensation steps. The results are further significant improvements of the 4D gated cardiac PET images. The much improved gated cardiac PET image quality increases the visibility of anatomical details of the heart, which can be explored to provide more accurate estimation of the cardiac motion vector field and cardiac contractility.

Keywords 4D gated cardiac PET • 4D image reconstruction methods • Respiratory and cardiac motion estimation and compensation

B.M.W. Tsui (✉) • T. Feng • J. Wang • J. Xu • S.L. Zimmerman • T.H. Schindler
Department of Radiology, Johns Hopkins Medical Institute, Baltimore, MD, USA
e-mail: btsui1@jhmi.edu

M.R. Abraham
Department of Medicine, Johns Hopkins Medical Institute, Baltimore, MD, USA

© The Author(s) 2016   3
Y. Kuge et al. (eds.), *Perspectives on Nuclear Medicine for Molecular Diagnosis and Integrated Therapy*, DOI 10.1007/978-4-431-55894-1_1

1.1   Introduction

The development of quantitative image reconstruction in medical imaging, including emission computed tomography (ECT) and x-ray CT [1, 2], has recently shifted from three-dimensional (3D) to four-dimensional (4D), i.e., the inclusion of the time dimension. There are two major goals for this development. First is to reduce reconstructed image artifacts due to patient motion. In particular, compensation of involuntary patient motion, e.g., respiratory motion, that causes resolution loss has received much attention [3–6]. Second is to improve the temporal resolution of dynamic images for improved detection of global and regional motion abnormalities [7, 8]. An important application is gated myocardial perfusion (MP) ECT imaging. Despite extensive research in other imaging modalities over the last two decades, MP ECT, especially gated SPECT and more recently PET, has continued to be the major biomedical imaging technique for the assessment of MP in clinical practice. The potential of extracting additional quantitative information, such as abnormalities from existing data without additional clinical studies, radiation dose or discomfort to the patients, has great significance in biomedical imaging [9–13].

The long-term goal of the study is to integrate the two aforementioned goals of the current quantitative 4D imaging reconstruction methods, i.e., to improve the quality and quantitative accuracy of the 4D cardiac gated MP PET images while reducing the blurring caused by respiratory motion (RM) and cardiac motion (CM). This is in addition to compensation of other image degrading factors, e.g., statistical noise, photon attenuation and scatter, and collimator-detector blur, to improve both spatial and temporal resolution. In this work, we present the development of a data-driven RM estimation method and quantitative 4D statistical image reconstruction methods that compensate for RM and CM separately, and for dual respiratory and cardiac (R&C) motion for improved lung and cardiac PET imaging. We hypothesize that by applying a statistical 4D image reconstruction method that accurately compensates for RM and CM and other image degrading factors, we would be able to minimize image artifacts caused by the image degrading factors, improve image resolution and reduce image noise. This would result in two significant clinical benefits, i.e., (a) reduction of false positives and false negatives for improved diagnosis, and (b) reduction of imaging time and/or radiation dose to the patient.

In addition, the much improved 4D gated cardiac PET image quality increases the visibility of details of cardiac structures. The information can be explored in a feature-based motion estimation method to determine the cardiac motion vector field and cardiac contractility.

1.2 Materials and Methods

1.2.1 Data-Driven Respiratory Motion Detection and Gating Method

There are two general approaches to obtain respiratory gated PET data [14]. One is to use an external tracking device that directly measures a RM surrogate [3, 15]. The other is to derive RM information from the acquired data [16–19]. These data-driven RM detection methods can avoid the cost and effort and directly provide a surrogate RM signal. We developed two data-driven methods that estimated the RM from $^{13}NH_3$ and ^{18}F-FDG cardiac gated list-mode PET data. In Fig. 1.1a, b, the $^{13}NH_3$ images show more liver uptake than the ^{18}F-FDG images. Our data-driven method for the $^{13}NH_3$ was based on the total counts in each consecutive short segment (200–500 ms) of PET data. For the ^{18}F-FDG, RM signal was extracted based on the axial center-of-mass of the short segment PET data. Figure 1.1c shows the relative RM gating signal amplitude as a function of time obtained from the $^{13}NH_3$ list-mode data. The estimated RM signal compared well with that obtained from an external tracking device. It was used to divide the RM into multiple respiratory gates. The respiratory gated image data were used to estimate the motion vector field of the RM and incorporated in the 4D image reconstruction method to achieve motion compensation.

From the estimated RM signal in Fig. 1.1c, we divided the list-mode data into six equal-count respiratory frames, each of which is further divided into eight cardiac-gated frames using the ECG R-wave markers. The result was a full set of dual six-frame respiratory gated and eight-frame cardiac-gated dataset. We then applied the RM compensation method described in Sect. 1.2 to the six-frame respiratory-gated dataset.

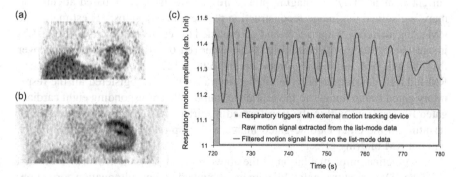

Fig. 1.1 Sample respiratory-gated projection images from (**a**) $^{13}NH_3$ cardiac and (**b**) ^{18}F-FDG cardiac images. (**c**) Comparison of a RM signal derived from an external tracking device and from the total count variation of the short segment projections of the $^{13}NH_3$ cardiac PET data

1.2.2   4D PET Image Reconstruction Methods with Attenuation, and Respiratory and Cardiac Motion Compensation

The 4D PET image reconstruction methods used in this study were applied to the respiratory-gated and cardiac-gated projection data. Specifically, for the 4D PET image reconstruction method with dual R&C motion compensation, we divided the acquired list-mode data into six equal-count respiratory frames each with eight cardiac-gated frames as described in Sect. 1.2.1. Image reconstructions without attenuation correction were performed on this dataset to estimate the RM in lung PET studies and both RM and CM in cardiac PET studies. A special feature of our method was the modeling of the RM-induced deformations of the PET image and CT-based attenuation map in RM estimation and during PET image reconstruction for accurate and artifact-free attenuation corrected PET images.

1.2.2.1   4D PET Image Reconstruction with Respiratory Motion and Attenuation Compensation

We developed a 4D PET image reconstruction method with RM and attenuation compensation to improve the image quality of ^{18}F-FDG PET images for improved small lung lesion detection [20, 21]. First, a reference respiratory gated frame was chosen from the six equal-count respiratory frames. Then the PET image at the reference frame and the RM from the reference frame to the other respiratory-gated PET frames were estimated by minimizing the Poisson log-likelihood function. As shown in Fig. 1.2, the RM-induced deformations of both the PET image and CT-based attenuation map were modeled in the RM estimation and during PET image reconstruction. Our method is applicable to respiratory-gated PET data from current clinical PET/CT imaging procedures with only one CT-based attenuation map. We solved the image reconstruction problem in two steps: (1) estimated the RM using an iterative approach, and (2) modeled the estimated RM in a 4D OS-EM image reconstruction algorithm [21] that achieved 6 ~ 10 times acceleration over the 4D ML-EM algorithms proposed by others [22, 23]. The final estimated RM-induced deformations were applied to transform and registered all the respiratory gated frame images to the reference frame. The corresponding eight cardiac-gated frames from within the transformed respiratory-gated frames were summed resulting in the eight cardiac-gated image with respiratory compensation, that is, without RM blurring effect.

  In a practical implementation of the above method [24], the RM was estimated from the 4D respiratory- gated PET images obtained without attenuation correction. The estimated RM was used in the 4D image reconstruction shown in Fig. 1.2 without further update. It provided respiratory-gated attenuation effect that matches the respiratory-gated PET images for accurate attenuation compensation.

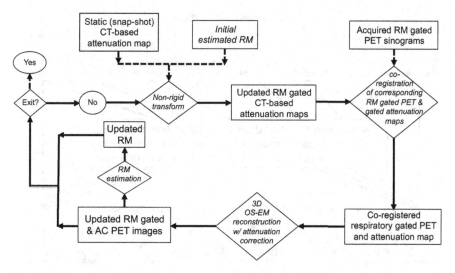

Fig. 1.2 A flowchart of the 4D image reconstruction method with RM and attenuation compensation. A snap-shot CT image was acquired from which a static attenuation map was derived. A reference respiratory gated frame was chosen. The updated PET image at the reference frame and the RM from the reference frame to the other respiratory-gated PET frames were jointly estimated by minimizing the log-likelihood function

1.2.2.2   4D Image Reconstruction with Cardiac Motion Compensation

In CM compensation, a reference frame was chosen from the eight-frame cardiac-gated images. As shown in Fig. 1.3, a B-spline non-rigid transformation and registration was applied to each cardiac-gated image and registered it to the reference frame and summed. The procedure was repeated at different cardiac-gated frames in the cardiac cycle to form the CM compensated gated cardiac image set.

1.2.2.3   4D Image Reconstruction with Dual Respiratory and Cardiac Motion Compensation

The 4D image reconstruction with dual R&C motion compensation was achieved by combining the RM and CM compensation described in Sects. 1.2.2.1 and 1.2.2.2. After estimating the accurate RM and respiratory gated attenuation maps based on Sect. 1.2.2.1, 48-frame dual R&C gated images were obtained. For each cardiac gate, the RM compensation described in Sect. 1.2.2.1 was used. The result was RM compensated cardiac-gated images. Cardiac motion compensation was achieved by applying the same approach in Sect. 1.2.2.2. The resultant eight-frame gated cardiac images shown in Fig. 1.3 thus included both RM and CM compensation.

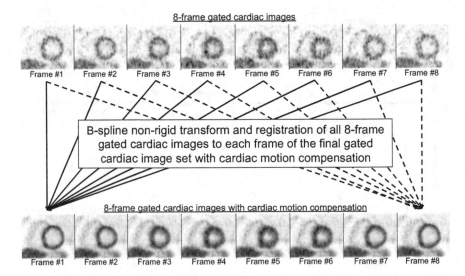

Fig. 1.3 In the CM compensation, a B-spline non-rigid transformation and registration was applied to each cardiac-gated image and registered it to the reference frame and summed

1.2.3 Evaluation of the 4D PET Image Reconstruction with Respiratory and Attenuation Compensation

We evaluated the 4D image reconstruction method with respiratory and attenuation compensation to two clinical applications. They were the detection of small lung lesions and the improvement of image quality in gated cardiac PET images. In the lung lesion detection study, we used realistic simulated 4D respiratory gated lung PET projection data. In the gated cardiac study, patient data from a ^{13}NH$_3$ MP PET study and a ^{18}F-FDG cardiac PET study were used. The goal was to assess the reduction of image resolution from blurring due to RM.

1.2.3.1 Evaluation Using Realistic Simulated PET Study with Small Lung Lesions

We evaluated the 4D PET image reconstruction with respiratory and attenuation compensation method using a realistic Monte Carlo (MC) simulated PET dataset from the 4D XCAT (eXtended CArdiac Torso) phantom [25]. The 4D XCAT phantom is an extension of the 4D NCAT (Nurbs-based CArdiac Torso) phantom [26], which provides realistic models of the anatomical structures of the entire human body based on the visible human data [27]. In addition, the 4D XCAT phantom includes realistic models of normal RM based on respiratory-gated CT data [28], and normal cardiac motion based on tagged MRI data. The cardiac motion model in the new 4D XCAT is based on state-of-the-art high-resolution cardiac-gated CT and tagged MRI data [29]. A 4D activity distribution phantom that modeled the uptake of the PET tracer in the different organs and a corresponding 4D attenuation coefficient distribution phantom that modeled the attenuation of different organs at the 511 keV photon energy were generated based on the 4D XCAT phantom. In addition, three small lung lesions with increased activity uptakes were inserted at different locations in the lung. The 4D activity distribution also served as the truth in the quantitative evaluation study.

Realistic respiratory-gated PET projection data were generated from the 4D activity and attenuation distributions using a combined SimSET [30] and GATE [31] MC simulation software that took advantage of the high efficiency of the former in computing the photon transport in the voxelized phantom and the ability of the latter to model the complex detector geometry and imaging characteristics of a clinical GE PET system [32]. The 4D PET image reconstruction method with RM and attenuation compensation was applied to the simulated RM-gated projection data. The results were compared to those obtained with conventional 3D and 4D image reconstruction methods without motion compensation.

1.2.3.2   Evaluation Using Data from Clinical Gated Cardiac PET Studies

We also evaluated the clinical efficacy of the 4D image reconstruction method with RM and attenuation compensation using clinical $^{13}NH_3$ MP PET and ^{18}F-FDG cardiac PET data. A GE Discovery VCT (RX) PET/CT system was used in the patient studies. Prior to the PET scan, a low-dose CT scan was acquired from the patient. In the $^{13}NH_3$ MP PET study, ~370 MBq of $^{13}NH_3$ was infused intravenously as a bolus over 10 s. List-mode PET data were acquired for 20 min. In the ^{18}F-FDG cardiac PET study of a different patient, ~370 MBq of ^{18}F-FDG was administered through IV injection. A list-mode PET data acquisition was performed ~60 min post injection. The 4D image reconstruction method with RM and attenuation compensation as described in Sect. 1.2.1 were applied to the acquired list-mode data. The resultant MP PET and cardiac PET images were compared to those obtained with the conventional image reconstruction method without RM compensation. Specifically, they were evaluated for improved lung lesion detection from the reduction of resolution loss due to RM blur.

1.2.4   Evaluation of the 4D PET Image Reconstruction Method with Dual Respiratory and Cardiac Motion Compensation

The evaluation of the 4D PET image reconstruction method with dual R&C motion compensation was performed on the same clinical $^{13}NH_3$ MP PET and ^{18}F-FDG cardiac PET datasets used in Sect. 1.2.3.2. Here, the goal was to assess the improvement of the quality of the gated cardiac PET images in terms of image resolution and image noise.

1.3 Results and Discussion

1.3.1 Improvement of Small Lung Lesion Detection with Respiratory and Attenuation Compensation

We evaluated the 4D PET image reconstruction with respiratory and attenuation compensation method using a realistic simulated PET dataset from the 4D XCAT phantom [19, 20] and the Monte Carlo (MC) method as described in Sect. 1.2.3. The method included RM detection using the data-driven gating method as described in Sect. 1.2.1. The results are shown in Fig. 1.4. The activity distribution of the 4D XCAT phantom with three small lung lesions is shown in Fig. 1.4a. The reconstructed PET images without RM compensation in Fig. 1.4b show the resolution loss due to RM blur. Also the reconstructed images with RM and attenuation compensation using the known RM from the 4D XCAT phantom (Fig. 1.4c) and using the estimated RM (Fig. 1.4d) were compared. The results indicate the effectiveness of the RM estimation method and the 4D image reconstruction

(a)   (b)   (c)   (d)

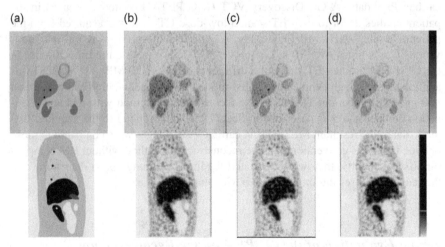

Fig. 1.4 Results from a simulation study to evaluate the 4D PET image reconstruction with respiratory and attenuation compensation for improved lung lesion detection. A realistic MC simulated PET dataset from the 4D XCAT phantom was used. A sample (*Top row*) coronal slice and (*Bottom row*) sagittal slice through the lung showing three small lung nodules. (**a**) Activity distribution of the 4D XCAT phantom. Reconstructed images obtained from using (**b**) the 3D ML-EM method with no RM compensation, and the 4D ML-EM method (**c**) with modeling of the true RM from the 4D XCAT phantom, and (**d**) with the RM estimation described in Sect. 1.2.1

method with RM and attenuation compensation to reduce resolution loss due to RM blur and to improve small lung lesion detection in lung PET images.

1.3.2   Improvement of Gated Cardiac PET Images with Respiratory Motion and Attenuation Compensation

We applied the 4D image reconstruction method with RM and attenuation compensation to the clinical $^{13}NH_3$ MP PET and ^{18}F-FDG cardiac PET datasets described in Sect. 1.2.3.2. The results are shown in Figs. 1.5 and 1.6, respectively. Figures 1.5a

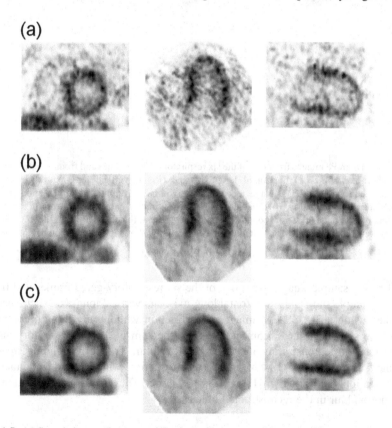

Fig. 1.5 (a) Sample images from one of the six respiratory-gated frames and from selected sample (*Left*) short-axis, (*Middle*) horizontal long-axis, and (*Right*) vertical long-axis slice images obtained using a 3D OS-EM image reconstruction without any motion compensation from a $^{13}NH_3$ MP PET study. (b) The sum of all six respiratory gated images from (a) showing the effect of RM blur. (c) Corresponding sample images as in (b) obtained using the 4D OS-EM image reconstruction with RM and attenuation compensation showing the reduction of RM motion blur in the reconstructed images

(a)

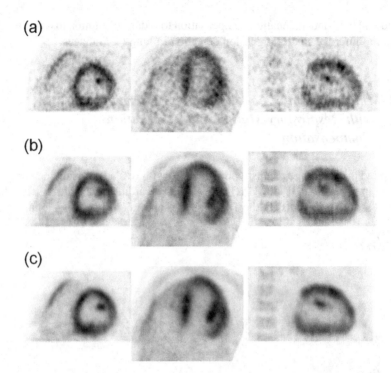

(b)

(c)

Fig. 1.6 (a) Sample images from one of the six respiratory-gated frames and from selected sample (*Left*) short-axis, (*Middle*) horizontal long-axis, and (*Right*) vertical long-axis slice images obtained using a 3D OS-EM image reconstruction without any motion compensation from a ^{18}F-FDG cardiac PET study. (b) The sum of all six respiratory-gated frames from (a) showing the effect of RM blur. (c) Corresponding sample images as in (b) obtained using the 4D OS-EM image reconstruction with RM and attenuation compensation showing the reduction of RM motion blur in the reconstructed images

and 1.6a are sample images from one of the six respiratory-gated frames and from selected sample short-axis, horizontal long-axis, and vertical long-axis slice images obtained using a 3D OS-EM image reconstruction without any motion compensation are shown. Figures 1.5b and 1.6b are the sum of all six respiratory-gated frame images demonstrating the effect of RM blur. The corresponding images obtained using the 4D OS-EM image reconstruction with RM and attenuation compensation are shown in Figs. 1.5c and 1.6c. They show the reduction of RM motion blur in the reconstructed images.

1.3.3 Improvement of Gated Cardiac PET Images with Dual Respiratory and Cardiac Motion Compensation

We applied the 4D image reconstruction method with dual R&C motion compensation to the clinical $^{13}NH_3$ MP PET and ^{18}F-FDG cardiac PET datasets described in Sect. 1.2.3.2. The results are shown in Figs. 1.7 and 1.8, respectively. Figures 1.7a and 1.8a and sample images from one of the eight cardiac-gated frames and from selected sample short-axis, horizontal long-axis, and vertical long-axis slice images obtained using a 3D OS-EM image reconstruction without motion compensation. Figures 1.7b and 1.8b show the corresponding images obtained using the 4D OS-EM image reconstruction with dual R&C motion compensation. They show the significant improvement in image quality in terms of improved image resolution from RM compensation and much lower image noise level from the CM compensation.

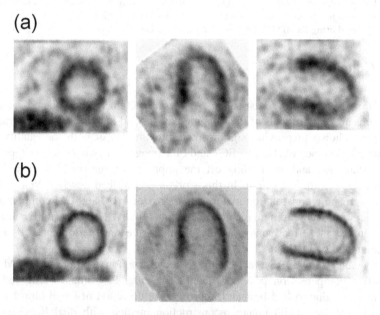

(a)

(b)

Fig. 1.7 (**a**) Sample images from one of the eight cardiac gates from selected sample (*Left*) short-axis, (*Middle*) horizontal long-axis, and (*Right*) vertical long-axis slices images obtained using a 3D OS-EM with no motion compensation from a $^{13}NH_3$ MP PET study. (**b**) Corresponding images obtained using the 4D OS-EM with R&C motion compensation

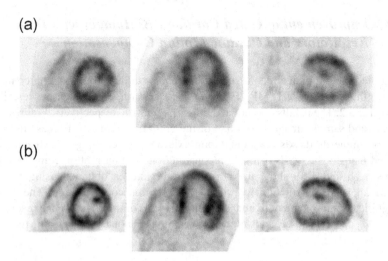

Fig. 1.8 (**a**) Sample images from one of the eight cardiac gates from selected sample (*Left*) short-axis, (*Middle*) horizontal long-axis, and (*Right*) vertical long-axis slices images obtained using a 3D OS-EM with no motion compensation from a ^{18}F-FDG cardiac PET study. (**b**) Corresponding images obtained using the 4D OS-EM with R&C motion compensation

1.4 Conclusions

Three-dimensional (3D) statistical image reconstruction methods using iterative algorithms and with models of the imaging physics and imaging system character-istics have shown to provide significant improvements in both the quality and quantitative accuracy of static SPECT and PET images. They have led to improved clinical diagnosis and, by trading off the improved image quality, for reduced patient dose and imaging time. In this work, we described newly developed 4D statistical image reconstruction methods that provided RM and CM compensation for further improvement in image quality and quantitative accuracy in PET images. We evaluated the effectiveness of the 4D image reconstruction methods using simulation and patient data.

Our results showed that a 4D image reconstruction method with RM and attenuation compensation provided quantitative lung PET images with reduced resolution loss due to RM blur and improved the detection of small lung lesions. We also evaluated a 4D image reconstruction method with dual R&C motion compensation using data from a clinical [13]NH$_3$ MP PET and a clinical ^{18}F-FDG cardiac PET study. The results showed 4D gated cardiac PET images with improved image resolution from RM compensation and much lower image noise level from the CM compensation.

The improved 4D gated cardiac PET images reveal anatomical details, such as the papillary muscle and interventricular sulcus, of the heart that were not possible with conventional 3D image reconstruction methods. The anatomical details allowed the development of feature-based myocardial motion vector estimation methods [33, 34] that overcame the aperture problem in traditional motion estimation methods. The accuracy of CM estimation will be further improved with continued improvement of the 4D image reconstruction methods and of the imaging characteristics in the next generation PET scanners that are coming into the market. It will allow extraction of new information about the contractility of the heart and provide additional diagnostic information for improved patient care.

References

1. Nehmeh SA, Erdi YE. Respiratory motion in positron emission tomography/computed tomography: a review. Semin Nucl Med. 2008;38(3):167–76.
2. Pretorius PH, King MA, Tsui BMW, LaCroix KJ, Xia W. A mathematical model of motion of the heart for use in generating source and attenuation maps for simulating emission imaging. Med Phys. 1999;26(11):2323–32.
3. McNamara JE, Pretorius PH, Johnson K, Mukherjee JM, Dey J, Gennert MA, et al. A flexible multicamera visual-tracking system for detecting and correcting motion-induced artifacts in cardiac SPECT slices. Med Phys. 2009;36(5):1913–23.
4. Chung A, Camici P, Yang G-Z, editors. List-mode affine rebinning for respiratory motion correction in PET cardiac imaging. Medical imaging and augmented reality. Berlin/Heidelberg: Springer; 2006.
5. Chen S, Tsui BMW. Evaluation of a new 4D PET image reconstruction method with respiratory motion compensation in a CHO study. J Nucl Med 2011: 150.
6. Chen S, Tsui BMW. Evaluation of a 4D PET image reconstruction method with respiratory motion compensation in a patient study. Society of nuclear medicine annual meeting. San Antonio; 2011: J Nucl Med. 2011. p. 2023.
7. Lee T-S, Higuchi T, Lautamäki R, Bengel F, Tsui BMW. Task-based evaluation of a 4D MAP-RBI-EM image reconstruction method for gated myocardial perfusion SPECT using a human observer study. Phys Med Biol. 2015;60:6789–809.
8. Lee T-S, Tsui BMW. Optimization of a 4D space-time gibbs prior in a 4D MAP-RBI-EMReconstruction method for application to gated myocardial perfusion SPECT. Proceeding of the fully three-dimensional image reconstruction meeting in radiology and nuclear medicine. 2009. p. 122.
9. Tang J, Lee T-S, He X, Segars WP, Tsui BM. Comparison of 3D OS-EM and 4D MAP-RBI-EM reconstruction algorithms for cardiac motion abnormality classification using a motion observer. IEEE Trans Nucl Sci. 2010;57(5):2571–7.
10. Tang J, Segars WP, Lee T-S, He X, Rahmim A, Tsui BMW. Quantitative study of cardiac motion estimation and abnormality classification in emission computed tomography. Med Eng Phys. 2011;33:563–72.
11. Gilland DR, Mair BA, Bowsher JE, Jaszczak RJ. Simultaneous reconstruction and motion estimation for gated cardiac ECT. IEEE Trans Nucl Sci. 2002;49(5):2344–9.
12. Mair BA, Gilland DR, Sun J. Estimation of images and nonrigid deformations in gated emission CT. IEEE Trans Med Imaging. 2006;25(9):1130–44.

13. Lee T-S, Tsui BMW. Evaluation of corrective reconstruction method for reduced acquisition time and various anatomies of perfusion defect using channelized hotelling observer for myocardial perfusion SPECT. IEEE nuclear science symposium and medical imaging conference record. 2010. p. 3523–6.
14. Dawood M, Buther F, Lang N, Schober O, Schafers K. Respiratory gating in positron emission tomography: a quantitative comparison of different gating schemes. Med Phys. 2007;34: 3067–6.
15. Klein GJ, Reutter BW, Ho MH, Reed JH, Huesman RH. Real-time system for respiratory-cardiac gating in positron tomography. IEEE Trans Nucl Sci. 1998;45:2139–43.
16. Chung A, Camici P, Yang G-Z. List-mode affine rebinning for respiratory motion correction in PET cardiac imaging. In: Medical imaging and augmented reality. Berlin: Springer; 2006. p. 293–300.
17. Büther F, Stegger L, Wübbeling F, Schäfers M, Schober O, Schäfers KP. List mode-driven cardiac and respiratory gating in PET. J Nucl Med. 2009;50:674–81.
18. Klein GL, Reutter BW, Huesman RH. Data-driven respiratory gating in list mode cardiac PET. J Nucl Med. 1999;40:113p.
19. Lamare F, Ledesma Carbayo MJ, Cresson T, Kontaxakis G, Santos A, Cheze Le Rest C, Reader AJ, Visvikis D. List-mode-based reconstruction for respiratory motion correction in PET using non-rigid body transformations. Phys Med Biol. 2007;52:[68].
20. Chen ST, Tsui BMW. Accuracy analysis of image registration based respiratory motion compensation in respiratory-gated FDG oncolgcial PET reconstruction. In: IEEE nuclear science symposium & medical imaging conference. Dresden; 2008. p. M06-417.
21. Chen S, Tsui BMW. Four-dmiensional OS-EM PET image reconstruction method with motion compensation. In: Fully three-dimensional image reconstruction in radiology and nuclear medicine. Beijing; 2009. p. 373–6.
22. Li TF, Thorndyke B, Schreibmann E, Yang Y, Xing L. Model-based image reconstruction for four-dimensional PET. Med Phys. 2006;33:1288–98.
23. Qiao F, Pan T, Clark JW, Mawlawi OR. A motion-incorporated reconstruction method for gated PET studies. Phys Med Biol. 2006;51:3769–83.
24. Chen S, Tsui BMW. Joint estimation of respiratory motion and PET image in 4D PET reconstruction with modeling attenuation map deformation induced by respiratory motion. J Nucl Med. 2010;51(supplement 2):523.
25. Segars WP, Sturgeon G, Mendonca S, Grimes J, Tsui BMW. 4D XCAT phantom for multimodality imaging research. Med Phys. 2010;37(9):4902–15.
26. Segars WP. Development of a new dynamic NURBS-based cardiac-torso (NCAT) phantom, PhD dissertation, The University of North Carolina, May 2001.
27. Segars WP, Tsui BMW. MCAT to XCAT: the evolution of 4-D computerized phantoms for imaging research. Proc IEEE. 2009;97(12):1954–68.
28. Segars WP, Mori S, Chen G, Tsui BMW. Modeling respiratory motion variations in the 4D NCAT Phantom. In: IEEE medical imaging conference. 2007. p. M26-356.
29. Segars WP, Lalush D, Frey EC, Manocha D, King MA, Tsui BMW. Improved dynamic cardiac phantom based on 4D NURBS and tagged MRI. IEEE Trans Nucl Sci. 2009;56:2728–38.
30. Lewellen TK, Harrison RL, Vannoy S. The simset program. In: Monte Carlo calculations in nuclear medicine, Medical science series. Bristol: Institute of Physics Publication; 1998. p. 77–92.
31. Jan S, et al. GATE: a simulation toolkit for PET and SPECT. Phys Med Biol. 2004; 49(19):4543.
32. Shilov M, Frey EC, Segars WP, Xu J, Tsui BMW. Improved Monte-Carlo simulations for dynamic PET. J Nucl Med Suppl. 2006;47:197.
33. Wang J, Fung GSK, Feng T, Tsui BMW. A papillary muscle guided motion estimation method for gated cardiac imaging. In: Nishikawa RM, Whiting BR, Hoeschen C, editors. Medical imaging 2013: physics of medical imaging, Proc. of SPIE, vol. 8668. Washington: SPIE; 2013. p. 86682G.
34. Wang J, Fung GSK, Feng T, Tsui BMW. An interventricular sulcus guided cardiac motion estimation method. Conference record of the 2013 I.E. nuclear science symposium and medical imaging conference, Seoul, 2013;October 27–November 2. p. 978–84.

Chapter 2
The Need for Quantitative SPECT in Clinical Brain Examinations

Hidehiro Iida, Tsutomu Zeniya, Miho Yamauchi, Kazuhiro Koshino, Takashi Temma, Satoshi Iguchi, Makoto Yamazaki, Junichiro Enmi, Naoya Kondo, Nobutoku Motomura, and Jyoji Nakagawara

Abstract This report describes details of the requirements and practical procedures for quantitative assessments of biological functional parametric images of the brain using ^{123}I-labeled tracers and clinical SPECT systems. With due understanding of the physics and the biological background, this is considered achievable even under clinical environments, provided that data are appropriately acquired, processed, and analyzed. This article discusses how potential hurdles have been overcome for quantitatively assessing quantitative functional parametric images in clinical settings, with successful examples that provided additional clinically useful information.

Keywords SPECT • Quantitation • ^{123}I-labeled radiopharmaceuticals • Reconstruction • Functional imaging

2.1 Introduction

Current clinical practice using SPECT relies largely on the interpretation of qualitative images reflecting physiologic functions. However, a quantitative analysis could provide further information to assist in the interpretation of disease status and treatment decisions. Methodological progress has made a quantitative determination of physiological functions through imaging feasible for brain scans, including parameters like the cerebral blood flow (CBF) and cerebral flow reactivity (CFR) after pharmacological vasodilatation and also neuro-receptor functions and others.

H. Iida (✉) • T. Zeniya • M. Yamauchi • K. Koshino • T. Temma • S. Iguchi • M. Yamazaki • J. Enmi • N. Kondo
Department of Investigative Radiology, National Cerebral and Cardiovascular Center Research Institute, 5-7-1, Fujishiro-dai, Suita City, Osaka 565-8565, Japan
e-mail: iida@ri.ncvc.go.jp

N. Motomura
Toshiba Medical Systems Corporation, 1385 Shimoishigami, Toshigi, Otawara City, Japan

J. Nakagawara
Department of Neurosurgery, Comprehensive Stroke Imaging Center, National Cerebral and Cardiovascular Center, 5-7-1, Fujishiro-dai, Suita City, Osaka 565-8565, Japan

© The Author(s) 2016   17
Y. Kuge et al. (eds.), *Perspectives on Nuclear Medicine for Molecular Diagnosis and Integrated Therapy*, DOI 10.1007/978-4-431-55894-1_2

The usefulness of such data has generally been limited to research due to the logistical complexity of quantitative examinations. Extensive work has then been carried out to make quantitative study doable in clinical environments, and some relevant study protocols are today generally accepted in clinical institutions in Japan.

Statistics show that 20 % of all SPECT clinical scans, namely approximately 20,000 scans annually, are carried out for the brain, mostly on patients with neurological (67 %) and cerebral vascular diseases (33 %), which is a much larger number than in other countries. Quantitative assessments of CBF (mostly with CFR) using ^{123}I-iodoamphetamine (IMP) comprise 5.6 % of all SPECT scans. Further, software programs assisting in the diagnosis are utilized with most brain scans, employing statistical analysis such as the 3D-SSP of Minoshima and others [1–5].

^{123}I-IMP and other ^{123}I-labeled tracers such as ^{123}I-iomazenil and ^{123}I-FP-CIT are approved for clinical use and can be employed in a quantitative analysis for demonstrating biological parametric images. Attenuation correction and scatter correction are necessary factors when conducting quantitative studies. Additional unique error of septal penetration is present when employing ^{123}I-labeled radiopharmaceuticals.

With SPECT scans there is the advantage over PET in the availability of the necessary scanner in clinical institutions. Availability of radiopharmaceuticals is another factor which would make conducting of such clinical research simple and straightforward. Standardization of the techniques is essential to be able to generate quantitative functional images that are consistent among institutions and SPECT scanners. This is important particularly when applying diagnosis-assisting software programs, to ensure consistent results independent of the SPECT devices installed at different institutions. The ability to refer to and compare results from different institutions or databases created at different institutions also requires that quantitative and reproducible results are needed.

This article describes how an integrated system was developed to enable a quantitative assessment of images of biological functions consistent among institutions in clinical setting with ^{123}I-labeled radiopharmaceuticals. To achieve this we describe the physics and technical background needed for the quantitation. Application and verification of the developed software packages as clinical diagnostic tools, and how users have been supported, will also be discussed for ^{123}I-IMP, ^{123}I-IMZ, and ^{123}I-FP-CIT examinations.

2.2 Requirements for Quantitative Reconstructions in SPECT

2.2.1 Scatter Correction

It is commonly accepted that the scatter and attenuation occurring in an object are the two major error factors with SPECT, and these need to be compensated for in the quantitative imaging. One technique to estimate the scatter distribution is to acquire projection data for additional energy windows in addition to the main window that covers the main peak. Selecting two additional windows below and above the main peak, the so-called triple-energy window (TEW) [6] method, is a commonly applied technique, in which acquired counts of the lower and upper windows are subtracted from those of the main window, and the reconstruction is then performed using the scatter-subtracted projection data. An advantage of this technique is that the procedures automatically compensate for the photons penetrating the collimator (see below).

An alternative approach is based on estimating the scatter from the scatter-uncorrected reconstructed images using the attenuation coefficient distribution. A formulation like the Klein-Nishina formula is commonly applied to simulate the scatter projection for a given tracer distribution and is termed the single scatter simulation (SSS) method [7]. This calculation can also be performed by Monte Carlo simulation (MCS), where simplification is effective to accelerate the calculations and ensure minimal loss of accuracy [8]. One further simplified approach is also feasible, by referring to the emission and attenuation data available in the projection domain; this was originally proposed by Meikle et al. [9] and was further optimized for ^{99m}Tc [10], ^{201}Tl [11, 12], and ^{123}I [13] in our group. A scatter fraction is empirically defined for a radioisotope as a function of the attenuation factor, which is then used to scale the simulated scatter distribution. This is the transmission-dependent convolution subtraction (TDCS) method and is applied to the geometric mean projection data. A number of verification studies have been carried out to ensure the accuracy of this method, but it must be noted that accuracy with the SSS and MCS theoretical methods is often limited because a number of factors are not taken into account. Our earlier work by a careful Monte Carlo simulation demonstrated that a non-negligible amount of scatter originates from outside objects such as the detector and scanner itself [14] and that this may be a source of errors if not taken into account.

With the software developed by our group for quantitative SPECT reconstruction (QSPECT), we have incorporated MCS- and TDCS-based scatter correction methods, and extensive work has shown support for this in the verification of the TDCS method for brain SPECT examinations. Due to the robustness and applicability when combined with other correction procedures, all results in the following will be with the TDCS scatter correction.

2.2.2 Septal Penetration in the Collimator

In addition to scatter and attenuation, ^{123}I has a further error arising from penetrating photons generated by high-energy gamma rays (>500 keV) emitted from the ^{123}I. These penetrating photons cause a down-scatter through the collimator and escaping photons from the scintillator, resulting in non-negligible levels of bias in

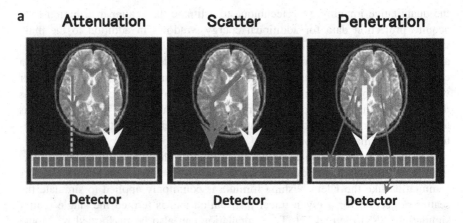

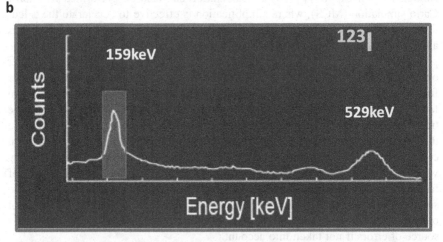

Fig. 2.1 (**a**) Error sources which need to be compensated for in quantitative reconstruction of brain SPECT images, attenuation, scatter, and photon penetration. (**b**) Energy spectrum for ^{123}I in a typical LEHR collimator. The significantly high background signal is a source of errors, caused by the high-energy photons emitted by the ^{123}I itself

the energy spectrum and therefore an offset in the projection data for the selected energy window (see Fig. 2.1).

Here it must be noted that the magnitude of the offset in the projection data due to the penetrating photons varies dependent on the collimator. With typical low-energy collimator sets, this represents a large amount, due to the thin walls of such collimators, while with typical ^{123}I-specifically designed collimator, the amount of offset is suppressed, due to thicker collimator walls. An example of a comparison of projection data obtained from two collimator sets of a typical low-energy high-resolution collimator (LEHR-para) and a ^{123}I-specific low-medium-energy general-purpose collimator (LMEGP-para) from one vendor is shown in Fig. 2.2. Collimator penetration is clearly visible with LEHR-para, but

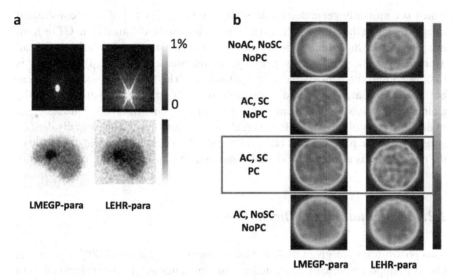

Fig. 2.2 (**a**) Typical projection data for a syringe-shaped phantom (*left*) and for a striatum phantom from Radiology Support Devices (Long Beach, LA, USA) (*right*) measured with ^{123}I-dedicated LMEGP-para and conventional LEHR-para collimator sets. (**b**) Reconstructed images for a uniform cylindrical phantom filled with ^{123}I-solution with and without attenuation correction (AC), scatter correction (SC), and photon penetration correction (PC). Different amounts of photon penetration are clearly visible as a high background outside the phantom on the projection data. In the projection data of the striatum phantom, striatum-to-whole brain ratio is also altered due to the penetrating photons. The reconstructed images also became different when not compensated. An appropriate correction procedure is important to compensate for the penetration for each set of the collimator

not with LMEGP-para for a ^{123}I-syringe and also on the striatal brain phantom (Fig. 2.2a). This difference causes the different reconstructed images of uniform cylindrical phantoms (Fig. 2.2b). It is important to note that the counts are decreased in the center of the cylindrical phantom when the attenuation correction is not applied to the data obtained with LMEGP-para collimator, while the decreased counts in the center is not visible with LEHR-para. The TEW technique is effective to compensate for the penetrating high-energy photons. With the scatter correction performed by the TEW technique, these penetrating photons are automatically compensated for. This is practical and effective, but at the expense of increased statistical noise.

In the QSPECT software, the penetration component is determined empirically for a collimator, as an extension of the TDCS scatter correction, as described in an earlier report [13].

2.2.3   Attenuation Correction

The Chang method [15] is the most common approach for attenuation correction (AC) in brain SPECT. This method utilizes an attenuation coefficient (μ) map which is commonly generated by detecting the head contours of the reconstructed images to which the AC is applied. The μ map can also be obtained from CT or from images of other modalities. The AC factors are then estimated for each pixel as an average over the 360° views with the attenuation coefficient (μ) map and is multiplied into the non-AC reconstructed images. The Chang method is empirical but the results are considered acceptable in most brain examinations. For the quantitative reconstruction, a uniform μ map is feasible if errors < 5 % are accepted in the deep parts of the brain. However, absolute values have to be carefully defined so as to make the pixel counts of the reconstructed images independent of the size of the object. This is also the case if a CT-based μ map is utilized in the reconstruction.

2.2.4 Attenuation Coefficient Map

Two possibilities are given to define the attenuation μ map in QSPECT software. One is to import externally generated attenuation μ maps, typically calculated from the Hounsfield unit (HU) images generated from a CT scan. Careful attention is needed to correct for the beam hardening effects when converting the attenuation map assessed with the continuous and rather low-energy photons to the quantitative HU and μ values corresponding to photons with single energy included in the energy window. Another possibility is to generate a homogeneous μ map by detecting the head contours. Extensive efforts have been made to provide the best accuracy in the head-contour detection algorithm, and a threshold was determined from the sinogram rather than the projection or the reconstructed images, and sine wave constraint was applied to the scatter-uncorrected data when defining the edge of the sinogram. Reconstruction was made for the filtered sinogram, and a threshold was applied again to determine the head contour, ensuring that an accurate head contour is generated. An empirically defined attenuation coefficient which effectively included the contribution of the bone value was then applied [13].

An attenuation coefficient map is utilized for the attenuation correction during the OSEM procedures and also for the scatter and penetration correction prior to the reconstruction if one utilizes one of the SSS, MCS, or TDCS methods for scatter correction. This attenuation coefficient map was utilized during the OSEM procedures as well as for the scatter and penetration correction prior to the reconstruction, by using the TDCS method as discussed earlier.

2.2.5 Implementation of the Collimator Aperture Model

It has been shown that implementation of a collimator aperture during the forward projection process on the three-dimensional domain makes the SPECT reconstruction more accurate [16]. Effects of this are increased, resulting in improved contrast and also suppression of statistical noise. The collimator aperture model shown in

Fig. 2.4 was implemented with the QSPECT reconstruction software for both the geometric mean and normal projection data. See further below.

2.2.6   SPECT Reconstruction

Two methods are known to quantitatively reconstruct images in the brain SPECT which will be discussed here. The filtered back projection (FBP) method is the one and has been the standard for reconstruction. For the FBP, the scatter correction has to be applied to the projection data before the reconstruction, and TEW is a well-established technique compensating for the septal penetration during the reconstruction. An attenuation correction is performed after the reconstruction in most cases based on the Chang method with an edge detection technique to generate homogeneous μ maps. The use of CT-based attenuation coefficient images is also possible, but selection of the absolute μ values needs careful consideration, and there are no published reports on how consistent results can be obtained with this technique with different equipment arrangements. A preliminary study carried out in Europe [17] showed unacceptable levels of variation and inconsistencies among sites. The reasons for the inconsistencies are unknown, but it was suggested that further careful evaluations are needed to standardize the detailed procedures. Although the FBP approach is straightforward and has been considered a standard, the method is limited when implementing new functionality to maximize the accuracy and image quality.

An alternative reconstruction method for SPECT is based on the maximum-likelihood expectation maximization (MLEM) algorithm, in which images are calculated with iterative procedures. Attenuation can be implemented in the forward projection process, so that the calculated reconstructed images are corrected for attenuation. The *ordered-subset maximum-likelihood expectation maximization* (OSEM) method is often utilized to accelerate convergence, as will be discussed later in this article. It must be noted that the TEW-based scatter correction includes correction also for the penetration, while currently the existing simulation-based scatter correction method does not include a penetration correction, and thus requires further development.

The QSPECT software employs the OSEM approach. A schematic representation of the process of the reconstruction in QSPECT software is shown in Fig. 2.3. Systematic errors arise due to neglecting higher μ values in the skull, but the effect is within ± 5 % in the middle part of the brain and also in other areas outside the cerebral tissue [13]. The following three formulations were implemented in the program. Suitable formulation can then be selected to best fit each clinical protocol.

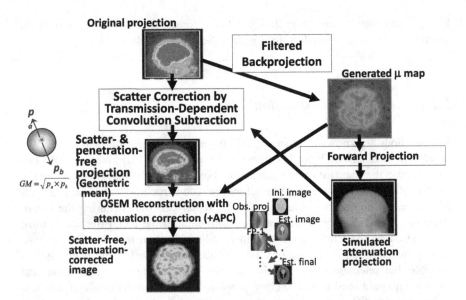

Fig. 2.3 Diagram illustrating the quantitative reconstruction protocol implemented in the QSPECT reconstruction software. The emission data are initially reconstructed with filtered back projection (top right image) to allow the brain outline to be determined and the μ map for the attenuation correction to be determined by assigning a uniform attenuation coefficient value of 0.1603 cm^{-1} to the detected brain volume. The μ map is forward projected to provide the attenuation projections for the scatter correction to calculate scatter- and penetration-compensated projection. The scatter correction is carried out using TDCS method; thus, the projection data becomes geometric mean data. Then, OSEM reconstruction is applied with the attenuation correction to generate the attenuation and scatter corrected images. The collimator aperture correction (APC) can also be applied in the reconstruction process using Eq. (2.2) (Figure is from Iida et al. [28])

2.2.6.1 OSEM on 2D Domains for the Pre-scatter Corrected Geometric Mean Projection

The first formulation is essentially identical to the one also described in earlier studies [9–11, 13]. Reconstruction is performed for each two-dimensional tomographic slice, with the projection corrected for scatter before the reconstruction. The pixel counts of the reconstructed image λ_j^{n+1} are calculated from the counts of the previous image λ_j^n. The scatter compensated projection data by the TDCS method [18] was applied, and the formulation for the geometric mean projection data is given as follows:

$$\lambda_j^{n+1} = \frac{\lambda_j^n}{\sum\limits_{i \in S_n} c_{ij}} \sum\limits_{i \in S_n} \frac{c_{ij} y_i}{\left(\sum\limits_k c_{ik} \lambda_k^n\right) \exp(-\mu L_i)} \tag{2.1}$$

where y_i is the count in the projection data corrected for the scatter and the collimator penetration, c_{ij} is a factor for the contributions from the projection pixel to the image pixel, $\exp(-\mu L_i)$ is the net attenuation factor for each of the geometric mean projections. Note that the projection data has to be corrected before the reconstruction calculations, eg by the TDCS scatter correction.

2.2.6.2 OSEM on 3D Domains for the Pre-scatter Corrected Geometric Mean Projection

This formulation includes the collimator aperture correction, and the reconstruction is carried out nearly wholly in a three-dimensional domain. The scatter compensated projection data by the TDCS method [18] was applied, giving the formulation for the geometric mean projection data as follows:

$$\lambda_j^{n+1} = \frac{\lambda_j^n}{\sum\limits_{i \in S_n} c_{ij} w_{ij}} \sum\limits_{i \in S_n} \frac{c_{ij} w_{ij} y_i}{\left(\sum\limits_k c_{ik} w_{ik} \lambda_k^n\right) \exp(-\mu L_i)} \tag{2.2}$$

where w_{ij} represents the collimator dependent blurring of the spatial resolution shown in Fig. 2.4. Note that the projection data has to be corrected for the scatter before the reconstruction calculations as in the eq. 2.1 in which y_i is the geometric mean projection data already corrected for scatter by means of the TDCS method, and c_{ij} represents the calculation of the geometric mean.

2.2.6.3 OSEM on 3D Domains Including the Scatter Correction Process

This formulation includes the scatter correction process during the reconstruction as follows:

$$\lambda_j^{n+1} = \frac{\lambda_j^n}{\sum\limits_i c_{ij} w_{ij}} \sum\limits_{i \in S_n} \frac{c_{ij} w_{ij} y_i}{\left\{\sum\limits_k c_{ik} w_{ik} \lambda_k^n \exp\left(-\sum\limits_m \mu_{ikm} l_{ikm}\right)\right\} + s_i} \tag{2.3}$$

The scatter projection at the i-th iteration, s_i, has to be estimated at each iteration either by the SSS or MCS methods from the i-th reconstructed images. It is also possible to use the TEW-based scattered projection for s_i. In QSPECT, an

Fig. 2.4 The model for collimator aperture correction implemented in the QSPECT reconstruction software. Spatial resolution was assumed to decrease linearly with the distance from the collimator with an initial value. The contribution weights, w_{ij}, calculated from this model were implemented in Eqs. (2.2) and (2.3), which compensated for the blurring effects due to the collimator aperture

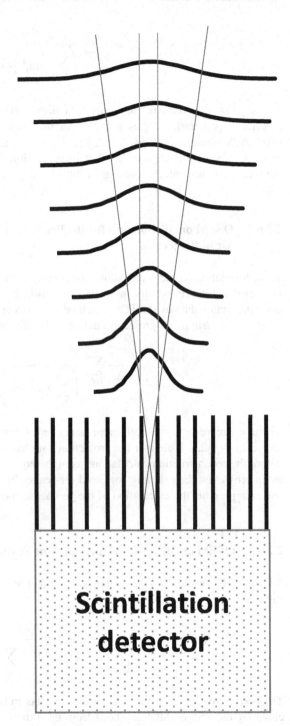

accelerated MCS [8] is implemented. Consequently, y_i it is not necessarily the geometric mean but may be the normal projection.

2.2.7 Calibration to Bq/mL

The QSPECT program is designed so that the pixel values correspond to the radioactivity concentration, the cps/mL. An experiment with a syringe filled with a ^{123}I-labeled radioactive pharmaceutical of known radioactivity gives a calibration factor to convert the pixel counts to the absolute radioactivity concentration which has units of Bq/mL. The accuracy of the absolute quantitation was ± 10 % for ^{123}I in uniform cylindrical phantoms provided that the diameter is less than 16 cm. For the future, this feature could be of use in internal dosimetry quantitation of radiotherapy agents such as ^{177}Lu peptides.

2.2.8 Dead Time Count Loss

The counting rate performance should be sufficiently high in clinical SPECT scanners, e.g., count losses <1 % up to a counting rate of 70 kcps. This would hold for ^{99m}Tc and other commonly used SPECT radiopharmaceuticals, but may not in ^{123}I-labeled tracers. The true counting rate of the system could be much higher than the observed rate for the given main window, attributed to the incidence of a large amount of penetrating photons originated from the high-energy gamma rays (>500 keV). Particularly, low-energy dedicated collimators such as LEHR collimators can accept large amounts of penetrating photons, and there may be a significant counting loss at counting rates much below 70kcps. Errors could be mostly in phantom experiments but may be smaller in clinical scans. It is however important to confirm the maximum counting rate that maintains the linearity of the SPECT counts to the true radioactivity.

2.3 Phantom Experiments

A number of studies have been carried out to evaluate the adequacy of the QSPECT reconstruction programs. The experiments were on geometrically shaped phantoms such as cylindrical phantoms and also on phantoms simulating the cerebral blood flow distribution and striatum structure with realistic head contours and skull structures. These phantom experiments are useful in validating the reconstruction procedures and also to ensure quality control of the data acquisition procedures.

2.3.1 Uniform Cylindrical Phantom

The cylindrical phantom gives information of how uniform images are obtained for uniform distributions of radioactivity. Image homogeneity could be degraded by several factors in relation to inappropriate corrections for attenuation, to scatter and penetration, and also to the insufficient quality control. The quality control includes the procedures for adjusting and correcting for inhomogeneous sensitivity, mistuned position linearity, misaligned center of rotation, large attenuations in the head holder, and other factors. Experiments to confirm the homogeneity for uniform phantom are highly suggested to ensure that the regional activity quantitation is not suffered from one of error factors mentioned above. However, it should be noted that inappropriate definition of the head contour and inconsistently defined attenuation coefficient values in relation to the presence of the skull may not be evaluated from the uniform cylinder phantom experiment.

2.3.2 3D Brain Iida Phantom for CBF Quantitation

Geometrically shaped phantoms are limited in simulating realistic head contours, the presence of the bone and trachea, and also the realistic radioactivity distribution. Therefore, dedicated brain-simulating phantoms are often desired to evaluate the overall accuracy of reconstructed images in realistic situations. We have developed a three-dimensional brain phantom (Iida phantom) that simulates the CBF distribution in cortical gray matter, with bone, trachea, and realistic head contours [19]. As shown in Fig. 2.5, accuracy of the QSPECT software can be evaluated by referring regional radioactivity concentration on the reconstructed images with those of design images of this phantom. This experiment would be useful if one wish to evaluate the accuracy of reconstructed images for multicenter clinical studies using SPECT techniques.

Differences in the spatial resolution have to be assessed when comparing SPECT images acquired from different SPECT systems, because the differences in the spatial resolution causes different quantitative values due to the partial volume effect [20]. Hoffman 3D phantoms [21] was utilized to assess and to compensate for the different spatial resolution in the cerebral FDG uptake images acquired at different institutions using different PET systems on healthy volunteers [20]. The Iida brain phantom is also useful to evaluate and equalize the spatial resolution of SPECT images obtained from different sites and probably better suited to SPECT, due to its importance in the determination of head contour in SPECT scans. Yamauchi et al. [22] demonstrated that equalization of the spatial resolution significantly reduced the inter-institutional variation of the normal database of rest- and acetazolamide-CBF images among three institutions. The Iida brain phantom may be better suited than the 3D Hoffman phantom when one intends to

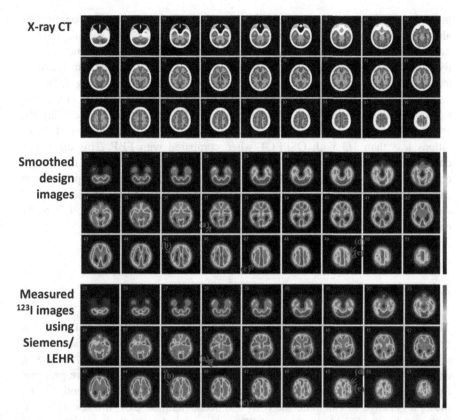

Fig. 2.5 (*Top*) X-ray CT images of the developed phantom, which contain water and bone-equivalent liquid in the cortical gray matter and bone components of the phantom, (*Middle*) digital design of the gray matter area of the phantom after smoothing with a 16 mm full-width at half maximum Gaussian filter, and (*Bottom*) SPECT images of the phantom filled with ¹²³I solution in the gray matter compartment and K₂HPO₄ solution in the bone compartment. All images are aligned to the digital design. The SPECT images showed good agreement with the digitally designed images. Spots shown with *arrows* (**a–e**) demonstrated are examples which indicated good agreement between the digital design and ¹²³I-SPECT images (Figure is from Iida et al. [19])

assess attenuation or scatter-related variations among different PET/SPECT scanners.

2.3.3   Striatum Phantom for Dopamine Transporter Imaging

For dopamine transporter imaging using ¹²³I-FP-CIT, a phantom simulating the striatum uptake of ¹²³I-FP-CIT with homogeneous background in the whole brain region (Radiology Support Devices, Long beach, LA, USA) was utilized to evaluate the accuracy and also to calibrate the inter-institutional variations in multicenter evaluations in the EU [23]. The QSPECT reconstruction program was also evaluated using this phantom to assess the accuracy of the specific binding ratio (SBR) values [24], by referring the values calculated from the true radioactivity in the striatum compartments relative to the whole-brain background concentration. Results demonstrated that the SBR values measured using QSPECT software agreed well with those determined from the true radioactivity concentrations. Variation was less than 1/3 of those with FBP reconstruction including the attenuation corrections. This suggested smaller inter-institutional/inter-vendor variations less than 1/3 with QSPECT when compared with FBP. This difference corresponds to the decline of both sensitivity and specificity from 97 to 78 % in our preliminary simulation study. It is therefore of a paramount importance to establish an accurate reconstruction methodology in order to provide a good diagnostic performance in clinical settings. Further careful evaluation is to be carried out.

2.3.4 QSPECT Program Packages

The program package of QSPECT uses a wrapper written in JAVA to run several programs written in C language for Microsoft Windows systems and also includes programs for reconstructing SPECT images, co-registering images, re-slicing, calculating functional images, and printing summary logs. Packages are prepared for the given data processing protocols for the given radiopharmaceuticals. Of those, a package to calculate the rest- and acetazolamide-CBF images with ^{123}I-IMP and the specific binding ratio (SBR) values with the distribution volume ratio (DVR) images with ^{123}I-FP-CIT have been utilized to support clinical diagnosis. The programs are also utilized to support clinical research.

2.4 Adequacy and Impact in Clinical Scans

2.4.1 Dopamine Transporter Function (SBR Quantitation) Using ^{123}I-FP-CIT

Figure 2.6 shows an example of an image of a ^{123}I-FP-CIT scan on a young healthy volunteer (29 years old, male) acquired using a three-head SPECT camera from Toshiba (Tochigi, Japan) fitted with a LHR-fan collimator. The reconstruction was carried out according to Eq. (2.2), which includes the TDCS scatter correction for the geometric projection data and the collimator aperture correction. It can be seen that the head contour was well delineated, as indicated by the red arrows. This is attributed to the carefully designed algorithm: the contour detection with the sine function constraint on the sonogram prior to the scatter correction. With the

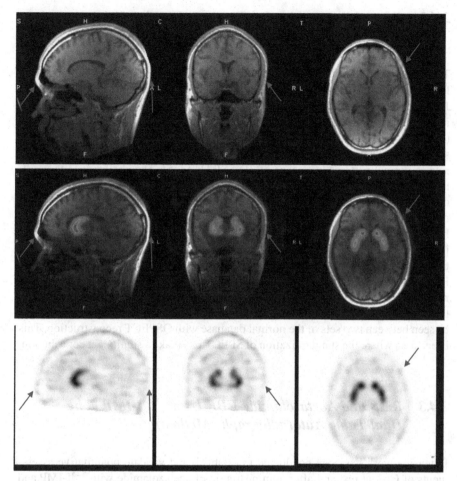

Fig. 2.6 An example of an image of ^{123}I-FP-CIT for a healthy 29-year-old male volunteer. The scan was made using the Toshiba 9300R (three-head camera) fitted with an LMEGP-fan collimator. Reconstruction was carried out according to Eq. (2.2) and includes the collimator aperture correction. The head contour is well delineated using the edge detection method implemented in the QSPECT software, as shown with the *red arrows*

improved sensitivity and spatial resolution achieved using the triple head SPECT camera with a fan beam collimator designed for ^{123}I-nuclides, the collimator aperture model was effective to enhance and provide better striatum-to-background contrast with minimal enhancement of the background noise, though the SBR values essentially remained without changes. There may be lots of application areas where improved image quality can make contributions in clinical settings.

2.4.2   Central Benzodiazepine Receptor Imaging Using
           ^{123}I-IMZ (Neuron Damage/Residual)

The radiopharmaceutical ^{123}I-iomazenil (IMZ) is a radiopharmaceutical approved for clinical diagnosis to assess local neuronal damage in patients with epilepsy in Japan. There are also other applications to identify the presence of neuronal damage in the prefrontal areas of patients with neurological deficits after chronic ischemia (or Moyamoya disease) and traumatic brain injuries. We have aimed to highlight significantly damaged areas using ^{123}I-IMZ and SPECT in such patients by referring to normal patterns by means of 3D-SSP [1] [3, 5]. The challenge is to verify that identical data can be obtained from different SPECT systems installed in different institutions. Consistency is essential in order to utilize a common (normal) database rather than generating separate ones at each institution. At present, we have confirmed that a normal database for ^{123}I-IMZ generated at two independent institutions installed with different vendor SPECT systems showed smaller variations when QSPECT with AC, SC, and PC was utilized, as compared with vendor FBP reconstruction employing AC only. It was also observed that while vendor reconstruction provided different damage regions with the 3D-SSP analysis using the normal database generated at different institutions, only small differences could be seen between two sets of the normal database with QSPECT reconstruction. This is one area where the standardization of SPECT can make a significant contribution.

2.4.3   Rest- and Acetazolamide-CBF Using ^{123}I-IMP (The
           Dual-Table Autoradiography Method)

Extensive work has been conducted to establish and validate quantitative assessments of CBF at rest and after administration of acetazolamide with ^{123}I-IMP and dynamic SPECT using the QSPECT program packages (Fig. 2.7). At present, the QSPECT software packages have been shown to be able to handle the data obtained from most SPECT cameras fitted with parallel beam collimators (see Table 2.1). A total of more than 60,000 scans have been carried out in Japan between 2006 and January 2015, with 16,000 scans in 2014. The scans were mainly to assess the risk of hyper-perfusion after revascularization therapy in patients who are candidates for coronary artery stents and for coronary endarterectomy.

The ^{123}I-IMP has a high first-pass extraction fraction and is capable of assessing quantitative CBF values for a physiologically wide range of blood flows [25, 26]. The object was to make the quantitative assessment of the rest- and acetazolamide-CBF images from scans obtained in a single session, with two injections of ^{123}I-IMP at 30 min intervals, to establish the ischemic status in the scans of each patient. A sophisticated compartment model was applied (called dual-table ARG) [27] to make it possible for the stress CBF images to be calculated using table look-up procedures without the need for image subtraction. This method

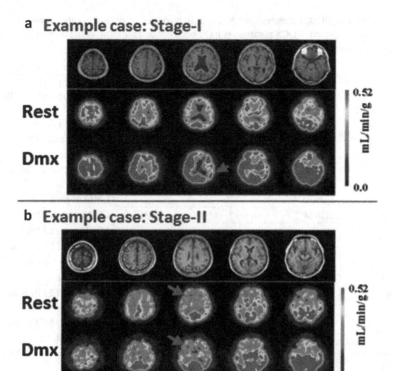

Fig. 2.7 MR and CBF images at rest and after acetazolamide stress assessed with ^{123}I-IMP and the dual-table ARG method on two typical low-risk patients (stage I) and a patient with high-risk (stage II) ischemia (Figure is from Iida et al. [28])

appeared not to result in increases in statistical noise and more importantly was able to provide quantitative CBF images with minimal errors and only little inconsistency between the rest- and acetazolamide-CBF assessments. A number of studies were carried out to verify the method in clinical settings, funded by the Ministry of Health, Labour and Welfare Research Foundation from the year of 2007 for 3 years as follows:

(a) There was a fairly good intra-institutional reproducibility of rest- and acetazolamide-CBF images for the same patient, approximately 10 % with 44 patients at nine institutions [28].
(b) Inter-institutional reproducibility of rest- and acetazolamide-CBF images was approximately 6 % in nine patients on 18 data points [29]. An example case is shown in Fig. 2.8.
(c) Consistent results for rest and acetazolamide CBF at rest and after acetazolamide in healthy volunteers among three institutions (a total of 32 healthy volunteers) [22].
(d) Agreement with PET scan results both on relative distribution and absolute values was shown in one institution for five patients [28].

Table 2.1 List of SPECT camera (3/8 NaI scintillator) and collimator combinations to which QSPECT can be applied. TDCS parameters have been defined for those systems prior to the first clinical examination

	SPECT camera		Collimator
Toshiba	GCA-9300	3/8inch	N2(LEHR fan), N1(LESHR fan). LEHR para
	GCA-7200		N2(LEHR fan), N1 (LESHR fan), LEHR para
			LEGP para
	ECAM		N2(LEHR fan), LMEGP para
	Symbia		LMEGP para
Siemens	ECAM	3/8inch	LEHR para, LMEGP para
	Symbia		LEHR para, LMEGP para
GE	Millennium VG	3/8inch	LEGP para, LEHR para
	Infinia		ELEGP para, LEHR para
Hitachi (Philips)	ADAC forte JET stream Philips BrightView Philips SKYLight	3/8inch	VXGP para
			CHR para, LEHR para, MEGP para
			LEGP para, MEGP para, VXHR para
Shimazu (Picker ADAC)	IRIX	3/8inch	LEGP para, LEHR para
	AXIS		LEGP para
	PRISM2000		LEHR para
	PRISM3000		LEGP para, LEHR para

This examination is one good example that demonstrates the contribution of quantitative SPECT in clinical settings. Results of 3D-SSP shown in Fig. 2.8 are helpful in understanding the severity of ischemia and the risk status in patients with major artery occlusion or stenosis. This would also contribute to evaluate a number of therapeutic trials in the future.

2.5 Quality Control of the SPECT Scanner

It must be noted that standardization of the quantitative SPECT examination requires detailed self-defined protocols, including for the procedures of the administration, blood sampling, instructions to patients and patient movement, QC of SPECT devices, SPECT acquisition workflow, data pre-processing, and QSPECT reconstruction. Active feedback to deal with possible adverse events related to above procedures at clinical institutions appeared to be effective to maintain the reliability of the clinical scan findings. From July 2009 till May 2011, 139 cases were defined as potentially posing problems or possibly resulting in adverse events

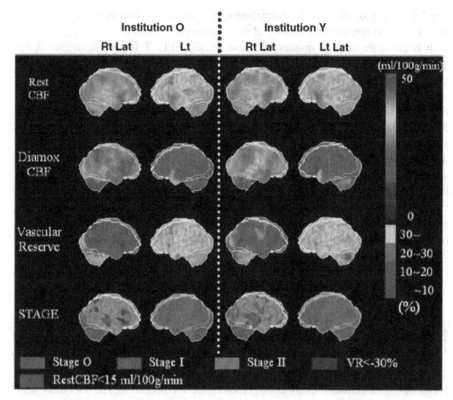

Fig. 2.8 Stereotactic extraction estimates based on the JET study (SEE-JET) images [4] of a patient obtained in institutions O and Y. The Rt Lat and Lt Lat indicate the right and left hemisphere outer lateral images, respectively. Cerebral blood flow at rest (rest CBF), CBF after the acetazolamide challenge (Diamox CBF), the cerebrovascular reserve (vascular reserve), and severity of hemodynamic cerebral ischemia (STAGE) are shown as three-dimensional cerebral surface images. Images are almost visually identical, from institutions O and Y (Figure is from Yoneda et al. [29])

at 67 institutions. Claims were mostly unexpected low CFR values or unexpectedly low or high absolute CBF values. The software package was designed to keep a record of the complete calculation process, and among the data obtained in this manner, the tissue time-activity curve (tTAC) analysis for sequential short frame dynamic images and dynamic projections appeared to be helpful to identify the sources of errors. Of the 139 cases identified, 64 (42 %) did not suggest errors in the data or in the calculation process, as the observed CFR or small CBF values could be confirmed from results of the tTAC analysis, both in the dynamic reconstructed images as well as in the projection data. In other studies, the tTAC analysis was able to identify errors in the blood radioactivity concentrations ($n = 26$), in the cross calibration procedures ($n = 25$), in the IMP administration ($n = 17$) due to the patient motion ($n = 11$), and other factors including insufficient SPECT QC ($n = 11$). Errors in the software program were not identified in any of the studies.

The feedback provided in the information to the clinical institution was evaluated to be effective to improve the quality of the examination results.

It is possible that the quality of reconstructed SPECT images is degraded by inaccurate reconstruction parameter settings in relation to the attenuation coefficients, accuracy of the head contour determination, inefficient statistical treatment, and also poor quality control (QC) of the SPECT device. It should be noted that there are no standard guidelines (like the NEMA standard) for reconstructed SPECT images, only for projection data. One contribution of the QSPECT reconstruction package is the ability to evaluate the image quality and accuracy on one domain with different systems. It was apparent that the engineers at the vendors should be encouraged to make effort to improve the quality of the reconstructed images rather than only on the projection data. Active feedback to the users at the clinical institutions is also essential to improve the quality of the examination in the quantitation. We also considered the FBP reconstruction with the scatter correction of Chang, for the scatter corrected-projection with TEW would be another possibility for standardization among different institutions. Systematic study has to be coordinated to validate the technique in multicenter settings.

2.6 Summary and Future Directions

The QSPECT package is able to reconstruct quantitative tomographic images from projection data acquired using commercial SPECT equipment. The adequacy was demonstrated with a series of phantom experiments. More importantly, the adequacy of images of biological functions and the use of stereotactic statistical analysis software were shown for some protocols in patient populations. Overall, this suggests the adequacy of using clinical SPECT devices for multicenter clinical studies. It is also possible to encourage the use of quantitative reconstruction with diagnosis-assisting software in clinical settings; this would enable an extension of the contribution of SPECT in evaluations of disease severity and so assist in decision making. Further systematic work should be designed to prove this concept for the various tracers in the various clinical settings.

References

1. Minoshima S, Frey KA, Koeppe RA, Foster NL, Kuhl DE. A diagnostic approach in Alzheimer's disease using three-dimensional stereotactic surface projections of fluorine-18-FDG PET. J Nucl Med. 1995;36(7):1238–48. Epub 1995/07/01.
2. Minoshima S, Giordani B, Berent S, Frey KA, Foster NL, Kuhl DE. Metabolic reduction in the posterior cingulate cortex in very early Alzheimer's disease. Ann Neurol. 1997;42(1):85–94. Epub 1997/07/01.
3. Mizumura S, Kumita S, Cho K, Ishihara M, Nakajo H, Toba M, et al. Development of quantitative analysis method for stereotactic brain image: assessment of reduced accumulation in extent and severity using anatomical segmentation. Ann Nucl Med. 2003;17(4):289–95. Epub 2003/08/23.
4. Mizumura S, Nakagawara J, Takahashi M, Kumita S, Cho K, Nakajo H, et al. Three-dimensional display in staging hemodynamic brain ischemia for JET study: objective evaluation using SEE analysis and 3D-SSP display. Ann Nucl Med. 2004;18(1):13–21. Epub 2004/04/10.
5. Ishii K, Kono AK, Sasaki H, Miyamoto N, Fukuda T, Sakamoto S, et al. Fully automatic diagnostic system for early- and late-onset mild Alzheimer's disease using FDG PET and 3D-SSP. Eur J Nucl Med Mol Imaging. 2006;33(5):575–83. Epub 2006/02/14.
6. Ichihara T, Ogawa K, Motomura N, Kubo A, Hashimoto S. Compton scatter compensation using the triple-energy window method for single- and dual-isotope SPECT. J Nucl Med. 1993;34(12):2216–21. Epub 1993/12/01.
7. Kadrmas DJ, Frey EC, Karimi SS, Tsui BM. Fast implementations of reconstruction-based scatter compensation in fully 3D SPECT image reconstruction. Phys Med Biol. 1998;43(4):857–73. Epub 1998/05/08.
8. Sohlberg A, Watabe H, Iida H. Acceleration of Monte Carlo-based scatter compensation for cardiac SPECT. Phys Med Biol. 2008;53(14):N277–85. Epub 2008/06/25.
9. Meikle SR, Hutton BF, Bailey DL. A transmission-dependent method for scatter correction in SPECT. J Nucl Med. 1994;35(2):360–7.
10. Narita Y, Eberl S, Iida H, Hutton BF, Braun M, Nakamura T, et al. Monte Carlo and experimental evaluation of accuracy and noise properties of two scatter correction methods for SPECT. Phys Med Biol. 1996;41(11):2481–96.
11. Iida H, Eberl S. Quantitative assessment of regional myocardial blood flow with thallium-201 and SPECT. J Nucl Cardiol. 1998;5(3):313–31.
12. Narita Y, Iida H, Eberl S, Nakamura T. Monte Carlo evaluation of accuracy and noise properties of two scatter correction methods for ^{201}Tl cardiac SPECT. IEEE Trans Nucl Sci. 1997;44:2465–72.
13. Iida H, Narita Y, Kado H, Kashikura A, Sugawara S, Shoji Y, et al. Effects of scatter and attenuation correction on quantitative assessment of regional cerebral blood flow with SPECT. J Nucl Med. 1998;39(1):181–9.
14. Hirano Y, Koshino K, Watabe H, Fukushima K, Iida H. Monte Carlo estimation of scatter effects on quantitative myocardial blood flow and perfusable tissue fraction using 3D-PET and (15)O-water. Phys Med Biol. 2012;57(22):7481–92. Epub 2012/10/30.
15. Chang L. A method for attenuation correction in radionuclide computed tomography. IEEE Trans Nucl Sci. 1978;25:638–43.
16. Frey EC, Tsui BMW. Collimator-detector response compensation in SPECT. In: Zaidi H, editor. Quantitative analysis in nuclear medicine imaging. Singapore: Springer US; 2006. p. 141–66.
17. Hapdey S, Soret M, Ferrer L, Koulibaly P, Henriques J, Bardiès M, et al. Quantification in SPECT: myth or reality ? A multicentric study. IEEE Nucl Sci Symp Conf Rec. 2004;5(3):3170–317.
18. Sohlberg A, Watabe H, Iida H. Three-dimensional SPECT reconstruction with transmission-dependent scatter correction. Ann Nucl Med. 2008;22(7):549–56. Epub 2008/08/30.

19. Iida H, Hori Y, Ishida K, Imabayashi E, Matsuda H, Takahashi M, et al. Three-dimensional brain phantom containing bone and grey matter structures with a realistic head contour. Ann Nucl Med. 2013;27(1):25–36.
20. Joshi A, Koeppe RA, Fessler JA. Reducing between scanner differences in multi-center PET studies. NeuroImage. 2009;46(1):154–9. Epub 2009/05/22.
21. Hoffman EJ, Cutler PD, Digby WM, Mazziotta JC. 3-D phantom to simulate cerebral blood flow and metabolic images for PET. IEEE Trans Nucl Sci. 1990;37:616–20.
22. Yamauchi M, Imabayashi E, Matsuda H, Nakagawara J, Takahashi M, Shimosegawa E, et al. Quantitative assessment of rest and acetazolamide CBF using quantitative SPECT reconstruction and sequential administration of (123)I-iodoamphetamine: comparison among data acquired at three institutions. Ann Nucl Med. 2014;28(9):836–50. Epub 2014/07/09.
23. Tossici-Bolt L, Dickson JC, Sera T, de Nijs R, Bagnara MC, Jonsson C, et al. Calibration of gamma camera systems for a multicentre European ^{123}I-FP-CIT SPECT normal database. Eur J Nucl Med Mol Imaging. 2011;38(8):1529–40.
24. Tossici-Bolt L, Hoffmann SM, Kemp PM, Mehta RL, Fleming JS. Quantification of [^{123}I]FP-CIT SPECT brain images: an accurate technique for measurement of the specific binding ratio. Eur J Nucl Med Mol Imaging. 2006;33(12):1491–9. Epub 2006/07/22.
25. Iida H, Akutsu T, Endo K, Fukuda H, Inoue T, Ito H, et al. A multicenter validation of regional cerebral blood flow quantitation using [^{123}I]iodoamphetamine and single photon emission computed tomography. J Cereb Blood Flow Metab. 1996;16(5):781–93. Epub 1996/09/01.
26. Iida H, Itoh H, Nakazawa M, Hatazawa J, Nishimura H, Onishi Y, et al. Quantitative mapping of regional cerebral blood flow using iodine-123-IMP and SPECT. J Nucl Med. 1994;35 (12):2019–30. Epub 1994/12/01.
27. Kim KM, Watabe H, Hayashi T, Hayashida K, Katafuchi T, Enomoto N, et al. Quantitative mapping of basal and vasareactive cerebral blood flow using split-dose (123)I-iodoamphetamine and single photon emission computed tomography. NeuroImage. 2006;33 (3):1126–35.
28. Iida H, Nakagawara J, Hayashida K, Fukushima K, Watabe H, Koshino K, et al. Multicenter evaluation of a standardized protocol for rest and acetazolamide cerebral blood flow assessment using a quantitative SPECT reconstruction program and split-dose ^{123}I-iodoamphetamine. J Nucl Med. 2010;51(10):1624–31.
29. Yoneda H, Shirao S, Koizumi H, Oka F, Ishihara H, Ichiro K, et al. Reproducibility of cerebral blood flow assessment using a quantitative SPECT reconstruction program and split-dose 123I-iodoamphetamine in institutions with different gamma-cameras and collimators. J Cereb Blood Flow Metab. 2012;32(9):1757–64.

Chapter 3
PET Imaging Innovation by DOI Detectors

Taiga Yamaya

Abstract Positron emission tomography (PET) plays important roles in cancer diagnosis, neuroimaging, and molecular imaging research. However potential points remain for which big improvements could be made, including spatial resolution, sensitivity, and manufacturing costs. Depth-of-interaction (DOI) measurement in the radiation sensor will be a key technology to get any significant improvement in sensitivity while maintaining high spatial resolution. We have developed four-layered DOI detectors based on our original light-sharing method. DOI measurement also has a potential to expand PET application fields because it allows for more flexible detector arrangement. As an example, we are developing the world's first, open-type PET geometry, "OpenPET," which is expected to lead to PET imaging during treatment. The DOI detector itself continues to evolve with the help of recently developed semiconductor photodetectors, often referred to as silicon photomultipliers (SiPMs). We are developing a SiPM-based DOI detector "X'tal cube" to achieve sub-mm spatial resolution, which is reaching the theoretical limitation of PET imaging. Innovation of SiPMs encourages our development of PET/MRI, which is attracting great notice in terms of smaller radiation exposure and better contract in soft tissues compared with current PET/CT.

Keywords PET • Depth-of-interaction • DOI • In-beam PET • Brain PET • SiPM • PET/MRI

3.1 Introduction

Positron emission tomography (PET) plays important roles in cancer diagnosis, neuroimaging, and molecular imaging research, but potential points remain for which big improvements could be made, including spatial resolution, sensitivity, and manufacturing costs. For example, the sensitivity of present PET scanners does not exceed 10 %. This means that more than 90 % of the gamma rays emitted from a subject are not utilized for imaging. Therefore, research on next generation PET technologies remains a hot topic worldwide.

T. Yamaya (✉)
Molecular Imaging Center, National Institute of Radiological Sciences, Chiba, Japan
e-mail: taiga@nirs.go.jp

© The Author(s) 2016   39
Y. Kuge et al. (eds.), *Perspectives on Nuclear Medicine for Molecular Diagnosis and Integrated Therapy*, DOI 10.1007/978-4-431-55894-1_3

The Imaging Physics Team at National Institute of Radiological Sciences (NIRS) has carried out basic studies on radiation detectors, data acquisition systems, image reconstruction algorithms, and data correction methods to improve image quality and quantity in nuclear medicine as well as to explore innovative systems.

A depth-of-interaction (DOI) detector, for which various methods have been studied [1–7], will be a key device to get any significant improvement in sensitivity while maintaining high spatial resolution (Fig. 3.1). In order to maintain enough detection efficiency, the scintillation crystals should be 2–3 cm long. In conventional detectors, the crystal thickness causes uncertainty in position identification, which results in degraded spatial resolution at the peripheral area of a field-of-view. On the other hand, DOI can reduce the parallax error while maintaining the efficiency.

We have developed four-layered DOI detectors based on a light-sharing method [8, 9]. One successful proof of concept was the "jPET" project, in which we developed brain prototype PET with our DOI detectors; almost uniform spatial resolution around 2 mm all over the field-of-view was obtained with iterative image reconstruction with geometrically defined system matrix [10]. We have also succeeded to upgrade the DOI detector to have better spatial resolution with cheaper production costs: successful identification of $32 \times 32 \times 4$ array of LYSO crystals sized in $1.45 \times 1.45 \times 4.5$ mm^3 with a 64ch flat panel PMT (H8500, Hamamatsu Photonics K.K., Japan) [11], which has enabled Shimadzu's new products of positron emission mammography.

DOI measurement also has a potential to expand PET application fields because it allows for more flexible detector arrangement. As an example, we are developing the world's first, open-type PET geometry, "OpenPET," which is expected to lead to PET imaging during treatment. In addition, flexible system design of OpenPET

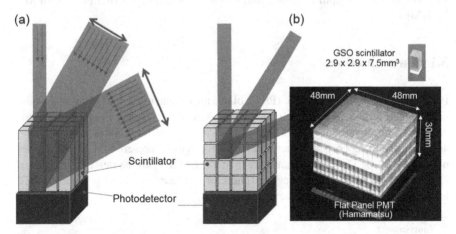

Fig. 3.1 Comparison between a conventional PET detector (**a**) and our depth-of-interaction (DOI) detector. The DOI detector (**b**) eliminates the parallax error, which is caused by the thickness of crystals in conventional 2D detectors

prototypes is enabling us to develop an innovative brain scanner "helmet-chin PET." The DOI detector itself continues to evolve with the help of recently developed semiconductor photodetectors, often referred to as silicon photomultipliers (SiPMs). We are developing a SiPM-based DOI detector "X'tal cube" to achieve sub-mm spatial resolution, which is reaching the theoretical limitation of PET imaging. Innovation of SiPMs encourages our development of PET/MRI, which is attracting great notice in terms of smaller radiation exposure and better contract in soft tissues compared with current PET/CT. By using our SiPM-based DOI detectors, we are developing a novel, high-performance, and low-cost brain PET/MRI to meet demands for earlier diagnosis of Alzheimer's disease. The key concept is a RF coil with DOI PET detectors, which has a potential to upgrade any existing MRI to PET/MRI. In this paper, an overview of above developments is shown.

3.2 The OpenPET: A Future PET for Therapy Imaging

OpenPET is our original idea to realize the world's first open-type 3D PET scanner for PET-image guided particle therapy such as in situ dose verification and direct tumor tracking. The principal of dose verification for particle therapy is based on the measurement of positron emitters which are produced through fragmentation reactions caused by proton or ^{12}C ion irradiation. Even with a full-ring geometry, the OpenPET has an open gap between its two detector rings through which the treatment beam passes, while conventional positron cameras applied to particle therapy imaging have been basically limited to planar imaging with lower detection efficiency [12–14]. Following our initial proposal of the dual-ring OpenPET (DROP) in 2008 (Fig. 3.2a) [15], we developed a small prototype in 2010 to show a proof of concept (Fig. 3.2b) [16]. In 2011, we also proposed the single-ring OpenPET (SROP), which is more efficient than DROP in terms of manufacturing cost and sensitivity [17]. We developed two small SROP prototypes in 2012 and 2013 (Fig. 3.2d, e) [18, 19], and we succeeded in visualizing a 3D distribution of beam stopping positions inside a phantom with the help of radioactive beams (^{11}C beam and ^{10}C beam) used as primary beams (Fig. 3.2f) [20]. Following these good results, in 2014, we have finally developed a whole-body prototype of DROP (Fig. 3.2g) [21].

The key technology which enabled OpenPET is our original, four-layered DOI detector. In order to measure radiations from the limited activity produced though fragmentation reactions, Zr-doped GSO (GSOZ), which contains less natural radioactivity, was chosen for the scintillators instead of Lu-based scintillators although timing performance was compromised. In order to compensate for the limited light yield, on the other hand, we used 64-channel, flat-panel PMTs with a super-bialkali photocathode (Hamamatsu R10552-100-M64), which had a 30 % higher quantum efficiency [22]. In order to enable stable in-beam PET measurement even under high background radiations, voltage divider circuits were designed so as to have

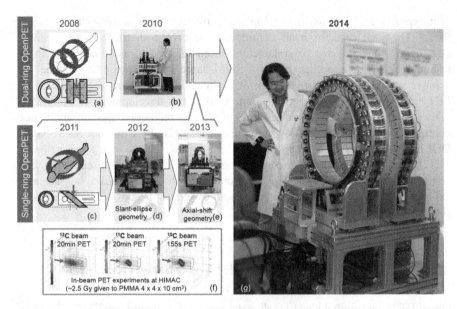

Fig. 3.2 Conceptual sketches and prototypes of the OpenPET geometries: the dual-ring OpenPET (DROP) (**a–b**) and the single-ring OpenPET (**c–e**). Following proofs-of-concept of in-beam imaging (**f**), a whole-body DROP was developed (**g**)

five times higher linearity. In order to avoid severe radiation damage, in addition, gain control ASICs were not implemented in the front-end circuits, and position analyzer circuits were placed with a 15-m cable extension. A data acquisition system was developed based on the single events collection.

The prototype consisted of two detector rings, and each detector ring had two subrings of 40 detectors. Each detector consisted of $16 \times 16 \times 4$ array of GSOZ ($2.8 \times 2.8 \times 7.5$ mm^3). The portable gantry had a compact design; each detector ring had a 940 mm outer diameter and 171 mm thickness for the detector inner bore of 640 mm diameter and 113 mm thickness.

3.3 The Helmet-Chin PET for Super High-Sensitive Brain Imaging

For a potential demand for brain molecular imaging, prototypes of brain dedicated PET scanners have been developed. However all previous developments are based on a cylindrical geometry [3, 10, 23–25], which is not the most efficient for brain imaging. Making the detector ring as small as possible is essential in PET, because sensitivity can be increased with a limited number of detectors. With appropriate DOI detectors, which reduce the parallax error caused by the thickness of the scintillators, spatial resolution can be maintained, or even improved by reducing the angular deviation effect. Therefore, we developed the world's first helmet-chin PET, in which DOI detectors are arranged to form a hemisphere, for compact, high-sensitivity, high-resolution, and low-cost PET imaging [26, 27].

Our basic idea relies on the evidence that the average sensitivity of a hemisphere PET is about 1.5-times higher than that of a cylinder PET of the same radius and height, while surface area is the same for both geometries (Fig. 3.3a, b). In addition, use of 12 % more detectors for "chin detectors," which are placed like a chin strap, improves sensitivity especially at the central area (Fig. 3.3c). In the prototype, 47 block detectors were used to form a hemisphere of 25 cm inner diameter and 50 cm outer diameter, and seven block detectors were used for the chin strap (Fig. 3.3d). The total number of detectors was about only 1/5 of that to be used in whole body PET. Each detector block was a four-layered DOI detector, which consisted of 1024 Zr-doped GSO crystals (2.8 mm × 2.8 mm × 7.5 mm) and a high-sensitivity type of 64-channel flat-panel PMT. The data acquisition system was

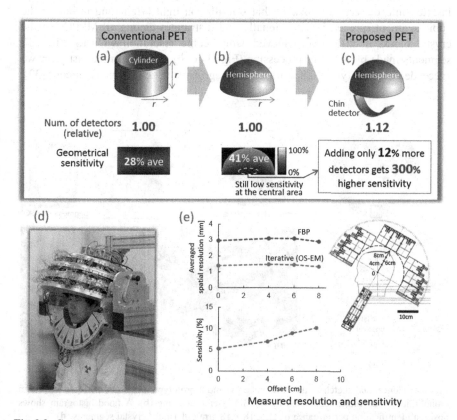

Fig. 3.3 Comparison between a conventional cylinder PET (**a**) and the proposed helmet-chin PET (**b, c**); the hemisphere detector arrangement obtains 1.5 times higher sensitivity, and adding only 12 % more detectors gets three times higher sensitivity at the central area. A prototype of the helmet-chin PET (**d**) succeeded in obtaining excellent sensitivity and resolution performance (**e**)

developed based on single event collection. An iterative reconstruction method with detector modeling was applied.

Measured sensitivity was 5 % at the cerebellum region and 10 % at the parietal region for a standard 400–600 keV energy window. Averaged FWHM of point sources was 3.0 mm (FBP) and 1.4 mm (iterative) (Fig. 3.3e).

3.4   The X'tal Cube: 0.8 mm Isotropic Resolution, a World Record

X'tal (crystal) cube is a future DOI detector we are developing. SiPMs, multi-pixel photon counters (MPPCs), are coupled on all sides of a scintillation crystal block, which is segmented into a 3D array of cubes [28] (Fig. 3.4a). Crystal segmentation is made by irradiating a laser to a monolithic crystal (Fig. 3.4b) [29]. No reflector is inserted into the crystal block so that scintillation light originating in one of the cubic segment spreads 3-dimensionally and distributes among all MPPCs on the crystal block. In 2012, we achieved 1-mm cubic resolution with $18 \times 18 \times 18$ segments made by 3D laser processing (Fig. 3.4c, d) [30, 31]. In the last year, we succeeded in identifying $(0.8 \text{ mm})^3$ crystal segments, which is a world record [32].

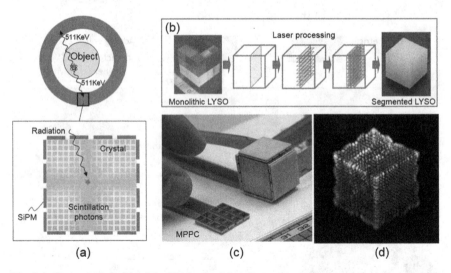

Fig. 3.4 Conceptual sketch of the X'tal cube (**a**) and a prototype X'tal cube detector (**c**) with a monolithic crystal block segmented by the 3D laser processing (**b**). A flood histogram shows position identification performance of $18 \times 18 \times 18$ array of 1 mm^3 crystal segments (**d**)

3.5 The Add-On PET: A PET Insert to Upgrade Existing MRI to PET/MRI

One of the major innovations made in recent years is combined PET/MRI (Fig. 3.5a) [33–46], but utilization of DOI measurement in PET detectors has not been studied well. DOI measurement, which allows for use of a smaller detector ring, is essential for PET in order to exploit the excellent potentials of PET imaging in terms of improved spatial resolution and sensitivity as well as reduced production costs of PET instrument. Therefore we proposed a new combined PET/MRI that makes full use of DOI measurement (Fig. 3.5b) [47, 48].

In order to make a PET detector ring as small as possible while placing electronic parts such as photodetectors and front-end circuits outside of a RF coil, PET detector modules were placed between spokes of the birdcage RF coil (Fig. 3.5c). For each detector module, electronic parts were covered with a Cu shielding box with a hole in front of the photodetectors, and scintillators were sticking out of the shielding box to allow their placement inside of the birdcage coil (Fig. 3.5e). In theory, the proposed birdcage coil integrated with PET detectors can be applied to any existing MRI as an additional choice of RF coils. For a proof of

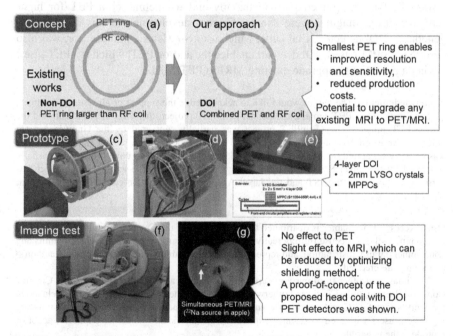

Fig. 3.5 Concept comparison between conventional PET/MRI (**a**) and the proposed add-on PET/MRI (**b**). A prototype (**c, d**) combined with DOI detector modules (**e**) was applied to 3T MRI (**f**) to demonstrate simultaneous PET/MRI imaging (**g**)

concept, we developed a full-ring prototype (four-layered arrays of 2.0 mm-LYSO with MPPCs) (Fig. 3.5d), which was applied to a 3T MRI (MAGNETOM Verio, Siemens) (Fig. 3.5f).

After evaluating interference between PET and MRI, no undesirable effect was seen in the PET imaging in terms of energy resolution and position identification. While a uniform static magnetic field was obtained, about a 20 % decrease in signal-to-noise ratio was observed in MR images; we suspected this was due to noise contamination from outside the MRI room. Although further optimization is required for shielding, we demonstrated a proof of concept of the proposed head coil with DOI PET detectors (Fig. 3.5g).

3.6 Conclusions

In PET, DOI measurement is a key technology to get significant improvement in sensitivity while maintaining high spatial resolution. DOI measurement also has a potential to expand PET application fields because it allows for more flexible detector arrangement. In this paper, two current developments, the OpenPET toward PET-image guided particle therapy and the helmet-chin PET for high-sensitive brain imaging, were shown. Current development status of the next-generation DOI detector X'tal cube, which uses SiPMs as a photosensor, was also described. SiPM-based DOI detector enabled the add-on PET, which is a PET insert having a potential to upgrade existing MRI to PET/MRI.

Acknowledgments The author would like to acknowledge the support of all research members engaged in the OpenPET project, the helmet-chin PET project, the X'tal cube project, and the add-on PET project. The OpenPET project was partially supported by the Grant-in-Aid for Scientists Research (A) of Kakenhi (22240065 and 25242052). The helmet-chin PET project was partially supported by ATOX Co., Ltd. (Tokyo, Japan). The X'tal cube project was partially supported by the Japan Science and Technology Agency (JST). The add-on PET project was partially supported by the JST and the Japan Agency for Medical Research and Development (AMED).

References

1. Carrier C, Martel C, Schmitt D, Leconte R. Design of a high resolution positron emission tomograph using solid state scintillation detectors. IEEE Trans Nucl Sci. 1988;35:685–90.
2. Yamamoto S, Ishibashi H. A GSO depth of interaction detector for PET. IEEE Trans Nucl Sci. 1998;45:1078–82.
3. Wienhard K, Schmand M, Casey ME, Baker K, Bao J, Eriksson L, et al. The ECAT HRRT: performance and first clinical application of the new high-resolution research tomograph. IEEE Trans Nucl Sci. 2002;49:104–10.
4. Yamashita T, Watanabe M, Shimizu K, Uchida H. High resolution block detectors for PET. IEEE Trans Nucl Sci. 1990;37:589–93.
5. Moses WW, Derenzo SE, Melcher CL, Manente RA. A room temperature LSO/PIN photodiode PET detector module that measures depth of interaction. IEEE Trans Nucl Sci. 1995;42:1085–9.
6. Miyaoka RS, Lewellen TK, Yu H, McDaniel DL. Design of a depth of interaction (DOI) PET detector module. IEEE Trans Nucl Sci. 1998;45:1069–73.
7. Shao Y, Silverman RW, Farrell R, Cirignano L, Grazioso R, Shah KS, et al. Design studies of a high resolution PET detector using APD arrays. IEEE Trans Nucl Sci. 2000;47:1051–7.
8. Murayama H, Ishibachi H, Uchida H, Omura T, Yamashita T. Depth encoding multicrystal detectors for PET. IEEE Trans Nucl Sci. 1998;45:1152–7.
9. Inadama N, Murayama H, Omura T, Yamashita T, Yamamoto S, Ishibashi H, et al. A depth of interaction detector for PET with GSO crystals doped with different amounts of Ce. IEEE Trans Nucl Sci. 2002;49:629–33.
10. Yamaya T, Yoshida E, Obi T, Ito H, Yoshikawa K, Murayama H. First human brain imaging by the jPET-D4 prototype with a pre-computed system matrix. IEEE Trans Nucl Sci. 2008;55:2482–92.
11. Tsuda T, Murayama H, Kitamura K, Yamaya T, Yoshida E, Omura T, et al. A four-layer depth of interaction detector block for small animal PET. IEEE Trans Nucl Sci. 2004;51:2537–42.
12. Pawelke J, Byars L, Enghardt W, Fromm WD, Geissel H, Hasch BG, et al. The investigation of different cameras for in-beam PET imaging. Phys Med Biol. 1996;41:279–96.
13. Iseki Y, Mizuno H, Futami Y, Tomitani T, Kanai T, Kanazawa M, Kitagawa A, Murakami T, Nishio T, Suda M. Positron camera for range verification of heavy-ion radiotherapy. Nucl Inst Methods Phys Res A. 2003;515:840–9.
14. Nishio T, Ogino T, Nomura K, Uchida H. Dose-volume delivery guided proton therapy using beam on-line PET system. Med Phys. 2006;33:4190–7.
15. Yamaya T, Inaniwa T, Minohara S, Yoshida E, Inadama N, Nishikido F, et al. A proposal of an open PET geometry. Phys Med Biol. 2008;53:757–73.
16. Yamaya T, Yoshida E, Inaniwa T, Sato S, Nakajima Y, Wakizaka H, et al. Development of a small prototype for a proof-of-concept of OpenPET imaging. Phys Med Biol. 2011;56:1123–37.
17. Tashima H, Yamaya T, Yoshida E, Kinouchi S, Watanabe M, Tanaka E. A single-ring OpenPET enabling PET imaging during radiotherapy. Phys Med Biol. 2012;57:4705–18.
18. Yoshida E, Tashima T, Wakizaka H, Nishikido F, Hirano Y, Inadama N, et al. Development of a single-ring OpenPET prototype. Nucl Inst Methods Phys Res A. 2013;729:800–8.
19. Yamaya T, Yoshida E, Tashima H, Nakajima Y, Nishikido F, Hirano Y, et al. A prototype of a novel transformable single-ring OpenPET. In: IEEE nuclear science symposium conference record. Piscataway: IEEE; 2013. M07-1.
20. Urakabe E, Kanai T, Kanazawa M, Kitagawa A, Noda K, Tomitani T, et al. Spot scanning using radioactive ^{11}C beams for heavy-ion radiotherapy. Jpn J Appl Phys. 2001;40:2540–8.
21. Yamaya T, Yoshida E, Tashima H, Inadama N, Nishikido F, Hirano Y, et al. Whole-body dual-ring OpenPET for in-beam particle therapy imaging. In: IEEE nuclear science symposium conference record. Piscataway: IEEE; 2014. M15-8.

22. Hirano Y, Nitta M, Inadama N, Nishikido F, Yoshida E, Murayama H, et al. Performance evaluation of a depth-of-interaction detector by use of position-sensitive PMT with a super-bialkali photocathode. Radiol Phys Technol. 2014;7:57–66.
23. Yamamoto S, Honda M, Oohashi T, Shimizu K, Senda M. Development of a brain PET system, PET-Hat: a wearable PET system for brain research. IEEE Trans Nucl Sci. 2011;58:668–73.
24. Majewski S, Proffitt J, Brefczynski-Lewis J, Stolin A, Weisenberger AG, Xi W, et al. HelmetPET: a silicon photomultiplier based wearable brain imager. In: IEEE nuclear science symposium conference record. Piscataway: IEEE; 2011. p. 4030–4.
25. Omura T, Moriya T, Yamada R, Yamauchi H, Saito A, Sakai T. Development of a high-resolution four-layer DOI detector using MPPCs for brain PET. In: IEEE nuclear science symposium conference record. 2012. p. 3560–3.
26. Tashima H, Ito H, Yamaya T. A proposed helmet-PET with a jaw detector enabling high-sensitivity brain imaging. In: IEEE nuclear science symposium conference record. 2013. M11-11.
27. Yamaya T, Yoshida E, Tashima H, Inadama N, Shinaji T, Wakizaka H, et al. First prototype of a compact helmet-chin PET for high-sensitivity brain imaging. J Nucl Med. 2015;56:317.
28. Yamaya T, Mitsuhashi T, Matsumoto T, Inadama N, Nishikido F, Yoshida E, et al. A SiPM-based isotropic-3D PET detector X'tal cube with a three-dimensional array of 1 mm3 crystals. Phys Med Biol. 2011;56:6793–807.
29. Moriya T, Fukumitsu K, Sakai T, Ohsuka S, Okamoto T, Takahashi H, et al. Development of PET detectors using monolithic scintillation crystals processed with sub-surface laser engraving technique. IEEE Trans Nucl Sci. 2010;57:2455–9.
30. Yoshida E, Hirano Y, Tashima H, Inadama N, Nishikido F, Moriya T, et al. Impact of the laser-processed X'tal cube detector on PET imaging in a one-pair prototype system. IEEE Trans Nucl Sci. 2013;60:3172–80.
31. Yoshida E, Tashima H, Hirano Y, Inadama N, Nishikido F, Muraya H, et al. Spatial resolution limits for the isotropic-3D PET detector X'tal cube. Nucl Inst Methods Phys Res A. 2013;728:107–11.
32. Munetaka N, Inadama N, Hirano Y, Nishikido F, Yoshida E, Tashima H, et al. The X'tal cube PET detector of isotropic (0.8 mm)^3 crystal segments. In: IEEE nuclear science symposium conference record. 2014. M04-1.
33. Shao Y, Cherry S. Simultaneous PET and MR imaging. Phys Med Biol. 1997;42:1965–70.
34. Slates RB, Farahani K, Shao Y, Marsden PK, Taylor J, Summers PE, et al. A study of artefacts in simultaneous PET and MR imaging using a prototype MR compatible PET scanner. Phys Med Biol. 1999;44:2015–27.
35. Catana C, Wu Y, Judenhofer MS, Qi J, Pichler BJ, Cherry SR. Simultaneous acquisition of multislice PET and MR images: initial results with a MR-compatible PET scanner. J Nucl Med. 2006;47:1968–76.
36. Pichler BJ, Judenhofer MS, Catana C, Walton JH, Kneilling M, Nutt RE, et al. Performance test of an LSO-APD detector in a 7-T MRI scanner for simultaneous PET/MRI. J Nucl Med. 2006;47:639–47.
37. Schlyer D, Vaska P, Tomasi D, Woody C, Maramraju S-H, Southekal S, et al. A simultaneous PET/MRI scanner based on RatCAP in small animals. In: IEEE nuclear science symposium conference record. 2007. p. 3256.
38. Schlemmer HP, Pichler BJ, Schmand M, Burbar Z, Michel C, Ladebeck R, et al. Simultaneous MR/PET imaging of the human brain: feasibility study. Radiology. 2008;248:1028–35.
39. Yamamoto S, Hatazawa J, Imaizumi M, Shimosegawa E, Aoki M, Sugiyama E, et al. A multi-slice dual layer MR-compatible animal PET system. IEEE Trans Nucl Sci. 2009;56:2706–13.
40. Yamamoto S, Imaizumi M, Kanai Y, Tatsumi M, Aoki M, Sugiyama E, et al. Design and performance from an integrated PET/MRI system for small animals. Ann Nucl Med. 2010;24:89–98.

41. Kwon SI, Lee JS, Yoon HS, Ito M, Ko GB, Choi JY, et al. Development of small-animal PET prototype using silicon photomultiplier (SiPM): initial results of phantom and animal imaging studies. J Nucl Med. 2011;52:572–9.
42. Maramraju SH, Smith SD, Junnarkar SS, Schulz D, Stoll S, Ravindranath B, et al. Small animal simultaneous PET/MRI: initial experiences in a 9.4 T microMRI. Phys Med Biol. 2011;56:2459–80.
43. Zaidi H, Ojha N, Morich M, Griesmer J, Hu Z, Maniawski P, et al. Design and performance evaluation of a whole-body ingenuity TF PET-MRI system. Phys Med Biol. 2011;56:3091–106.
44. Delso G, Fürst S, Jakoby B, Ladebeck R, Ganter C, Nekolla SG, et al. Performance measurements of the Siemens mMR integrated whole-body PET/MR scanner. J Nucl Med. 2011;52:1914–22.
45. Yoon HS, Ko GB, Kwon SI, Lee CM, Ito M, Chan Song I, et al. Initial results of simultaneous PET/MRI experiments with an MRI-compatible silicon photomultiplier PET scanner. J Nucl Med. 2012;53:608–14.
46. Lee B J, Grant A M, Chang C-M, Levin C S. MRI measurements in the presence of a RF-penetrable PET insert for simultaneous PET/MRI. Abstract Book of 2015 World Molecular Imaging Congress. 2015. SS 126.
47. Nishikido F, Obata T, Shimizu K, Suga M, Inadama N, Tachibana A, et al. Feasibility of a brain-dedicated PET-MRI system using four-layer detectors integrated with an RF head coil. Nucl Instr Methods A. 2014;756:6–13.
48. Nishikido F, Tachibana A, Obata T, Inadama N, Yoshida E, Suga M, et al. Development of 1.45-mm resolution four-layer DOI–PET detector for simultaneous measurement in 3T MRI. Radiol Phys Technol. 2015;8:111–9.

Chapter 4
Semiconductor Detector-Based Scanners for Nuclear Medicine

Wataru Takeuchi, Atsuro Suzuki, Yuichiro Ueno, Tohru Shiga, Kenji Hirata, Shozo Okamoto, Songji Zhao, Yuji Kuge, Naoki Kubo, Kentaro Kobayashi, Shiro Watanabe, Keiji Kobashi, Kikuo Umegaki, and Nagara Tamaki

Abstract Semiconductor detectors have the potential to improve the quantitative accuracy of nuclear medicine imaging with their better energy and intrinsic spatial resolutions than those of conventional scintillator-based detectors. The fine energy resolution leads to a better image contrast due to better scatter rejection. The fine intrinsic spatial resolution due to a pixelated structure leads to a better image contrast and lower partial volume effect. Their pixelated structures also improve the count-rate capability. The authors developed CdTe semiconductor detector-based positron emission tomography (CdTe-PET) and single-photon emission computed tomography (CdTe-SPECT) in order to test the potential of using semiconductor detectors in nuclear medicine. The physical performances of both systems were measured in several phantom experiments. The capability of using CdTe-PET

W. Takeuchi (✉) • A. Suzuki • K. Kobashi
Research and Development Group, Hitachi Ltd., 1-280, Higashi-Koigakubo Kokubunji-shi, Tokyo 185-8601, Japan
e-mail: wataru.takeuchi.rg@hitachi.com

Y. Ueno
Research and Development Group, Hitachi Ltd., 1-280, Higashi-Koigakubo Kokubunji-shi, Tokyo 185-8601, Japan

Faculty of Engineering, Hokkaido University, Sapporo, Japan

T. Shiga • N. Tamaki
Department of Nuclear Medicine, Graduate School of Medicine, Hokkaido University, Sapporo, Japan

K. Hirata • S. Okamoto • S. Zhao • K. Kobayashi • S. Watanabe
Graduate School of Medicine, Hokkaido University, Sapporo, Japan

Y. Kuge
Central Institute of Isotope Science, Hokkaido University Department of Integrated Molecular Imaging, Graduate School of Medicine, Hokkaido University, Sapporo, Japan

N. Kubo
Office of Health and Safety, Hokkaido University, Sapporo, Hokkaido, Japan

K. Umegaki
Faculty of Engineering, Hokkaido University, Sapporo, Japan

© The Author(s) 2016
Y. Kuge et al. (eds.), *Perspectives on Nuclear Medicine for Molecular Diagnosis and Integrated Therapy*, DOI 10.1007/978-4-431-55894-1_4

to measure the metabolic distribution of tumors was evaluated through scans of cancer patients and rat tumor models. The feasibility of using CdTe-SPECT for simultaneous dual-radionuclide imaging was evaluated through scans of phantoms and healthy volunteers. The results suggest that the prototype CdTe-PET can identify intratumoral metabolic heterogeneous distribution and that CdTe-SPECT can accurately acquire dual-radionuclide images simultaneously. Although there are still problems to be solved, semiconductor detectors will play significant roles in the future of nuclear medicine.

Keywords Semiconductor detector • Solid-state detector • CdTe • Intratumoral heterogeneity • Dual radionuclide

4.1 Introduction

Nuclear medicine plays a significant role in diagnosis, treatment planning, and treatment response evaluation. In particular, in oncology, biological imaging by positron emission tomography (PET) permits not only tumor detection but also gross tumor delineation and identification of biological heterogeneities [1, 2]. In the delineation of tumor boundaries by PET, achieving a good spatial resolution and quantitative accuracy are physical imaging concerns. The spatial resolution of the current PET images as used in clinical practice is 7–9 mm after reconstruction with many systems. The achievable spatial resolution depends primarily on the size of the detector elements. The typical PET scanner used in current clinical study is comprised of scintillation detectors 4×4 mm in size.

In nuclear cardiology and brain nuclear medicine, functional imaging by PET and single-photon emission computed tomography (SPECT) can measure the functional state of the myocardium and brain. Unlike PET, SPECT has the potential to enable simultaneous multi-radionuclide imaging. The scanning of multi-radionuclide pharmaceuticals will enable various kinds of functional images to be obtained without position error or time difference. The recent development of several cardiac SPECT systems that use solid-state detectors with a fine energy resolution [3–5] has led to simultaneous multi-radionuclide imaging recapturing the spotlight. A number of simultaneous multi-radionuclide imaging studies have been reported, especially for myocardial perfusion diagnosis [4, 5]. To enable accurate simultaneous multi-radionuclide imaging, a detector with a good energy resolution is necessary. In addition, improving the sensitivity of gamma-ray detection is also important for realizing simultaneous multi-radionuclide imaging with an appropriate dose of radiopharmaceuticals.

As mentioned above, the performance of nuclear medicine imaging depends on spatial resolution, energy resolution, and sensitivity. Semiconductor detectors, e.g., CdZnTe or CdTe detectors, provide improved energy resolution due to the direct conversion of gamma rays to charge carriers. This fine resolution leads to a better image contrast due to better scatter rejection. Semiconductor detectors also easily provide a pixelated structure that improves the count-rate capability and intrinsic spatial resolution. Flexibility in both sizing and a fine arrangement of semiconductor detectors is expected not only to improve the spatial resolution but also to obtain depth-of-interaction (DOI) information in PET and pixel-of-interaction in SPECT when the multidetector pixels are placed within each collimator hole. A high energy resolution is expected to reduce scattered components in detected signals and to improve the quantitative accuracy of the reconstructed images. These features of semiconductor detectors may lead to improved PET and SPECT images. The authors previously developed CdTe semiconductor detector-based PET (CdTe-PET) [1, 2] and SPECT (CdTe-SPECT) [6, 7]. The physical and clinical performances of the systems were evaluated through phantom, animal, and clinical studies.

4.2   Materials and Methods

4.2.1   Development and Performance Evaluation of Prototype CdTe-PET

4.2.1.1   Outline of CdTe-PET and Its Parameter Settings

CdTe-PET is a prototype semiconductor PET scanner for human brain imaging. This scanner is described in detail in a previous report [1]. In brief, the scanner uses CdTe detectors for dedicated three-dimensional emission scanning. It has a patient port with a diameter of 350 mm, a transaxial FOV of 310 mm, and an axial FOV of 250 mm. The size of a detector is $1.0 \times 4.0 \times 7.5$ mm. The detector channel is composed of two CdTe elements in the radial direction and two CdTe elements in the tangential direction. To utilize the depth-of-interaction (DOI) technique, three detector channels (six detectors) in the tangential direction are used. The transverse and axial spatial resolutions near the center are 2.3 and 5.1 mm, respectively. The energy resolution is 4.1 % at 511 keV (FWHM), which is superior to that of available scintillation detectors, e.g., 10–20 %. The long-term stability of the energy resolution of the CdTe detectors was assured by periodically resetting the bias [8]. No significant variances in the spectral peak position and energy resolution of the CdTe detectors were observed for over a year [9].

The energy of detected gamma rays is recorded in list-mode data. This data contains the energy information of two gamma rays in the coincidence detection. The size of an energy bin is 4 keV. Two energy windows, described below, were used. One energy window (390–540 keV) was used as a wide energy window (WEW), and another (494–540 keV) was used as a photopeak energy window (PEW). Sinogram data using both WEW and PEW were made by sorting the list-mode data by recorded energy. For all measured sinogram data and energy spectra, random coincidences were removed by using the delayed coincidence subtraction technique. The size of the sinogram data is 256 in the radial direction, 256 in the angular direction, 87 in the axial direction, and 44 in the oblique angular direction, i.e., ring difference. The matrix size of the reconstructed images is $256 \times 256 \times 87$ with voxels of $1.21 \times 1.21 \times 2.8$ mm.

To bring out the potential of CdTe detectors in human imaging, the main challenge to be solved is sensitivity. The effective atomic number of the CdTe is smaller than the scintillation detectors of the current PET scanner. The crystal size is also smaller than those detectors. To overcome the sensitivity problem, the following improvements were made.

To improve sensitivity, a novel signal processing method was developed [1]. The effective atomic number of the CdTe is 50, so the whole absorption rate of the 511-keV gamma ray is smaller than the current scintillation detectors, and a considerable amount of scattered gamma rays are generated and absorbed in nearby detectors. In the improved signal processing method, when the sum of the energy of two gamma rays detected in a neighborhood channel in a limited time window (64 ns) is around 511 keV, the record of the gamma rays detected at the opposing detector unit in the coincidence time window (14 ns) is checked for the coincidence detection. With this signal processing, the detector of our system is considered to be a continuous mass of CdTe from the viewpoint of sensitivity, although the position is determined digitally.

4.2.1.2 Image Reconstruction Method

A reconstruction system of the developed scanner coped with the sensitivity problem, avoiding unexpected statistical fluctuation in reconstructed images. To enable high-resolution imaging with a low amount of statistical data, we developed a reconstruction method that could suppress statistical noise without degrading the spatial resolution [1, 10]. The method is based on maximum a posteriori (MAP) [11] with median root prior (MRP) [12] and uses a resolution recovery technique [13, 14]. The method also uses an attenuation and normalization weighting technique. MRP assumes only local monotony and does not need any anatomical information such as MRI or CT images. MRP is also known as an effectual prior for reducing noise and preserving edge. Because of various incident angles and distances to detectors, reconstructed point source images blur into various shapes. To correct the point spread function (PSF), a 3-D image-space convolution technique was used [13]. The Gaussian kernel represents the PSF. The algorithm of the reconstruction method, named "point spread function correction with median root prior" (PSC-MRP), is shown in Eq. (4.1):

$$
\lambda_j^{k+1} = \frac{\lambda_j^k}{\left(1 + \beta \frac{\lambda_j^k - M_j}{M_j}\right) \cdot \left(\sum_i p_{ij} a_j n_j\right) \otimes G} \left(\sum_i p_{ij} \frac{y_i}{\sum_{j'} p_{ij'}\left(\lambda_{j'}^k \otimes G\right)}\right) \otimes G \quad (4.1)
$$

λ : pixelvalue (j = index, k = iteration)
y : obsereved data (i = index)
p : probability-matrix
a : attenuation-matrix
, where
n : normatlization-matrix
M : median of the neibourhodd
G : Gaussian-Kernel (*PSF*)
β : prior strength

The value y is measured data, and λ is emission image. The matrices p, a, and n represent probability (geometrical sensitivity), attenuation, and normalization (sensitivity of each detector), respectively. The value k is the number of iterations, and i and j are index numbers. The value β controls the effect of reducing noise, and M is a median of neighbor ($3 \times 3 \times 3$) voxels' values. The Gaussian kernel G represents the PSF. The PSFs were measured for a point source at different positions in a portion of the field of view. The G was parameterized to correct for point source location and to smooth for projection noise. When β is zero and G is not used, the reconstruction method equals attenuation and normalization weighted OSEM (ANW-OSEM) [15]. The numbers of subsets and iterations were 8 and 5, respectively.

4.2.1.3 Physical Performance Measurement

In accordance with the NEMA NU2-1994 standards [16], a count-rate performance experiment was conducted with CdTe-PET. In this evaluation, two energy windows (WEW and PEW described above) were used. The count-rate performance of CdTe-PET was measured with a standard 20-cm-inner-diameter, 20-cm-long phantom filled with water that contained a 3.7-kBq/cm^3 F-18 solution. The phantom was placed at the center of the FOV and scanned over ten half-lives. The performance was evaluated in WEW and PEW settings. The noise equivalent count rate (NEC2R) was calculated by NEC2R $= $ T*T/(T + S + 2*R) from the true (T) rate, scattered (S) rate, and random (R) rate. The random rate was multiplied by a factor of two because the random rate was evaluated by acquiring events in a delayed time window. The sensitivity of the scanner was also evaluated using the measurement data of count-rate performance.

4.2.1.4 Image Quality Evaluation

To evaluate the image quality of CdTe-PET with its energy window set to PEW, two kinds of experiments and studies, described below, were conducted.

Hoffman Phantom

A Hoffman phantom (filled with 9.1 kBq/ml F-18 solution) simulated the human brain was scanned for 10 min so as to equalize the measured count with the clinical situation. The data was reconstructed by (a) ANW-OSEM, (b) ANW-OSEM with post-reconstruction Gaussian filter (4-mm FWHM), and (c) PSC-MAP $\beta = 0.05$. The three images were compared visually.

Preclinical Evaluation with Rat Tumor Model

To evaluate the feasibility of visualizing intratumoral heterogeneity, a preclinical study using a rat tumor model was conducted. All animal care and experimental procedures were performed with the approval of the Laboratory Animal Care and Use Committee of Hokkaido University. Eight-week-old male Wistar-King-Aptekman/hok (WKAH) rats (Japan SLC, Inc.) were inoculated with a suspension of allogenic rat glioma cells (C6, 2×106 cells/0.2 ml) into the left calf muscle to generate glioma rat models. The rats were allowed free access to water and laboratory chow until the day before the experiment. When the tumors were 1–2 cm in diameter, the rats were fasted overnight. Under diethyl ether anesthesia, 200 kBq/g body weight of F-18-fluorodeoxyglucose (FDG) was intravenously injected into each rat. Fifty minutes after the injection of FDG, the rats were anesthetized with pentobarbital (50 mg/kg body weight, intraperitoneally). One hour after the FDG injection, each rat was scanned by CdTe-PET for 1 min. Then, images were reconstructed by PSC-MAP ($\beta = 0.05$). Four hours after the FDG injection, the rats were euthanized under deep pentobarbital anesthesia. The animals were sacrificed, and the whole tumors were quickly excised. Then, the excised tumors were frozen in isopentane/dry ice. The frozen tumor tissues were sectioned into slices for autoradiographic (ARG) imaging. The thickness of the sectioned slices was 0.15 mm. The number of slices was about 19. All of the sectioned slices were exposed to phosphor imaging plates (BAS-SR 2025, Fuji Photo Film Co., Ltd.) together with a set of calibrated standards. The autoradiographic exposure was performed for 12 h to detect the radioactivity of FDG. After the exposure, the imaging plates were scanned with a Fuji Bio-imaging Analyzer BAS-5000, and the units of the images were converted into a unit of Bq/ml by house-made software. All of the sectioned slices were integrated into a 3-D volume by using a slice-by-slice image registration technique. Then, the integrated 3-D ARG and PET images were compared.

Clinical Evaluation

As was previously reported [1, 2], patients with brain tumor or nasopharyngeal cancer injected FDG (340 MBq ca.) were scanned by CdTe-PET for 30 min. Then, images were reconstructed by PSC-MAP ($\beta = 0.05$). The patient volunteers gave written, informed consent in accordance with the Helsinki II Declaration. The study was approved by the ethics committees of both the Hokkaido University Graduate School of Medicine and Hitachi, Ltd. The capability of using CdTe-PET to measure the metabolic distribution of tumor was evaluated.

4.2.2 Development and Performance Evaluation of Prototype CdTe-SPECT

4.2.2.1 Outline of CdTe-SPECT

CdTe-SPECT is a prototype semiconductor SPECT system for human brain imaging. This system is described in detail in previous reports [6, 7]. In brief, CdTe-SPECT includes two detector heads. Each head consists of 192×96 detector pixels with a pitch of 1.4 mm, so the field of view of the detector head is 268×134 mm (tangential $\times$ axial). The size of each detector pixel is $1.2 \times 1.4 \times 5$ mm. The intrinsic energy resolution (FWHM) of the CdTe detector is 6.6 % at 140.5 keV, and the count-rate linearity is maintained at 200 kcps per head and under [9]. For high-sensitivity imaging, a wide aperture parallel-hole collimator (Fig. 4.1), which we call the "4-pixel matched collimator" (4-PMC), was previously developed [6, 7]. The hole size of the 4-PMC is matched to four detector pixels, that is, there are four (2×2) pixels per collimator hole. By contrast, the hole size of the standard parallel-hole collimator [9] is matched to one detector pixel, that is, a 1-pixel matched collimator (1-PMC). The specifications of both collimators are shown in Table 4.1. 4-PMC was designed to improve the sensitivity and spatial resolution in clinical SPECT imaging compared with 1-PMC. The sensitivities of 1-PMC and 4-PMC were 70 and 220 cps/MBq/head, respectively [7]. Therefore, 4-PMC has three times the sensitivity of 1-PMC. The rotation radius of the detector head is set to 130 mm for brain scans. In SPECT acquisition, each detector head is rotated by 360° over 3 min.

Fig. 4.1 Geometry of 4-PMC

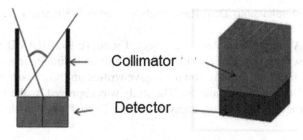

4-detector pixels per 1-hole

Table 4.1 Collimator specifications

Type	Hole pitch (mm)	Hole size (mm)	Hole length (mm)	Sensitivity (cps/MBq/head)
1-PMC	1.4	1.12	20.0	70
4-PMC	2.8	2.40	26.0	220

4.2.2.2 Image Reconstruction Method

The ordered subset expectation maximization (OSEM) (Hudson and Larkin 1994) including PSF and attenuation correction was used. The PSF of each collimator type was obtained by ray-tracing simulation [6, 7]. The attenuation factor of the gamma rays in a subject was approximated by an exponential function of the line integral from an image pixel to a detector pixel in an attenuation map. The projection image matrix size (tangential × axial) was 256×96 (pixel size $= 1.4 \times 1.4$ mm). The number of projection images was 120 over 360°. The reconstructed image matrix size $(x \times y \times z)$ was $256 \times 256 \times 96$ (pixel size $= 1.4 \times 1.4 \times 1.4$ mm). The numbers of subsets and iterations were 30 and 20, respectively. The reconstructed images were smoothed with a 14-mm FWHM Gaussian filter.

4.2.2.3 Performance Evaluation in Phantom Experiment and Clinical Study

Dual-Radionuclide Character-Shape Phantom

A character-shape dual-radionuclide phantom, which has three kinds of radioactivity, was scanned (Fig. 4.2). The activities are shown in Table 4.2. The photopeak energy windows for Tc-99m (141 keV) and I-123(159 keV) were 130–148 keV and 155–170 keV, respectively. An energy window-based scatter correction based on the triple energy window (TEW) method [17] was used. The measured energy spectrum and reconstructed images were evaluated.

Simultaneous Dual-Radionuclide Human Brain Study

A healthy volunteer was injected with Tc-99m HAS-D and I-123 IMP and then scanned by CdTe-SPECT for 21 min as a simultaneous dual-radionuclide brain study. The healthy volunteer gave written, informed consent in accordance with the Helsinki II Declaration. The study was approved by the ethics committees of both the Hokkaido University Graduate School of Medicine and Hitachi, Ltd. The

Fig. 4.2 Dual-radionuclide character-shape phantom

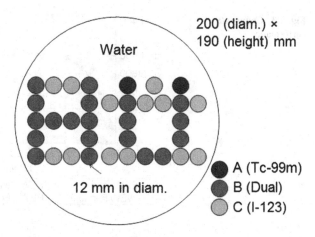

Table 4.2 Radioactivities of dual-radionuclide character-shape phantom

Kinds of vial	Tc-99m (kBq/ml)	I-123 (kBq/ml)
A (Tc-99m)	44.6	0
B (Dual)	49.3	115.5
C (I-123)	0	101

feasibility of using CdTe-SPECT for simultaneous dual-radionuclide study was evaluated.

4.3 Results and Discussion

4.3.1 Performance Evaluation of CdTe-PET by Phantom Experiment and Clinical Study

4.3.1.1 Physical Performance of CdTe-PET

Figure 4.3 shows the result of the count-rate performance examination. The left vertical axis is the count rate of "true" and "random." The right vertical axis is the noise equivalent count rate (NEC2R). The horizontal axis is the activity of the cylinder phantom. Table 4.3 shows the results for sensitivity, NECR, and scatter fraction. The sensitivity was 22.0 and 8.5 kcps/(kBq/ml) in WEW and PEW, respectively. The NECR at 7.4 kBq/ml was 45 and 25 kcps in WEW and PEW, respectively. The scatter fraction was 39 and 12 % in WEW and PEW, respectively. Comparing PEW with WEW, although the sensitivity was less than a half, the NECR was more than a half. The scatter fraction for PEW was less than a third of that for WEW.

Fig. 4.3 Count-rate performance

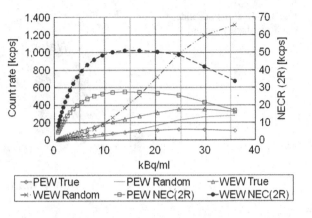

Table 4.3 Count-rate performances in each energy window

Energy window	WEW	PEW
Sensitivity [kcps/(kBq/ml)]	22.0	8.5
Peak NECR [kcps]	51	28
NECR at 3.7 kBq/ml [kcps]	32	18
NECR at 7.4 kBq/ml [kcps]	45	25
Scatter fraction [%]	39	12

4.3.1.2 Image Quality of CdTe-PET

Hoffman Phantom

Shown in Fig. 4.4 are images reconstructed by (a) ANW-OSEM, (b) ANW-OSEM with a Gaussian filter (4-mm FWHM), and (c) PSC-MAP $\beta = 0.05$. Even with filtering, images reconstructed by ANW-OSEM had speckle noise. The PSC-MAP image was not speckled and not blurred. Therefore, the edge between gray matter and white matter in the PSC-MAP image was well defined.

Preclinical Evaluation with Rat Tumor Model

The diameter of each tumor was ca. 16 mm. A 3-D ARG volume made by integrating 19 slices is shown in Fig. 4.5. The heterogeneous intratumoral FDG distribution in each tumor was visualized by both CdTe-PET and ARG (Figs. 4.5 and 4.6). CdTe-PET images were visually consistent with ARG (Fig. 4.6).

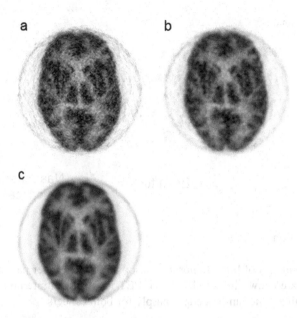

Fig. 4.4 Reconstructed image of Hoffman phantom. (**a**) ANW-OSEM, (**b**) ANW-OSEM + Gaussian filter, and (**c**) PSC-MAP (b = 0.05)

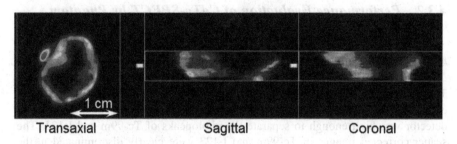

Fig. 4.5 Integrated 3-D ARG volume

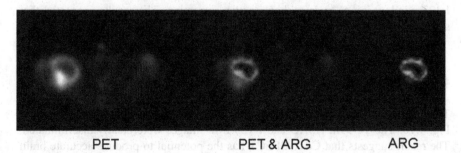

Fig. 4.6 Comparison of ARG and PET images. "PET + ARG" shows image fused by image registration method

Fig. 4.7 Clinical image
example of brain tumor
patient and nasopharyngeal
cancer patient

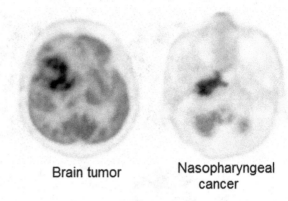

Brain tumor   Nasopharyngeal
                                    cancer

Clinical Evaluation

Reconstructed images of brain tumor and nasopharyngeal cancer patients scanned
by CdTe-PET are shown in Fig. 4.7. CdTe-PET identified intratumoral heterogeneity and visualized the tumor's edge sharply for both cancers.

4.3.2 Performance Evaluation of CdTe-SPECT by Phantom Experiment and Clinical Study

4.3.2.1 Dual-Radionuclide Character-Shape Phantom

The photopeaks of Tc-99m and I-123 were clearly discriminated in the measured
energy spectrum (Fig. 4.8). The energy resolution of the CdTe semiconductor
detector was high enough to separate the photopeaks of Tc-99m and I-123. The
scatter-corrected images of Tc-99m and I-123 were clearly discriminated in the
character-shape phantom image in Fig. 4.9. Because of the high-energy resolution
of the CdTe semiconductor detector, there was no Tc-99m contamination in the
I-123 window image even without scatter correction. The results suggested that
simultaneous Tc-99m and I-123 study by using CdTe-SPECT was feasible.

4.3.2.2 Simultaneous Dual-Radionuclide Human Brain Study

The result of a simultaneous Tc-99m and I-123 dual-radionuclide scan is shown in
Fig. 4.10. The Tc-99m HSAD and I-123 IMP images were clearly discriminated.
The result suggests that CdTe-SPECT has the potential to produce accurate brain

Fig. 4.8 Energy spectrum of dual-radionuclide character-shape phantom measurement

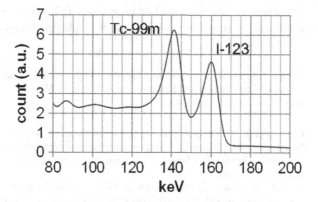

Fig. 4.9 Reconstructed image of dual-radionuclide character-shape phantom

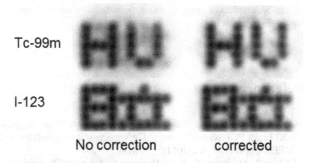

Fig. 4.10 Reconstructed image of simultaneous dual-radionuclide brain study

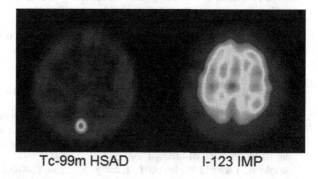

perfusion images (Tc-99m HSAD) and cerebral blood volume (Tc-99m HSAD) images simultaneously.

4.4 Conclusion

Prototype CdTe-PET and CdTe-SPECT systems were developed, and their performances were evaluated. The results suggest that CdTe-PET enables better identification of intratumoral metabolic distribution and that CdTe-SPECT will enable simultaneous dual-radionuclide brain study to become available clinically. Semi-conductor detectors have the potential to play a significant role in the future of nuclear medicine.

Acknowledgments This work was supported in part by the Creation of Innovation Centers for Advanced Interdisciplinary Research Areas Program, Ministry of Education, Culture, Sports, Science and Technology, Japan.

References

1. Morimoto Y, Ueno Y, Takeuchi W, Kojima S, Matsuzaki K, Ishitsu T, et al. Development of a 3D brain PET scanner using CdTe semiconductor detectors and its first clinical application. IEEE Trans Nucl Sci. 2011;58:2181–9.
2. Shiga T, Morimoto Y, Kubo N, Katoh C, Takeuchi W, Usui R, et al. A new PET scanner with semiconductor detectors enables better identification of intratumoral inhomogeneity. J Nucl Med. 2009;50:148–55.
3. Kubo N, Zhao S, Fujiki Y, Kinda A, Motomura N, Katoh C, et al. Evaluating performance of a pixel array semiconductor SPECT system for small animal imaging. Ann Nucl Med. 2005;19:633–9.
4. Bocher M, Blevis IM, Tsukerman L, Shrem Y, Kovalski G, Volokh L. A fast cardiac gamma camera with dynamic SPECT capabilities: design, system validation and future potential. Eur J Nucl Med Mol Imaging. 2010;37:1887–902.
5. Ko T, Utanohara Y, Suzuki Y, Kurihara M, Iguchi N, Umemura J, et al. A preliminary feasibility study of simultaneous dual-isotope imaging with a solid-state dedicated cardiac camera for evaluating myocardial perfusion and fatty acid metabolism. Heart Vessel. 2014. doi:10.1007/s00380-014-0578-4.
6. Suzuki A, Takeuchi W, Ishitsu T, Tsuchiya K, Ueno Y, Kobashi K. A four-pixel matched collimator for high-sensitivity SPECT imaging. Phys Med Biol. 2013;58:2199–217.
7. Suzuki A, Takeuchi W, Ishitsu T, Tsuchiya K, Morimoto Y, Ueno Y, et al. High-sensitivity brain SPECT system using cadmium telluride (CdTe) solid-state detector and 4-pixel matched collimator. Phys Med Biol. 2013;58:7715–31.
8. Seino T, Kominami S, Ueno Y, Amemiya K. Pulsed bias voltage shutdown to suppress the polarization effect for a CdTe radiation detector. IEEE Trans Nucl Sci. 2008;55:2770–4.
9. Tsuchiya K, Takahashi I, Kawaguchi T, Yokoi K, Morimoto Y, Ishitsu T, et al. Basic performance and stability of a CdTe solid-state detector panel. Ann Nucl Med. 2010;24:301–11.
10. Takeuchi W, Morimoto Y, Suzuki A, Matsuzaki K, Kojima S, Kobashi K, et al. Iterative reconstruction method using prior information and point spread function for high resolution CdTe PET scanner. J Nucl Med(Meeting abstract). 2008;49:388.

11. Green PJ. Bayesian reconstructions from emission tomography data using a modified EM algorithm. IEEE Trans Med Imaging. 1990;9:84–93.
12. Alenius S, Ruotsalainen U. Generalization of median root prior reconstruction. IEEE Trans Med Imaging. 2002;21:1413–20.
13. Reader AJ, Julyan PJ, Williams H, Hastings DL, Zweit J. EM algorithm system modeling by image-space techniques for PET reconstruction. IEEE Trans Nucl Sci. 2003;50:1392–7.
14. Panin VY, Kehren F, Michel C, Casey M. Fully 3-D PET reconstruction with system matrix derived from point source measurements. IEEE Trans Med Imaging. 2006;25:907–21.
15. Zaidi H. Quantitative analysis in nuclear medicine imaging. New York: Springer; 2006. p. 167–204.
16. NEMA. NEMA standards publication NU2-1994. 1994.
17. Ichihara T, Ogawa K, Motomura N, Kubo A, Hashimoto S. Compton scatter compensation using the triple-energy window method for single- and dual-isotope SPECT. J Nucl Med. 1993;34:2216–21.

Chapter 5
Kinetic Analysis for Cardiac PET

Yuuki Tomiyama and Keiichiro Yoshinaga

Abstract *Objective:* PET has the ability to evaluate functional information as well as visualization of radiotracer uptake. Compartmental model is a basic idea to analyze dynamic PET data. C-HED has been the most frequently used PET tracer for the evaluation of cardiac sympathetic nervous system (SNS) function. The washout of norepinephrine from myocardium is associated with increasing SNS activity in heart failure (HF). However, the existence of washout of ^{11}C-HED from the myocardium is controversial. Although "retention index" (RI) is commonly calculated to quantify the uptake of HED, RI is not purely able to distinguish washout parameter and uptake parameter. Therefore, in this study, we aimed to evaluate whether HED was washed out from the myocardium using compartment model analysis.

Material and Methods: We compared HED parameters in ten normal volunteers (32.4 ± 9.6 years) and nine HF patients (age: 57.3 ± 17.3 years, LVEF: 36.1 ± 16.7 %). Each subject underwent rest ^{11}C-HED PET. We estimated RI, inflow rate K1, and washout rate k2 using single-compartment model analysis using ^{11}C-HED PET.

Result: HF patients showed lower RI and inflow rate K1 compared to normal volunteers (RI: 0.06 ± 0.02 vs. 0.15 ± 0.03 min^{-1}, $p < 0.001$, K1: 0.14 ± 0.05 vs 0.20 ± 0.03 ml/min/g, $p < 0.001$). Washout rate k2 also significantly increased in HF patients (k2: 0.036 ± 0.026 vs. 0.016 ± 0.011 min^{-1}, $p = 0.041$).

Conclusion: HF patients showed reduced RI, reduced K1, and higher washout rate k2 compared to normal. This result may imply that HED PET is able to evaluate washout parameter using compartment model.

Keywords Compartment model analysis • ^{11}C-Hydroxyephedrine • Retention index • Sympathetic nervous system function

Y. Tomiyama (✉)
Department of Nuclear Medicine, Hokkaido University Graduate School of Medicine, Kita15 Nishi7, Kita-Ku, Sapporo 060-8638, Hokkaido, Japan
e-mail: tomiyamayuuki@frontier.hokudai.ac.jp

K. Yoshinaga
Department of Nuclear Medicine, Hokkaido University Graduate School of Medicine, Kita15 Nishi7, Kita-Ku, Sapporo 060-8638, Hokkaido, Japan

Molecular Imaging Research Center, National Institute of Radiological Sciences, 4-9-1 Anagawa, Inage-Ku, Chiba 263-8555, Japan

© The Author(s) 2016

Y. Kuge et al. (eds.), *Perspectives on Nuclear Medicine for Molecular Diagnosis and Integrated Therapy*, DOI 10.1007/978-4-431-55894-1_5

5.1 Introduction

Positron emission tomography (PET) is a powerful tool to evaluate functional information imaging as well as anatomical information [1, 2]. PET is the most reliable modality for assessing functional information, especially in cardiovascular imaging [3, 4]. When biomedical functions are analyzed using PET images, compartment model analysis is generally applied [5, 6]. Compartment model analysis enables to observe the pharmacokinetics of radiotracer in human body. Thus, we apply compartment model analysis to evaluating pharmacokinetics of ^{11}C-hydroxyephedrine (HED).

[11]C- HED has been the most frequently used PET tracer for the estimation of cardiac sympathetic nervous system (SNS) function [7–9]. In general, [11]C- HED data has been evaluated using the retention index (RI) [8]. RI is a parameter that can be calculated easily compared to other quantitative parameters. RI includes uptake and washout parameters. However, RI does not differentiate washout parameters from cardiac HED data. Cardiac washout parameter is widely used for evaluation of SNS function and increased cardiac washout is associated with cardiac events in heart failure (HF) [10]. Therefore, it would be important to evaluate the washout parameters using HED PET. Compartment model analysis might have a potential to evaluate precise pharmacokinetics of ^{11}C-HED and also has a potential to evaluate purely washout parameter [11].

In this study, we aimed to analyze HED uptake parameter and washout parameter using single-compartment model analysis in patients with HF.

5.2 Methods

5.2.1 Study Subjects

Ten healthy volunteers and nine HF patients participated in the current study. The healthy volunteers (ten men, 32.4 ± 9.6 years) had a low pretest likelihood of coronary artery disease (<5 %) based on risk factors [12]. HF patients were recruited from a group of patients who underwent HED PET for the assessment of sympathetic neuronal function. They were six men and three women (57.3 ± 17.3 years). The study was approved by the Hokkaido University Graduate School of Medicine Human Research Ethics Board. Written informed consent was obtained from all participants.

5.2.2 Positron Emission Tomography/Computed Tomography ^{11}C-HED PET/CT Imaging

^{11}C-HED was produced from ^{11}C-methyl iodide and metaraminol (free base) using standard methods with high purity and high specific activity [13].

All participants were instructed to fast overnight. PET/CT imaging was performed with a 64-slice PET/CT scanner (Biograph Siemens/CTI, Knoxville, TN, USA). A low-dose CT was performed for attenuation correction. The CT co-registered to standard orthogonal PET images was then re-sliced into series of short-axis, horizontal long-axis, and vertical long-axis images.

Immediately after the administration of 5 mCi(185 MBq) of intravenous ^{11}C-HED, participants underwent 40-min 3D list-mode PET acquisition. The images were reconstructed using filtered back correction with a12-mm Hann filter and were reconstructed into 23 frames (10×10 s; 1×60 s; 5×100 s; 3×180 s; 4×300 s) [14].

5.2.3 RI Estimation

RI is obtained by normalizing late phase of tracer activity concentrations (30–40 min) of left ventricular (LV) myocardium divided by the integral of the arterial input function (AIF). The time-activity curve was derived from a small circular region of interest in the left ventricular cavity (Fig. 5.1, [10]).

5.2.4 Compartment Model Analysis

Harms HJ et al. reported the single-tissue model was more robust than two-tissue compartment model and results obtained were similar to more precise models [11]. Thus, we used single-compartment model to evaluate ^{11}C-HED washout parameter.

In single-compartment model analysis, tracer kinetics are consisted by only two parameters, which are inflow rate K1 and washout rate k2 (Fig. 5.1, [6]). In this study, K1 and k2 were estimated using the nonlinear least squares method. This approach used AIF arterial input function and tissue activity carve (TAC) of LV myocardium [15, 16]. Distribution volume was also calculated [17]. The equation of distribution volume was inflow rate K1 divided by washout rate k2.

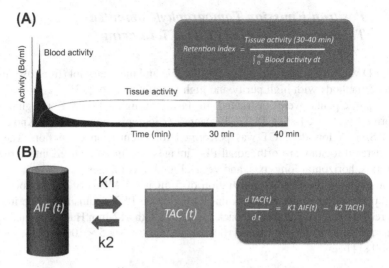

Fig. 5.1 Analysis methods of ^{11}C-hydroxyephedrine. (**a**) Calculation method of retention index: retention index was obtained by normalizing late activity concentrations of left ventricular myocardium divided by the integral of the arterial input function.(**b**) Single-tissue compartment model: single-tissue compartment model enables to monitor inflow rate K1 and washout rate k2 of radiotracer between arterial input function (AIF) and tissue activity curve (TAC). AIF and TAC were obtained from LV cavity and myocardial tissue, respectively

5.2.5 Statistical Analysis

Data are expressed as mean $\pm$ SD. The differences between the means of two volumetric results were examined using the unpaired two t-test. Fisher's exact tests were used for categorical variables. P-value of less than 0.05 was considered indicative of a statistically significant difference. Statistical calculations were carried out using JMP software version 12.0 (SAS Institute, Inc., Cary, NC).

5.3 Results

5.3.1 Subjects' Background

Table 5.1 summarizes the baseline characteristics of the volunteers and HF patients. HF patients also had laboratory data and echocardiography data. The HF patients were older than normal.

Table 5.1 The baseline characteristics

	Normal volunteers ($n = 10$)	Heart failure patients ($n = 9$)	P-value
Age (year)	32.4 ± 9.6	57.3 ± 17.3	<0.001
Sex (M/F)	10/0	6/3	0.09
Height (cm)	172.7 ± 8.8	162.2 ± 8.4	<0.001
Wight (kg)	68.2 ± 13.5	56.8 ± 17.4	<0.001
Laboratory data			
BNP (pg/ml)	–	633.7 ± 876.8	–
Plasma noradrenalin (pg/ml)	–	469.4 ± 317.7	–
Urinary noradrenaline (μg/day)	–	127.9 ± 54.5	–
Echocardiography			
LVEF (%)	–	36.1 ± 16.7	–
LVEDV (ml)	–	180.2 ± 95.2	–

Data expressed as mean ± SD. *BNP* brain natriuretic peptide, *LVEF* left ventricular ejection fraction, *LVEDV* left ventricular end-diastolic volume, *M* male, *F* female

Fig. 5.2 Difference of retention index between the heart failure and normal. Heart failure patients showed significantly decreased RI compared to normal volunteers

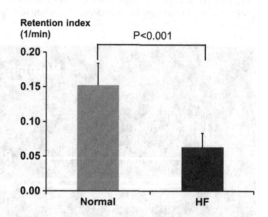

5.3.2 HED PET Data Normal Volunteers and HF Patients

HF patients significantly decreased RI compared to normal volunteers (0.060 ± 0.020 vs. 0.150 ± 0.032 1/min, $P < 0.001$, Fig. 5.2). In compartment model analysis, HF patients showed decreased inflow rate K1 (0.14 ± 0.03 vs. 0.20 ± 0.05 ml/min/g, $P = 0.004$, Fig. 5.3a) and reduced distribution volume (5.17 ± 2.93 vs. 22.4 ± 23.1 mL/g, $P = 0.04$, Fig. 5.3c). In addition, HF patients significantly increased washout rate k2 compared to normal volunteers (0.036 ± 0.026 vs. 0.016 ± 0.011 1/min, $P = 0.044$, Figs. 5.3b and 5.4.).

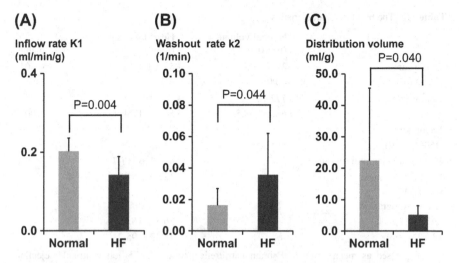

Fig. 5.3 Difference of parameters calculated using compartment model analysis. Heart failure patients showed significantly decreased inflow rate K1 and distribution volume (**a**, **c**). Heart failure patients also showed significantly decreased washout rate k1 (**b**)

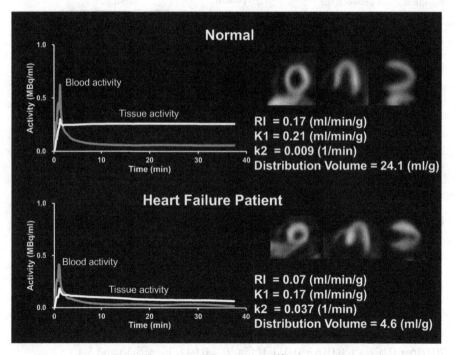

Fig. 5.4 Example of myocardial time activity curveswith[11]C-hydroxyephedrine. Heart failure patient's time-activity curve showed enhanced washout compared to normal volunteer's one

5.4 Discussion

HF patients showed decreased RI, inflow rate K1, and distribution volume compared to normal volunteers. In contrast, the HF patients increased washout parameter k2.

Many previous studies reported patients with imparted SNS function showed lower ^{11}C-HED uptake [8, 17]. Thus, the present data agree with previous reports.

In this study, HF patients showed significantly increased washout rate k2 compared to normal volunteers. Previous studies using ^{123}I-MIBG reported HF patient showed increased washout rate [10, 18]. Previous study also reported that washout parameter of ^{11}C-HED was well correlated with plasma and cardiac norepinephrine in experiments with rats [7]. Therefore, current data that HF patient showed increased washout rate may be considered to be appropriate.

5.4.1 Study Limitation

Our study had a small population and HF patients were significantly older than normal volunteers. Therefore, further investigations with larger and age-matched populations are required.

In addition, washout parameters were not compared to other clinical indexes. Comparison washout of ^{11}C-HED and other clinical parameter such as ejection fraction, laboratory parameter, and washout of ^{123}I-MIBG should be the next step.

5.5 Conclusion

In this study, we applied compartment model analysis to evaluating washout of ^{11}C-hydroxyephedrine (HED).

As a result, HF patients showed reduced RI, K1, and distribution volume and higher washout rate k2 compared to normal. This result may imply that HED PET is able to evaluate washout parameter using compartment model.

Conflicts of Interest None

Acknowledgments The authors thank Keiichi Magota, PhD; Ken-ichi Nishijima, PhD; Daisuke Abo, MSc; and Eriko Suzuki for their support for this study. This manuscript has been reviewed by a North American English-language professional editor Ms. Holly Beanlands. The authors also thank Ms. Holly Beanlands for critical reading of the manuscript.

This study was supported in part by grants from the Japanese Ministry of Education, Culture, Sports, Science and Technology (Category B, No. 23390294) and grants from the Innovation Program of the Japan Science and Technology Agency. Tomiyama was supported by postgraduate students' Travel Award Program by Hokkaido University. Dr. Yoshinaga is supported by the Imura Clinical Research Award (Adult Vascular Disease Research Foundation).

References

1. Yoshinaga K, Burwash IG, Leech JA, Haddad H, Johnson CB, deKemp RA, Garrard L, Chen L, Williams K, DaSilva JN, Beanlands RS. The effects of continuous positive airway pressure on myocardial energetics in patients with heart failure and obstructive sleep apnea. J Am Coll Cardiol. 2007;49:450–8.
2. Katoh C, Morita K, Shiga T, Kubo N, Nakada K, Tamaki N. Improvement of algorithm for quantification of regional myocardial blood flow using 15O-water with PET. J Nucl Med. 2004;45:1908–16.
3. Tomiyama Y, Manabe O, Oyama-Manabe N, Naya M, Sugimori H, Hirata K, Mori Y, Tsutsui H, Kudo K, Tamaki N, Katoh C. Quantification of myocardial blood flow with dynamic perfusion 3.0 Tesla MRI: validation with o-water PET. J Magn Reson Imaging. 2015;42(3):754–62.
4. Kikuchi Y, Oyama-Manabe N, Naya M, Manabe O, Tomiyama Y, Sasaki T, Katoh C, Kudo K, Tamaki N, Shirato H. Quantification of myocardial blood flow using dynamic 320-row multi-detector CT as compared with (1)(5)O-H(2)O PET. Eur Radiol. 2014;24:1547–56.
5. Yoshinaga K, Tomiyama Y, Suzuki E, Tamaki N. Myocardial blood flow quantification using positron-emission tomography: analysis and practice in the clinical setting. Circ J. 2013;77:1662–71.
6. Klein R, Beanlands RS, deKemp RA. Quantification of myocardial blood flow and flow reserve: technical aspects. J Nucl Cardiol. 2010;17:555–70.
7. Thackeray JT, Renaud JM, Kordos M, Klein R, Dekemp RA, Beanlands RS, DaSilva JN. Test-retest repeatability of quantitative cardiac 11C-meta-hydroxyephedrine measurements in rats by small animal positron emission tomography. Nucl Med Biol. 2013;40:676–81.
8. Schwaiger M, Kalff V, Rosenspire K, Haka MS, Molina E, Hutchins GD, Deeb M, Wolfe Jr E, Wieland DM. Noninvasive evaluation of sympathetic nervous system in human heart by positron emission tomography. Circulation. 1990;82:457–64.
9. Bengel FM, Ueberfuhr P, Ziegler SI, Nekolla S, Reichart B, Schwaiger M. Serial assessment of sympathetic reinnervation after orthotopic heart transplantation. A longitudinal study using PET and C-11 hydroxyephedrine. Circulation. 1999;99:1866–71.
10. Matsunari I, Aoki H, Nomura Y, Takeda N, Chen WP, Taki J, Nakajima K, Nekolla SG, Kinuya S, Kajinami K. Iodine-123 metaiodobenzylguanidine imaging and carbon-11 hydroxyephedrine positron emission tomography compared in patients with left ventricular dysfunction. Circ Cardiovasc Imaging. 2010;3:595–603.
11. Harms HJ, de Haan S, Knaapen P, Allaart CP, Rijnierse MT, Schuit RC, Windhorst AD, Lammertsma AA, Huisman MC, Lubberink M. Quantification of [(11)C]-meta-hydroxyephedrine uptake in human myocardium. EJNMMI Res. 2014;4:52.

12. Diamond GA, Forrester JS. Analysis of probability as an aid in the clinical diagnosis of coronary-artery disease. N Engl J Med. 1979;300:1350–8.
13. Rosenspire KC, Haka MS, Van Dort ME, Jewett DM, Gildersleeve DL, Schwaiger M, Wieland DM. Synthesis and preliminary evaluation of carbon-11-meta-hydroxyephedrine: a false transmitter agent for heart neuronal imaging. J Nucl Med. 1990;31:1328–34.
14. Allman KC, Wieland DM, Muzik O, Degrado TR, Wolfe Jr ER, Schwaiger M. Carbon-11 hydroxyephedrine with positron emission tomography for serial assessment of cardiac adrenergic neuronal function after acute myocardial infarction in humans. J Am Coll Cardiol. 1993;22:368–75.
15. Katoh C, Yoshinaga K, Klein R, Kasai K, Tomiyama Y, Manabe O, Naya M, Sakakibara M, Tsutsui H, deKemp RA, Tamaki N. Quantification of regional myocardial blood flow estimation with three-dimensional dynamic rubidium-82 PET and modified spillover correction model. J Nucl Cardiol. 2012;19:763–74.
16. Mori Y, Manabe O, Naya M, Tomiyama Y, Yoshinaga K, Magota K, Oyama-Manabe N, Hirata K, Tsutsui H, Tamaki N, Katoh C. Improved spillover correction model to quantify myocardial blood flow by 11C-acetate PET: comparison with 15O-H 2O PET. Ann Nucl Med. 2015;29:15–20.
17. Schafers M, Dutka D, Rhodes CG, Lammertsma AA, Hermansen F, Schober O, Camici PG. Myocardial presynaptic and postsynaptic autonomic dysfunction in hypertrophic cardiomyopathy. Circ Res. 1998;82:57–62.
18. Boogers MJ, Borleffs CJ, Henneman MM, van Bommel RJ, van Ramshorst J, Boersma E, Dibbets-Schneider P, Stokkel MP, van der Wall EE, Schalij MJ, Bax JJ. Cardiac sympathetic denervation assessed with 123-iodine metaiodobenzylguanidine imaging predicts ventricular arrhythmias in implantable cardioverter-defibrillator patients. J Am Coll Cardiol. 2010;55:2769–77.

Part II
Biomarker and Molecular Probes

Chapter 6
How Far Are We from Dose On Demand of Short-Lived Radiopharmaceuticals?

Giancarlo Pascali and Lidia Matesic

Abstract PET radiopharmaceuticals are currently produced using a centralized approach, which makes sustainable the distribution to few imaging centers of an only small set of tracers (virtually only [^{18}F]FDG). However, a wider set of structures have demonstrated a potential applicability for imaging in a specific manner several disease condition. In order to allow this wider and more personalized use of PET imaging, the production paradigms need to be changed. In this contribution we will explain how Dose-On-Demand systems can be conceptualized and what are the challenges that are still to be overcome in order for such approach to be of widespread utility.

Keywords Dose On Demand • Microfluidics • PET • Radiochemistry

6.1 Introduction

The clinical production of radiopharmaceuticals or radiotracers for positron-emitting tomography (PET) is currently performed in centralized locations such as commercial radiopharmacies or some dedicated radiochemistry facilities. Generally, these facilities contain a cyclotron to produce the PET radioisotope and laboratories furnished with lead-shielded hot cells containing automated radiosynthesis modules to produce the radiotracer. Quality control equipment is also required to validate and confirm the purity of the radiotracer prior to its dispatch to the imaging centers.

The majority of radiotracer production facilities synthesize [^{18}F]FDG, the gold standard for detecting a variety of cancers. Nowadays, [^{18}F]FDG can be produced in a large batch, making it relatively affordable. Portions can then be dispatched and transported by road or air to the relevant hospital owing to the half-life of fluorine-18 (110 min).

G. Pascali (✉) • L. Matesic
ANSTO LifeSciences, Cyclotron building 81, Missenden Rd, Camperdown, NSW 2050, Australia
e-mail: gianp@ansto.gov.au

© The Author(s) 2016   79
Y. Kuge et al. (eds.), *Perspectives on Nuclear Medicine for Molecular Diagnosis and Integrated Therapy*, DOI 10.1007/978-4-431-55894-1_6

A major challenge in clinical PET radiochemistry is that there are a greater number of hospitals or PET clinics than there are PET radiotracer production facilities. Furthermore, the demand for new clinical PET radiotracers is low due to the cost of production in a centralized location. New PET radiotracers are overwhelmingly used for research purposes only.

To overcome this obstacle, a decentralized approach has been envisaged [1]. Here, scientists could produce their radiotracer of interest in-house, economically and on demand, leading to a concept that we have defined as Dose On Demand (DOD). This short review will cover the important aspects of DOD and detail the journey toward the DOD of short-lived radiopharmaceuticals.

6.2 DOD Features

The current production approach of PET radiotracers imposes several limitations and challenges for guaranteeing the most efficient organization of imaging studies [2]. A possible way to improve this situation would require a system for which the type and the quantity of the produced tracer is defined and directly handled by an as final as possible user (e.g., hospital pharmacy, imaging laboratory). This system should implement the reduction to the minimum possible of the amounts of radioactivity and chemicals needed in the preparation, added to an overall simplification of the production process. Such conceptual process can be defined as "Dose On Demand" (*DOD*) [3, 4, 5]: the operation of producing a radiopharmaceutical in the shortest time possible, using the minimum amount of chemicals and radioactivity strictly needed for the production of the single (or few) imaging dose (s) required.

This approach, exemplified in Fig. 6.1, would provide several benefits to the overall PET community. Firstly, it will hand over *flexibility* in the application directly to the hospital/imaging center, which can decide on a patient basis which tracer to produce and when; this could also happen in small regional centers, thus not forcing anymore interested patients to commute long distances to the few useful imaging hospitals. This flexibility will also allow the utilization of rare or research tracers to be facilitated, as in this system the small amounts of chemicals and radioactivity needed for a DOD production would be economically sustainable for a single imaging center. Secondly, while a fault in production from a centralized approach will have impact on a large number of patients, a *fault* in one DOD system will have an impact limited to the patients utilizing those doses only. Lastly, due to the *reduction* in raw materials needed (as well as related topics, e.g., safety, storage) and the redistribution of running costs over more institutes, the imaging doses will result in a reduced cost and in tracers' availability to a wider population.

In order to realize a DOD process, few requirements can be envisaged.

Firstly, the production needs to be implemented on an automated instrument that can implement preset operations, as well as allowing remote interaction of the operator for minor modifications (i.e., "Automation"). In addition, it has to have

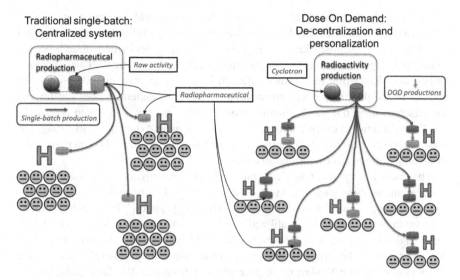

Fig. 6.1 Comparison between traditional centralized approach and DOD

real-time monitoring and audit trail capabilities for monitoring and trending purposes. Secondly, the instrument used needs to be able to handle small aliquots of reagents, from fractions to hundreds of μL (i.e., "Discretization") with accuracy and repeatability. The handling operations comprise moving, merging, mixing, heating, and similar processes. In other words, the instrument has to be capable to give a defined "chemical history" to any given aliquot of reagents used (that can be different among several aliquots). Thirdly, the processes implemented need to be serially repeatable with minimum operator intervention ("Restarting"). This can be achieved by substituting single-use parts in the system or by cleaning it using validated procedures. A final peculiarity that contributes to achieving DOD is the need to use the minimum amount of chemicals ("Reduction"), which would maximize the atom efficiency of the process, as well as allow an acceptable sacrifice in employing single-use parts or realize a faster cleaning of the system.

If all these requirements can be respected in a process system, a DOD production can be implemented and can be used to produce several doses of the same tracer or of different tracers, using the same system and minimal operator interventions.

6.3   Early Examples Conducible to DOD

The possibility to tailor the production of nuclear medicine (NM) tracers as much as possible to the needs of the final user has always been present, and indeed some example of approaches that can be linked to DOD concept can be found in early and current practices.

Generators of radioactive raw nuclides have been widely used (e.g., ^{99m}Tc, ^{68}Ga) [6]; the elution of the desired radionuclide is generally done upon demand and followed by simple chemical reactions (generally performed directly in the same NM department) to obtain the final radiopharmaceutical. This approach respects the Restarting requirement, though limited to the raw nuclide production and not to the pharmaceutical preparation; however, it generally does not respect the Discretization nor the Reduction requirements, as it is difficult to separately handle the amount of chemicals needed for a single patient (i.e., in the μLs range). It sometimes respects the Automation requirement, but in most NM departments, these preparations are performed manually.

The use of very *short half-life* nuclides can be natively defined as a DOD application, as their handling must be done shortly before their use in imaging. Typical examples are the production of [^{15}O]-H$_2$O [7] and [^{13}N]-NH$_3$ [8]; shortly after production, the systems utilized can be restarted easily due to their simple setup and the fast decay of process wastes. However, also in this case, these processes cannot be properly defined as DOD since they generally respect the Automation and the Restarting requirements, but neither the Discretization nor the Reduction (i.e., no difference if the production is used for one or several contemporary patients). ^{11}C chemistry [8] also falls within the use of very short half-life nuclides as more productions can be run on the same machine on the same day. However, also in this case, the typical systems used can be even less defined as DOD, due to its relatively longer half-life (compared to ^{15}O and ^{13}N).

Currently, the approach that most resembles DOD is represented by the *cassette-based* systems. In this case, Automation and Restarting requirements can be easily achieved; Discretization and Reduction are generally not pursued, because nowadays these systems are used for single-batch productions, but the principles underlying cassette philosophy could be used to project single-use/single-dose cassettes. In fact, these systems are basically very compact macrofluidic systems; this understanding clarifies how *microfluidic* concepts can be the ones that should allow a full implementation of DOD in radiopharmaceutical production.

6.4   DOD Proof-of-Principle Examples

6.4.1   Minicyclotron/Minichemistry/MiniQC

The Biomarker Generator (BG75), made by ABT Molecular Imaging, is a small (0.37 m × 1.25 m) self-shielded 7.5 MeV cyclotron coupled to an aseptic single-use card-based automated chemical production module and an automated module for quality control. The BG75 was initially used for the DOD production of [^{18}F] fluoride and [^{18}F]FDG [9]. Using the computer's software, the operator is able to select whether the [^{18}F]fluoride or [^{18}F]FDG is to be produced. For the production of [^{18}F]fluoride (~1 mCi/min at 5 μA), the process is complete once the product is delivered into the specified vial. Alternatively, for the production of [^{18}F]FDG, the software prompts the operator to prepare the tracer-specific Dose Synthesis Card (DSC) and the chemistry and quality control modules while the cyclotron is preparing the [^{18}F]fluoride. The radiosynthesis is then completed on the DSC, including relevant purification, and dispensed into a shielded, sterile syringe or vial. An aliquot of the product is removed for quality control (pH determination, acetonitrile and ethanol residual solvent determination, radiochemical identity and purity, Kryptofix 2.2.2. determination, and a filter integrity test), which is automatically performed by the system, without any operator input.

The BG75 has been able to consistently produce a 10–13 mCi dose of [^{18}F]FDG at 40 min intervals up to six times per day, with products meeting the required USP limits for release [9]. To date, other DOD radiotracers synthesized using the BG75 include Na[^{18}F]F [10] and [^{18}F]FMISO [11, 12].

6.4.2   Continuous Flow Microfluidics

Interestingly, proof-of-concept studies have been recently conducted into the production of [^{18}F]FLT using the cyclotron component of the BG75 system and the Advion NanoTek microfluidic system [13]. Between 70 and 80 mCi of [^{18}F]fluoride were produced by the minicyclotron and the radiosynthesis was subsequently performed under continuous-flow microfluidic conditions to yield [^{18}F]FLT in sufficient quantity and purity for clinical trials. The number of radiochemists using a microfluidic approach has been steadily accumulating in recent years. This may be related to the advantages of microfluidic systems over traditional automated radiochemistry modules, which include a decrease in the amount chemical reagents used, shorter reaction times, greater radiochemical yields, the ability to use solvents under supercritical conditions, and reduced radiation exposure to the operator due to the lower amounts of radioactivity used. The NanoTek Microfluidic Synthesis System by Advion was the first commercially available continuous-flow microfluidic system. The system comprises a concentrator module to azeotropically evaporate the [^{18}F]fluoride from the cyclotron and subsequently reconstitute the isotope into the appropriate solvent; a pump module containing two syringe pumps and loops to store chemical precursors and a reactor module, which contains a syringe pump and loop to house the isotope along with thermostatted slots to store up to four microreactors, where the radiochemical reactions occur.

The previous example of the production of [^{18}F]FLT is the latest in a growing list of radiotracers prepared using the NanoTek system. The first instance was the production of [^{18}F]fallypride for use in micro-PET studies [14]. Initially, the radiochemical optimization of [^{18}F]fallypride was conducted by dispensing 10 μL solutions of the tosyl-fallypride precursor and [^{18}F]fluoride complex into the microreactor at 10 μL/min to obtain 1–1.5 mCi doses of [^{18}F]fallypride. These optimization reactions were performed sequentially and could be considered an early form of DOD. Once the optimal radiochemical conditions were determined, the authors were able to prepare a dose of [^{18}F]fallypride sufficient for human injection (15 mCi) by increasing the volume of the two solutions from 10 μL to

200 μL. The authors also alluded to the fact that multiple high doses of [^{18}F] fallypride could be produced using the same microreactor. Soon after, Pascali et al. [15] described the sequential radiolabeling of ethyl-ditosylate and propyl-ditosylate in the NanoTek system using the same solution of [^{18}F]fluoride complex and swapping the precursor between productions by emptying and refilling the precursor loop with a different substrate. These examples of DOD demonstrated the economical use of the [^{18}F]fluoride solution to yield two radiotracers on the same day. The authors also sequentially prepared several injectable doses of [^{18}F]CB102, a cannabinoid type 2 receptor agonist, for small animal PET imaging, suggesting that freshly prepared doses using a DOD approach were superior to a batch solution to be used over a certain shelf life.

To further evaluate the robustness and reliability of a DOD approach, Pascali et al. were able to produce three sequential doses of three different [^{18}F] fluorocholines with a total processing time of 13–15 min for each dose, including SPE purification [5]. While this example includes a modification to the NanoTek system to incorporate SPE purification, typically, the radiochemical outputs are purified externally to the NanoTek system, particularly HPLC purification. Recent examples include the preparation of [^{18}F]FPEB [16], whereby the radiosynthesis occurred in the NanoTek and the reaction output was sent to a vial preloaded with water and pre-concentrated onto an Oasis HLB Light SPE cartridge to remove DMSO present in the reaction mixture. The cartridge was eluted with acetonitrile and water before being transferred to a GE TRACERlab F$_X$F$_N$ synthesis unit to conduct semi-preparative HPLC purification and formulation. Additionally, the Tau imaging agent, [^{18}F]T807, was produced with the same modifications [17]. Three consecutive >100 mCi productions of [^{18}F]T807 were performed for validation purposes, and [^{18}F]T807 became the first example of human use of a radiopharmaceutical prepared by continuous-flow microfluidics.

The NanoTek system has been modified recently to include HPLC and SPE purification [18]. By utilizing the cable harnessing of the system, a custom-made electrical board was engineered whereby additional switches and analog signals could be added and be controlled by the NanoTek software to activate externally powered devices and record external signals (e.g., detectors), if applicable. This customized system was able to produce 1- or 2-step radiotracers such as [^{18}F] CB102, [^{18}F]fluoroethylcholine [18], [^{18}F]MEL050 (melanin targeting) [19], [^{18}F] fallypride, and [^{18}F]PBR111 (TSPO receptor) [20], in a DOD manner. Similarly, [^{18}F]FMISO has been produced by integrating a HPLC system to the NanoTek through a six-port valve [21]. By fine-tuning the HPLC conditions for [^{18}F]FMISO, the authors were able to eliminate the requirement for SPE.

6.4.3   Peptide Labeling

While microfluidic systems have mainly been utilized to radiolabel small mole-cules, reports of peptide or protein radiolabeling using microfluidics are limited.

Early work in this area featured the direct [^{18}F]radiolabeling of bombesin derivatives (with 7–8 amino acid residues) that had been modified to incorporate trimethylammonium or triarylsulfonium leaving groups [22]. The peptides could be radiolabeled reproducibly, suggesting a possible DOD approach; however, due to the harsh temperature conditions required for radiolabeling, this method would be unsuitable for protein radiolabeling. An alternative route to radiolabel a peptide is through the use of a prosthetic group as an indirect radiolabeling method. [^{18}F]SFB [23] and even, the most abundantly used PET tracer, [^{18}F]FDG [24] have been utilized as prosthetic groups for the radiolabeling of peptides. Although both prosthetic groups were synthesized on macroscale equipment, the subsequent peptide radiolabeling was performed under microfluidic conditions. In each case, the peptide was radiolabeled in a shorter period of time, in higher radiochemical yield (RCY), and using a smaller quantity of the peptide compared to conventional radiolabeling techniques. Only recently has the first microfluidic radiosynthesis of a prosthetic group and the ensuing peptide radiolabeling been reported [25]. Here, the [^{18}F]F-Py-TEP prosthetic group was prepared in the first microreactor of an Advion NanoTek system from [^{18}F]fluoride and the corresponding precursor. After exiting the microreactor, the [^{18}F]F-Py-TEP was transferred to a second microreactor, where it reacted with a model peptide containing free amines. Once again, the peptide coupling was faster than conventional methods and obtained in higher RCY. These accounts all imply that the DOD of radiolabeled peptides for molecular imaging is currently being explored and may be employed in the future.

6.4.4 Solid-Phase Approaches

Although the use of microfluidic conditions is leading to radiochemical reactions being completed in less time than traditional approaches, to further decrease the overall radiochemical processing times, new methods are required to decrease or eliminate the time taken to process and activate the starting [^{18}F]fluoride. One option is to trap the [^{18}F]fluoride onto a resin and subsequently perform on-resin radiofluorinations, thus eliminating the need for azeotropic evaporations and re-solubilization of the [^{18}F]fluoride complex. Reusable polymer-supported phosphazenes have been investigated as suitable resins to perform the [^{18}F]fluoride trapping and radiofluorination [26]. The PS-P$_2$^{tBu} resin was able to trap >99% of [^{18}F]fluoride, with no leaching of activity was observed when the column was subsequently dried with helium gas. It was found that substrates with sulfonate leaving groups resulted in the highest RCY when subjected to on-column radiofluorination. The same phosphazene resin could be recycled at least three times using the same substrate, or at least two times using a different substrate, which implies that the DOD production of radiotracers is possible through solid-phase radiofluorination.

Other work in this area includes a continuous-flow system comprising a polystyrene-imidazolium-chloride (PS-Im$^+$Cl$^-$) monolith which traps [^{18}F]fluoride [27]. A solution of base and the relevant precursor could then be flowed through the

PS-Im^{+}[^{18}F]F^{-} monolith into a preheated microfluidic chip where the radiochemical reaction takes place. The advantage of this method is that the entire process is performed in continuous flow and the microfluidic platform has a very small footprint compared to current processes.

6.4.5 Droplet Systems

An interesting extension in the field of microfluidic radiochemistry is through the use of droplets. Also sometimes referred to as segmented flow chemistry, it features droplets (nL- μL) which are separated by an immiscible carrier fluid, similar to oil droplets in water. Droplets can be thought of as individual nano- or microreactors and can be used to aid radiolabeling optimization, whereby each droplet is the result of a predetermined set of reaction parameters. Droplets consisting of approximately 120 nL were formed during the coupling of [^{18}F]FSB with an anti-prostate stem cell antigen diabody [28]. Using a 5 μL sample of the diabody solution was sufficient to screen over 100 different reaction conditions using the droplets, and hence, the optimal reaction conditions were determined rapidly with minimal use of the precious diabody solution. Droplet systems have also been utilized in electrowetting-on-dielectric (EWOD) devices. In EWOD systems, droplets are sandwiched between two plates; the bottom plate consists of electrode pads to manipulate the movement of the droplets throughout the microchip, while the top plate electrically grounds the droplets. The EWOD chip was first used in the synthesis of [^{18}F]FDG [29], but its use has more recently expanded to include [^{18}F]FLT [30], [^{18}F]fallypride [31], and [^{18}F]SFB [32]. While the EWOD chip produces these radiolabeled molecules in comparable, if not greater, RCY than previously, drawbacks of the system include off-chip purification and the potential for radioactivity and volatile side products to escape since the chip is exposed to air. It is envisaged that with advances in technology, the EWOD chip could be further automated, be disposable, and lead to scientists producing their desired radiotracer on demand.

6.5 Challenges and Future of DOD

As it can be seen, a perfect DOD system is still not existent, but several data are available demonstrating that such approach should represent the reality in the next future. However, to witness this paradigmatic change, several challenges need to be fronted, and they will represent the future of DOD research in radiopharmaceutical production.

One of the biggest challenges is to understand whether one only system could achieve the desired spread of operations that a DOD process should implement. This should cover not only the production steps but also the switching of chemicals, cleaning, and priming steps. It is very likely that these systems will be based on micronized approaches (e.g., microfluidics, nanodroplets), but understanding which *philosophy* they should implement is still under discussion. For example, a system can be projected to implement several different preexisting routes, which would lead to different products in different quantities, or, on the contrary, be represented by a fixed framing to which flexibly interface single-use components/modules (i.e., similar to microcassettes) to build up the desired process. Another possibility might also be represented by the possibility to use the exact same system into which different chemicals are delivered, depending on the production needs. All these options are amenable to deliver a DOD system, but the choice of one or the other will drive the final performance and actual ease/flexibility of use.

Even once the underlying philosophy is clarified, some technical problems are still unsolved or partially addressed. *Purification* of the finished product represents probably the most important issue, and while there are several excellent systems to perform chemical reactions, there is a notable lack in miniaturization of purification methods or their interfacing with micronized chemistry systems. Some research is now available on micro-chromatographic systems [33], mainly facilitated by the advancements of monolith polymers [34] that can be easily integrated with micron-sized channels/reservoirs [35]. These solutions allow the reduction of inherent void volumes, therefore improving the atom efficiency in the purification process. Also, similar solutions may be useful for the cases in which a simple solid-phase extraction (SPE) would be sufficient to purify the relevant molecule [36, 37]. Polymer chemistry advancement possibly represents the field where useful innovations can have a relevant impact on miniaturized purifications. As an example, molecularly imprinted polymers (MIP) represent a promising approach that would allow to streamline the selective separation of the molecule of interest and its efficient elution [38]. MIP structures are prepared by building the polymer pores around a desired template molecule; once the template is removed, the material acquires selectivity of shape and electronic interaction (i.e., with functional groups of polymer) for the desired molecule [39]. MIP systems are in fact also referred as "synthetic receptors."

Another innovation that would be generally useful in radiochemistry but particularly applicable to DOD systems (due to their preferred micronized nature) is the use of supported precursors. These systems should be projected in such a way that the labeling reaction is the only event that would make the molecular structure to become free from the solid support bond. In this way, no other complex organic species will be present in the resulting mixture, and only simple filtration and reformulation steps would be required in order to retrieve the radiopharmaceutical. Some systems based on supported sulfonates [40] or triazene [41] have been reported up to date, and patent literature also refers to examples of supported ionic precursors (e.g., iodonium compounds) [42]. However, none of these systems have demonstrated a preferential use compared to traditional methods, probably because of the mismatch between the support active surface and reagent accessibility to it. The use of micronized systems could be beneficial in solving this mismatch, and indeed the use of sulfonate precursors supported on a monolith structure grown directly in a microfluidic chip gave satisfying yields of radiofluorination [43].

A further modification to this approach, which would facilitate the respect of DOD requirements, could be the use of *reversibly* linked precursors. In this concept, the precursor should form a bond (e.g., covalent coordination) with the support material, and as usual, the labeling reaction should be able to selectively cleave the structure from the support; however, in a second "recycling" step, a change in conditions will allow the recovery of the precursor out of the system and offer a support free to be reversibly functionalized again with a different precursor. A recent paper reported the catalysis by TiO_2 nanoparticles in radiofluorinating a tosylate precursor [44]; interestingly enough, the authors suspect that the process is catalyzed due to selective coordination of the tosylate moiety with the titania surface, therefore opening to the idea of a reversible functionalization of metal nanoparticles with several different precursors prior to radiolabeling. Another possibility, drawn from the field of self-healing materials, might be the use of reversible click reactions, a nice example of which is represented by the 1,2,4-triazoline-3,5-dione chemistry (TAD) moieties. This structure reacts in a reversible way (using different temperatures, Fig. 6.2) with indoles through an ene click reaction [45]; however, it undergoes fast Diels-Alder reactions with dienes and is

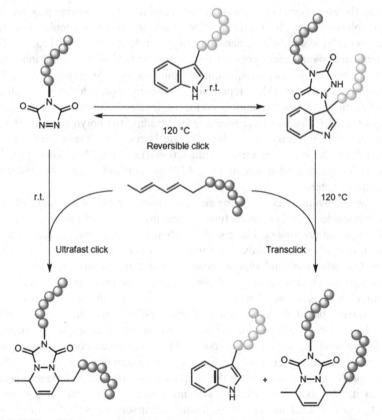

Fig. 6.2 TAD residue in reversible click-chemistry transformations (Taken from [45])

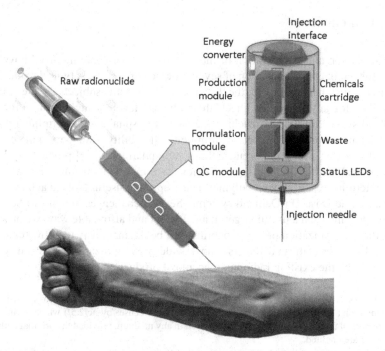

Fig. 6.3 Idealized concept for a DOD system, used to inject directly in the patient the desired radiopharmaceutical

widely used in biology for its capacity to bind irreversibly tyrosine residues [46]. Such an approach could be very useful in DOD processes aimed at protein labeling, for which radiolabeled prosthetic groups enabling click chemistry are now widely employed [47].

Another important point to clarify is whether DOD systems should produce product vials (as in the traditional approach), a syringe/cartridge dose, or even directly deliver the radiopharmaceutical preparation into the vein of the subject (see Fig. 6.3). Though currently unlikely, the possibility to overcome the concept of product vial is very appealing on the base of flexibility, atom efficiency, and procedure streamlining. Therefore, an outstanding challenge is represented by modifying the regulators' view [48, 49] on the requirements needed to prepare injectable radiopharmaceuticals for human use, in order to allow easier and more personalized modalities of dose delivery. One of the ways to achieve such result is represented by the change in quality control (QC) paradigms; in fact, the traditional way to produce a separate vial for QC [50] should be overtaken by the possibility of realizing a DOD process whose precise control and monitoring would represent itself a guarantee of good-quality end product.

6.6 Conclusions

Miniaturization and optimization of the biochemical hardware involved have created a substantial personalization of several medical practices. A typical example of this trend that has improved the treatment of diabetic subjects is the current possibility for any person to check their glucose levels using a straightforward handheld system, instead of reaching the nearest hospital and performing a proper blood examination. This level of simplicity, flexibility, and personalization is currently lacking in the important field of radiopharmaceutical production. However, several studies are starting to demonstrate that new chemical technologies (e.g., microfluidics, high-tech polymers) can represent useful tools to achieve what we can define Dose-On-Demand systems. Several challenges are still to be faced before reaching such a useful target in an efficient and affordable way; we however think that the realization of this capability will be the main way to allow the use of rare and disease dedicated tracers whose widespread utilization is currently hindered [51] by the existing radiopharmaceutical production paradigms.

References

1. Keng PY, Esterby M, van Dam RM. Emerging technologies for decentralized production of PET tracers. In: Positron emission tomography – current clinical and research aspects. 2012. doi:10.5772/1280
2. Satyamurthy N. Electronic generators for the production of positron-emitter labeled radio-pharmaceuticals where would PET be without them? Clin Positron Imaging. 1999;2:233–53.
3. Wang M-W, Lin W-Y, Liu K, Masterman-Smith M, Kwang-Fu Shen C. Microfluidics for positron emission tomography probe development. Mol Imaging. 2010;9:175–91.
4. Arima V, Pascali G, Lade O, et al. Radiochemistry on chip: towards dose-on-demand synthesis of PET radiopharmaceuticals. Lab Chip. 2013;13:2328–36.
5. Pascali G, Nannavecchia G, Pitzianti S, Salvadori PA. Dose-on-demand of diverse 18F-fluorocholine derivatives through a two-step microfluidic approach. Nucl Med Biol. 2011;38:637–44.
6. Knapp FF (Russ., Mirzadeh S. The continuing important role of radionuclide generator systems for nuclear medicine. Eur J Nucl Med. 1994;21:1151–65.
7. Welch MJ, Kilbourn MR. A remote system for the routine production of oxygen-15 radio-pharmaceuticals. J Label Compd Radiopharm. 1985;22:1193–200.
8. Miller PW, Long NJ, Vilar R, Gee AD. Synthesis of 11C, 18F, 15O, and 13N radiolabels for positron emission tomography. Angew Chem Int Ed Engl. 2008;47:8998–9033.

9. Awasthi V, Watson J, Gali H, Matlock G, McFarland A, Bailey J, Anzellotti A. A "dose on demand" biomarker generator for automated production of [(18)F]F(-) and [(18)F]FDG. Appl Radiat Isot. 2014;89:167–75.

10. Awasthi V, Gali H, McFarland A, Anzellotti A. Automated manufacture of Na[18F]F at the University of Oklahoma Health Sciences Center (OUHSC). Dose on-demand and imaging studies. J Nucl Med. 2014;55:1243.

11. Anzellotti A, Bailey J, Ferguson D, McFarland A, Bochev P, Andreev G, Awasthi V, Brown-Proctor C. Automated production and quality testing of [18F]labeled radiotracers using the BG75 system. J Radioanal Nucl Chem. 2015;305:387–401.

12. Anzellotti A, Yuan H. Automated manufacture of [18F]FMISO in the BG 75 system. Synthesis and purification using solid phase extraction. J Nucl Med. 2015;56:1001.

13. Gali H, Nkepang G, Galbraith W, Hammond K, Awasthi V, Collier TL. Preparation of [F-18] FLT using an ABT compact cyclotron and continuous flow microfluidics. J Label Compd Radiopharm. 2015;58 Suppl 1:S362.

14. Lu S, Giamis AM, Pike VW. Synthesis of [F]fallypride in a micro-reactor: rapid optimization and multiple-production in small doses for micro-PET studies. Curr Radiopharm. 2009;2:49–55.

15. Pascali G, Mazzone G, Saccomanni G, Manera C, Salvadori PA. Microfluidic approach for fast labeling optimization and dose-on-demand implementation. Nucl Med Biol. 2010;37:547–55.

16. Liang SH, Yokell DL, Jackson RN, Rice PA, Callahan R, Johnson KA, Alagille D, Tamagnan G, Collier TL, Vasdev N. Microfluidic continuous-flow radiosynthesis of [(18)F] FPEB suitable for human PET imaging. Medchemcomm. 2014;5:432–5.

17. Collier T, Yokell D, Rice P, Jackson R, Shoup T, Normandin M, Brady T, El Fakhri G, Liang S, Vasdev N. First human use of the tau radiopharmaceutical [18F]T807 by microfluidic flow chemistry. J Nucl Med. 2014;55:1246.

18. Pascali G, Berton A, DeSimone M, Wyatt N, Matesic L, Greguric I, Salvadori PA. Hardware and software modifications on the Advion NanoTek microfluidic platform to extend flexibility for radiochemical synthesis. Appl Radiat Isot. 2014;84:40–7.

19. Matesic L, Kallinen A, Wyatt NA, Pham TQ, Greguric I, Pascali G. [18F]Fluorination optimisation and the fully automated production of [18F]MEL050 using a microfluidic system. Aust J Chem. 2015;68:69–71.

20. Matesic L, Kallinen A, Greguric I, Pascali G. Dose-on-demand production of multiple 18F-radiotracers on a microfluidic system. J Label Compd Radiopharm. 2015;58 Suppl 1:S22.

21. Zheng M-Q, Collier L, Bois F, Kelada OJ, Hammond K, Ropchan J, Akula MR, Carlson DJ, Kabalka GW, Huang Y. Synthesis of [(18)F]FMISO in a flow-through microfluidic reactor: development and clinical application. Nucl Med Biol. 2015;42:578–84.

22. Selivanova SV, Mu L, Ungersboeck J, Stellfeld T, Ametamey SM, Schibli R, Wadsak W. - Single-step radiofluorination of peptides using continuous flow microreactor. Org Biomol Chem. 2012;10:3871.

23. Richter S, Bouvet V, Wuest M, Bergmann R, Steinbach J, Pietzsch J, Neundorf I, Wuest F. (18)F-Labeled phosphopeptide-cell-penetrating peptide dimers with enhanced cell uptake properties in human cancer cells. Nucl Med Biol. 2012;39:1202–12.

24. Bouvet VR, Wuest F. Application of [18F]FDG in radiolabeling reactions using microfluidic technology. Lab Chip. 2013;13:4290–4.

25. Cumming RC, Olberg DE, Sutcliffe JL. Rapid 18 F-radiolabeling of peptides from [18 F] fluoride using a single microfluidics device. RSC Adv. 2014;4:49529–34.

26. Mathiessen B, Zhuravlev F. Automated solid-phase radiofluorination using polymer-supported phosphazenes. Molecules. 2013;18:10531–47.

27. Ismail R, Irribaren J, Javed MR, Machness A, Michael van Dam R, Keng PY. Cationic imidazolium polymer monoliths for efficient solvent exchange, activation and fluorination on a continuous flow system. RSC Adv. 2014;4:25348.

28. Liu K, Lepin EJ, Wang M-W, et al. Microfluidic-based 18F-labeling of biomolecules for immuno-positron emission tomography. Mol Imaging. 2011;10:168–76.

29. Keng PY, Chen S, Ding H, et al. Micro-chemical synthesis of molecular probes on an electronic microfluidic device. Proc Natl Acad Sci U S A. 2012;109:690–5.

30. Javed MR, Chen S, Kim H-K, Wei L, Czernin J, Kim C-JCJ, van Dam RM, Keng PY. Efficient radiosynthesis of 3'-deoxy-3'-18F-fluorothymidine using electrowetting-on-dielectric digital microfluidic chip. J Nucl Med. 2014;55:321–8.
31. Javed MR, Chen S, Lei J, Collins J, Sergeev M, Kim H-K, Kim C-J, van Dam RM, Keng PY. High yield and high specific activity synthesis of [18F]fallypride in a batch microfluidic reactor for micro-PET imaging. Chem Commun (Camb). 2014;50:1192–4.
32. Chen S, Javed MR, Kim H-K, Lei J, Lazari M, Shah GJ, van Dam RM, Keng P-Y, Kim C-JCJ. Radiolabelling diverse positron emission tomography (PET) tracers using a single digital microfluidic reactor chip. Lab Chip. 2014;14:902–10.
33. Ali I, Aboul-Enein HY, Gupta VK. Nanochromatography and nanocapillary electrophoresis. 2009. doi:10.1002/9780470434925
34. Ghanem A, Ikegami T. Recent advances in silica-based monoliths: preparations, characterizations and applications. J Sep Sci. 2011;34:1945–57.
35. Wouters B, De Vos J, Desmet G, Terryn H, Schoenmakers PJ, Eeltink S. Design of a microfluidic device for comprehensive spatial two-dimensional liquid chromatography. J Sep Sci. 2015;38:1123–9.
36. Zhou D, Chu W, Peng X, McConathy J, Mach RH, Katzenellenbogen JA. Facile purification and click labeling with 2-[18F]fluoroethyl azide using solid phase extraction cartridges. Tetrahedron Lett. 2015;56:952–4.
37. Fedorova O, Kuznetsova O, Stepanova M, Maleev V, Belokon Y, Wester H-J, Krasikova R. A facile direct nucleophilic synthesis of O-(2-[18F]fluoroethyl)-l-tyrosine ([18F]FET) without HPLC purification. J Radioanal Nucl Chem. 2014;301:505–12.
38. Turiel E, Martín-Esteban A. Molecularly imprinted polymers for sample preparation: a review. Anal Chim Acta. 2010;668:87–99.
39. Haupt K, Mosbach K. Molecularly imprinted polymers and their use in biomimetic sensors. Chem Rev. 2000;100:2495–504.
40. Brown LJ, Bouvet DR, Champion S, et al. A solid-phase route to18F-labeled tracers, exemplified by the synthesis of [18F]2-Fluoro-2-deoxy-D-glucose. Angew Chemie. 2007;119:959–62.
41. Riss PJ, Kuschel S, Aigbirhio FI. No carrier-added nucleophilic aromatic radiofluorination using solid phase supported arenediazonium sulfonates and 1-(aryldiazenyl)piperazines. Tetrahedron Lett. 2012;53:1717–9.
42. Brady F, Luthra S, Robins E. Solid-phase fluorination of uracil and cytosine. 2006. US 10/538,904.
43. Ismail R, Machness A, van Dam RM, Keng P-Y. Solid-phase [18F]fluorination on a flow-through glass microfluidic chip. In: 16th int. conf. miniaturized syst. chem. life sci. 2012. Okinawa, Japan, p. 629–631
44. Sergeev ME, Morgia F, Lazari M, Wang C, van Dam RM. Titania-catalyzed radiofluorination of tosylated precursors in highly aqueous medium. J Am Chem Soc. 2015;137:5686–94.
45. Billiet S, De Bruycker K, Driessen F, Goossens H, Van Speybroeck V, Winne JM, Du Prez FE. Triazolinediones enable ultrafast and reversible click chemistry for the design of dynamic polymer systems. Nat Chem. 2014;6:815–21.
46. Ban H, Nagano M, Gavrilyuk J, Hakamata W, Inokuma T, Barbas CF. Facile and stabile linkages through tyrosine: bioconjugation strategies with the tyrosine-click reaction. Bioconjug Chem. 2013;24:520–32.
47. Kim DW. Bioorthogonal click chemistry for fluorine-18 labeling protocols under physiologically friendly reaction condition. J Fluor Chem. 2015;174:142–7.
48. Salvadori AP. Radiopharmaceuticals, drug development and pharmaceutical regulations in Europe. Curr Radiopharm. 2015;1:7–11.
49. VanBrocklin FH. Radiopharmaceuticals for drug development: United States regulatory perspective. Curr Radiopharm. 2015;1:2–6.
50. Yu S. Review of 18F-FDG synthesis and quality control. Biomed Imaging Interv J. 2006;2: e57.
51. Reilly RM, Lam K, Chan C, Levine M. Advancing novel molecular imaging agents from preclinical studies to first-in-humans phase I clinical trials in academia – a roadmap for overcoming perceived barriers. Bioconjug Chem. 2015;26:625–32.

Chapter 7
Advantages of Radiochemistry in Microliter Volumes

Pei Yuin Keng, Maxim Sergeev, and R. Michael van Dam

Abstract Positron emission tomography (PET) provides quantitative 3D visualization of physiological parameters (e.g., metabolic rate, receptor density, gene expression, blood flow) in real time in the living body. By enabling measurement of differences in such characteristics between normal and diseased tissues, PET serves as vital tool for basic research as well as for clinical diagnosis and patient management. Prior to a PET scan, the patient is injected with a short-lived tracer labeled with a positron-emitting isotope. Safe preparation of the tracer is an expensive process, requiring specially trained personnel and high-cost equipment operated within hot cells. The current centralized manufacturing strategy, in which large batches are prepared and divided among many patients, enables the most commonly used tracer (i.e., [^{18}F]FDG) to be obtained at an affordable price. However, as the diversity of tracers increases, other strategies for cost reduction will become necessary. This challenge is being addressed by the development of miniaturized radiochemistry instrumentation based on microfluidics. These compact systems have the potential to significantly reduce equipment cost and shielding while increasing diversity of tracers produced in a given facility. The most common approach uses "flow-through" microreactors, which leverage the ability to precisely control reaction conditions to improve synthesis times and yields. Several groups have also developed "batch" microreactors which offer significant additional advantages such as reduced reagent consumption, simpler purifications, and exceptionally high specific activity, by reducing operating volumes by orders of magnitude. In this chapter, we review these "batch" approaches and the advantages of using small volumes, with special emphasis on digital microfluidics, in which reactions have been performed with volumes as low as ~1 µL.

Keywords Microfluidics • Radiosynthesis • Positron emission tomography (PET) • Electrowetting-on-dielectric (EWOD) • Microscale chemistry

P.Y. Keng • M. Sergeev • R.M. van Dam (✉)
Crump Institute for Molecular Imaging and Department of Molecular and Medical Pharmacology, David Geffen School of Medicine, University of California, Los Angeles, CA, USA
e-mail: mvandam@mednet.ucla.edu

© The Author(s) 2016   93
Y. Kuge et al. (eds.), *Perspectives on Nuclear Medicine for Molecular Diagnosis and Integrated Therapy*, DOI 10.1007/978-4-431-55894-1_7

7.1 Introduction

7.1.1 Radiosynthesis of Positron Emission Tomography Tracers

Positron emission tomography (PET) is an extremely powerful, noninvasive diagnostic imaging technology capable of measuring a plethora of biological processes in vivo [1]. In research, PET can provide dynamic information about normal or diseased states of a living organism and, in the clinic, can provide information that is critical for diagnosis, selection of therapy, or monitoring response to therapy. In some cases, PET can detect biochemical changes associated with disease before any anatomical changes can be observed [2].

PET requires injection of a tracer labeled with a positron-emitting isotope, such as fluorine-18, nitrogen-13, oxygen-15, carbon-11, or a radiometal. Fluorine-18 possesses physical and nuclear properties that are particularly desirable for radiolabeling and imaging [3]. For example, the low positron energy and range ensure high-resolution imaging while minimizing radiation exposure to the patient. In addition, the 110 min half-life is sufficiently long for multistep synthesis, transport to the imaging site, and imaging over extended periods.

Due to the hazard of working with radioactive materials, a specialized infrastructure of automated radiosynthesizers operating in radiation-shielded "hot cells" by expert personnel is required. Due to the high costs, a couple of tracers (including 2-[^{18}F]fluoro-2-deoxy-D-glucose, [^{18}F]FDG) are currently produced in a "satellite" manner. Radiopharmacies manufacture large batches that are subdivided among many patients within a local area to leverage economies of scale and offer the compound at an affordable price. As the diversity of PET tracers used in medical care and research increases, opportunities to share costs are reduced, and alternative innovative approaches are needed to reduce the high cost of each batch.

A particularly promising approach is the development of miniaturized radiosynthesizers based on microfluidic technology that can enable dramatic reductions in the cost of equipment and the amount of radiation shielding needed. An additional innovation is the concept of disposable "cassettes," which allows each synthesizer to make a wide range of tracers simply by using different cassettes, rather than being dedicated to production of a single tracer [4].

7.1.2 Microfluidics for Radiosynthesis

It has been well established that the geometry of microfluidic devices offers many advantages for the synthesis of short-lived radiopharmaceuticals [5–7]. In particular, the small dimensions enable improved control of reaction conditions via rapid mixing and efficient heat transfer, leading to faster reactions and improved selectivity, thus higher yields.

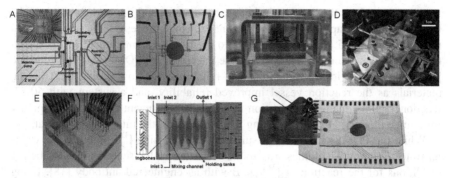

Fig. 7.1 Batch microfluidics devices for synthesis of PET tracers: (**a**) PDMS chip with 40 nL reactor (Adapted from reference [14] with permission from AAAS). (**b**) Scaled-up PDMS chip with 5 μL reactor (Adapted from reference [15], Copyright © 2010 by the Society of Nuclear Medicine and Molecular Imaging, Inc.). (**c**) Chemically inert polydicyclopentadiene (pDCPD) polymer chip with 5 μL reactor (Reproduced from reference [56]). (**d**) Chemically inert pDCPD chip with 60 μL reactor (Reproduced with permission from reference [50], Copyright © 2010 John Wiley & Sons, Ltd.). (**e**) PDMS chip for optimizing radiolabeling reaction in variable volume droplets (~100 nL) (Reproduced with permission from reference [59], Copyright © 2015 IOP Publishing). (**f**) PDMS chip for radiometal labeling with 25 μL reaction volume (Reproduced with permission from reference [19], Copyright © 2013 Elsevier, Inc.) (**g**) EWOD chip with reaction volume ranging from 2 to 17 μL

Most commonly in the field of radiochemistry, these devices are based on "flow-through" microreactors, where reactions occur by flowing reagent streams through mixers and preheated capillary tubes or microchannels. Numerous groups have demonstrated the radiosynthesis of [^{18}F]FDG in polymer chips [8], glass chips [9], and capillary tubes [10]. This technology has been commercialized (e.g., Advion Biosciences "NanoTek" and Scintomics "μ-ICR"), and dozens of different radio-tracers labeled with F-18, C-11, N-13, and Tc-99 m have been demonstrated [11]. Recent advances have enabled the integration of solvent exchange processes [12, 13], which previously were accomplished via bulky, off-chip subsystems.

Because it is important that flow-through systems are completely filled with liquid in order to achieve accurate fluid handling, typical operating volumes are comparable to macroscale systems (i.e., >500 μL). Another class of microfluidic device based on small (<50 μL) volumes known as "batch" microreactors have also been used for radiochemistry (Fig. 7.1). These devices are particularly attractive for radiochemistry because all synthetic steps including solvent exchange can be integrated into a single chip and because small volumes can reduce reagent consumption, enhance reaction kinetics, improve specific activity, reduce radiolysis, and simplify purification, as described below.

7.1.3   Platforms for Microliter Volume Synthesis

The first batch microfluidic synthesis of [^{18}F]FDG was demonstrated in a polydimethylsiloxane (PDMS) chip with 40 nL reaction volume [14]. Microvalves were used to close the reactor during reaction steps, and the permeability of the PDMS enabled escape of vapor for solvent exchange processes. By scaling up the reactor volume to 5 μL, it was possible to produce mCi amounts of [^{18}F]-labeled tracers [15]. Unfortunately, due to adverse interaction of PDMS with [^{18}F]fluoride [16], radioactivity losses were high and reliability was low. Using inert plastic materials as the reaction vessel improved reliability, and a system with 50 μL reaction volume enabled production of tracers of sufficient quantity and quality for human imaging [17], establishing the relevance of the micro-batch format.

While the PDMS chip was not suitable for processing [^{18}F]fluoride, the capability to react small volumes was found to be useful for screening radiolabeling conditions for the reaction of [^{18}F]SFB with an engineered antibody [18]. Using <100 nL per droplet, many reaction conditions could be tested, and then the whole batch could be labeled once optimal conditions were found. A quasi-continuous-flow PDMS chip using small volumes (25 μL) has also been used for radiolabeling peptides and proteins with radiometals such as Ga-68 and Cu-64 [19]. The small volume enabled improved stoichiometry of the label and ligand, dramatically improving the labeling yield and potentially avoiding the need for extensive purification.

Recently, our group demonstrated successful radiosynthesis of [^{18}F]FDG and other molecules using another type of batch microfluidic device based on the digital manipulation of droplets between two parallel plates [20, 21] known as electrowetting-on-dielectric (EWOD). Droplets are controlled by on-chip electrodes (Fig. 7.2), eliminating the need for bulky valve actuators, pumps, and radiation shielding as is needed in the approaches mentioned above. A wide range of reagents and reaction conditions can be used on these EWOD microchips because they are constructed from inert and thermally stable materials (glass substrate, metallic electrode layer, inorganic dielectric layer, and fluoropolymer layer). Because droplets are surrounded by gas, evaporation and solvent exchange can readily be performed on the chip. Resistive heating, temperature sensing for precise temperature control, and impedance sensing for measuring electrical properties of liquid can all be integrated on the chip without the need of additional bulky hardware [22].

Using this platform, our laboratory has reported the successful synthesis of [^{18}F] FDG [20], 3-[^{18}F]fluoro-3′-deoxy-fluorothymidine ([^{18}F]FLT) [23], [^{18}F]fallypride [24], and N-succinimidyl 4-[^{18}F]fluorobenzoate ([^{18}F]SFB) [25] with radiochemical yields of 22 ± 8 % ($n = 11$), 63 ± 5 % ($n = 5$), 65 ± 6 % ($n = 7$), and 19 ± 8 % ($n = 5$), respectively. The final ^{18}F-labeled compounds passed all quality control tests required by the United States Pharmacopeia for injection into humans and have been successfully used in preclinical PET. The syntheses of [^{18}F]FDG and [^{18}F]FLT on a simplified EWOD chip have also been reported by others [26, 27]. These results suggest that the EWOD-based synthesizer can meet the requirements for on-demand production of diverse PET tracers to meet preclinical or clinical needs.

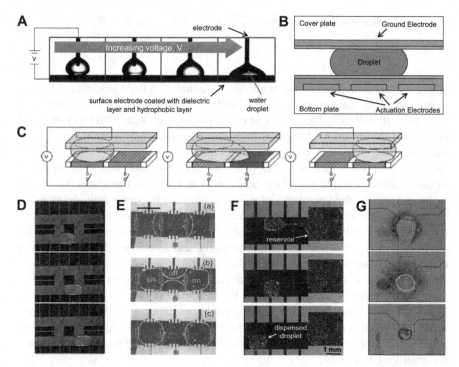

Fig. 7.2 Structure and operation of EWOD microfluidic chips. (**a**) Illustration of the "electrowetting" effect. (**b**) Schematic of typical EWOD device with droplet sandwiched between the two plates. (**c**) Applying a local field to one end of the droplet using a small control electrode (typically 1 or 2 mm square) can generate a force on the droplet in a direction toward the activated electrode (Diagram courtesy of Robin Garrell). This force enables several operations, including (**d**) droplet transport along a predetermined path, (**e**) droplet splitting, and (**f**) droplet dispensing from an on-chip reservoir. Incorporation of specialized heating electrodes permits additional operations such as (**g**) evaporation of solvent. ((d) is reproduced with permission from reference [60] (Copyright © 2004 American Chemical Society), (e) is reproduced with permission from reference [61] (Copyright © 2003 IEEE), (f) is reproduced from reference [62] with permission of The Royal Society of Chemistry.)

7.2 Advantages of Radiosynthesis at the Microliter Scale

7.2.1 Miniaturization and Disposability

Perhaps the most significant potential advantage of batch microfluidics in the field of radiochemistry is the potential to integrate the entire synthesis, purification, and formulation apparatus into an extremely compact system. Size of the components that need to be shielded (because they contain or contact radioactivity) has a tremendous impact on the amount of radiation shielding needed. For a constant thickness "shell" of shielding, t, the volume (and weight and cost) of the shielding scale is

$$\text{Shielding volume} \sim (r+t)^3 - r^3 = (3r^2t + 3rt^2 + t^3)$$
$$= 3r^2t\left(1 + \frac{t}{r} + \frac{1}{3}\frac{t^2}{r^2}\right)$$

where r is the dimension of the synthesizer. Assuming a fixed shielding thickness where $t \ll r$, the scale factor is proportional to r^2. Thus, moving from macroscale systems with ~20-inch dimensions to microfluidic chips with ~2-inch dimensions can reduce the needed shielding 100-fold. This reduction could make it practical for radiochemistry chips to be used in benchtop situations instead of needing to operate them in specialized facilities equipped with hot cells and mini cells to shield radiation, thus removing one of the bottlenecks in PET tracer production.

Integrating the fluid pathways of a radiosynthesizer into a microfluidic chip has other advantages as well. If the chip can be made to be very inexpensive, the entire fluid pathway can be discarded after each synthesis run, eliminating the need for developing and validating a cleaning protocol and associated documentation or cleaning the system on a daily basis. This concept of disposability is increasingly being used in macroscale synthesizers to simplify setup, cleanup, and compliance with cGMP manufacturing guidelines for PET tracers that are used in humans [4]. Disposable cassettes also provide flexibility: with a single synthesizer instrument, the operator can choose to install different disposable cassettes (with different pre-configured fluid path configurations) along with matching reagent kits to make different PET tracers [4].

7.2.2   Reduced Radiolysis

Radiolysis is the process of chemical bond cleavage caused by radiation. Molecules of a PET probe undergo irradiation from both the starting [^{18}F]fluoride (external radiolysis) and from other radiolabeled molecules (autoradiolysis) [28–30], which can lead to reduction in the yield of the probe and the formation of radioactive side products. The mechanism of damage is believed to be related to the formation of radical species in the solvent by high-energy particles [29]. While the final injectable formulation can be stabilized against autoradiolysis with addition of radical scavengers (e.g., ethanol) to preserve radiochemical purity [30], this is not generally possible at earlier stages during the radiosynthesis process.

Fluorine-18 emits positrons with high energy ($E_{max} = 0.633$ MeV) that cause ionization of the solvent while dissipating their kinetic energy along their travel range. The range is up to ~2.4 mm, but due to the tortuous path they follow, the distribution of final displacements of positrons from their origin is characterized by a smaller range (i.e., full width at one third maximum ~1 mm) [31]. When the reaction vessel dimensions (e.g., vial, flask, or Eppendorf tube: ~10 mm) are much greater than this range, each positron deposits all of its energy into the solvent, leading to extensive radiolysis (Fig. 7.3a).

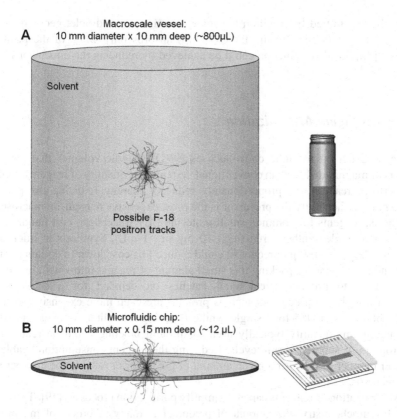

Fig. 7.3 Illustration of radiolysis suppression. (**a**) Possible positron tracks from decay of a fluorine-18 atom at the center of a conventional macroscale reaction vessel. Because the positron range is significantly less than the reactor dimensions, the positron will deposit all of its energy into the solvent, where it causes radiolysis. This is true of decay events happening throughout the vial. (**b**) In contrast, in an EWOD microfluidic chip, one dimension of the solvent volume is very thin compared to the positron range. Thus, a significant portion of the possible tracks are mostly or entirely outside the droplet. Thus, most positrons will escape the solvent after having only deposited a small fraction of their energy in the solvent, reducing radiolysis

Rensch et al. have shown via simulations and experiments that the degree of radiolysis is geometry dependent [3]. In vessels for which at least one dimension is significantly smaller than the positron range (e.g., capillary tubing or EWOD chips), there is significantly reduced radiolysis because positrons can escape the solvent before depositing very much of their energy (Fig. 7.3b). For example, the solvent within a 100 μm diameter capillary reactor absorbs only 10 % of the energy of positrons emitted from within the solvent, and a planar droplet geometry with 100 µm height (similar to the EWOD chip) absorbs only 40 % of the positron energy [32]. Further reduction could be achieved by reducing the dimensions.

7.2.3 Reagent Minimization

Because batch microfluidic chips such as EWOD handle volumes that are 2–3 orders of magnitude less than conventional systems, the quantity of reagents needed to perform reactions is proportionately reduced, thereby reducing the per-run reagent cost. Generally the precursor is the most expensive reagent. In macroscale synthesis, reagents for common small-molecule PET tracers can cost hundreds of US$ for a single synthesis run (e.g., 10 mg in ~1 mL). Synthesis in microliter volumes (e.g., 10–100 µg precursor) could reduce this cost down to dollars per run (depending on costs of packing this small amount of reagent into vials), making it economical to produce even small batches on demand for a single user. Biomolecule-based precursors such as proteins are even more expensive, costing up to thousands of US$ for a single synthesis. Using microliter volumes, the 100 s of micrograms quantity typically used for protein labeling could be reduced to microgram or submicrogram levels. Reducing the reagent consumption enables a greater number of runs per a given amount of precursor or reduces the cost per run of precursor.

Minimization of reagents can also simplify purification processes [19]. Typically in ^{18}F-radiochemistry, the amount of precursor is many of orders of magnitude higher than the amount of [^{18}F]fluoride to ensure the fluorination reaction occurs as rapidly as possible. For example, in the synthesis of [^{18}F]FDG, one typically uses about 40 µmol of mannose triflate [33], compared to the 600 pmol of [^{18}F]fluoride ion in a 1000 mCi batch, representing an excess of 5 orders of magnitude. Even accounting for typical final specific activity, the amount of [^{19}F]fluoride + [^{18}F] fluoride is about 60–600 nmol, meaning there is still an excess of about 2–3 orders of magnitude of precursor compared to ([^{18}F] + [^{19}F])FDG. This means that at the end of the synthesis, there are vast amounts of unreacted (or hydrolyzed) precursor that must be separated from a much smaller amount of the desired product. Because of the high amounts or precursor, large reaction volume, and the chemical similarity between precursor (native or hydrolyzed) and product, long semi-preparative HPLC purification times may be needed, resulting in a large solvent volume in the purified product. While suitable for patient use, these large volumes can be problematic for imaging in small animals, where the tracer must be sufficiently concentrated to inject enough radioactivity for imaging (typically 100–200 µCi) within the maximum recommended injection volume to avoid physiological per- turbation (e.g., <100 µL for mice). Using smaller amounts of reagents in microfluidic formats, several groups have demonstrated that analytical-scale HPLC is sufficient for purification [24, 34], resulting in more concentrated final formulation. Purification has also been successfully performed with on-chip structures similar to typical macroscale Sep-Pak cartridges [35–37].

Reduced amount of reagents may also simplify the quality control (QC) testing that is needed prior to injection in humans. In general, the reduced amounts of reagents and solvents will lead to reduced amounts of residual impurities after the purification process. An interesting prospect of using extremely tiny volumes is that if the total amount of reagent added is below the injectable limits set by various regulatory agencies, then a test for the absence of that particular chemical may become unnecessary.

7.2.4 High Specific Activity

The specific activity (SA) of a PET tracer (e.g., labeled with fluorine-18) is defined as the ratio of the number of ^{18}F-labeled molecules to the total number of ^{18}F-labeled and ^{19}F-labeled molecules and is typically reported in units of radioactivity per mass (e.g., Ci/μmol). For a certain desired injected dose (e.g., 10 mCi for humans), the higher the SA, the lower the mass that is injected.

High SA of a PET tracer is important for several reasons. First, because many PET tracers are based on pharmacologically active compounds, only a very low mass should be injected to avoid eliciting a pharmacological response. Second, for tracers that target low-abundance receptors (e.g., in neurological imaging), injecting lower mass avoids saturation or high occupancy of the receptors. This is especially important in small animal imaging, in which significantly higher radioactivity is injected (per mass of the animal) compared to human subjects to achieve sufficient image quality with the higher resolution (smaller voxel size) scanners that are used for animals [38]. Third, high SA may improve image quality by increasing the proportion of targets occupied by radioactive forms of the tracer while reducing competitive interactions of the nonradioactive forms. Other reasons to maximize SA are related to the logistics of PET tracer production. Often, tracers need to be transported from the radiopharmacy where they are produced to the imaging center. Because of the radioactive decay during this transport time, the SA is reduced by a factor of 2 for each half-life, and a high initial SA is needed to ensure sufficient SA at the time of imaging.

For fluorine-18, the maximum theoretical SA is 1710 Ci/μmol; however, the actual SA of the final tracer is significantly lower, typically 1–10 Ci/μmol [39]. This means the number of fluorine-18 atoms is dwarfed (~200–2000X) by the number of fluorine-19 contaminant atoms. Some of the fluorine-19 contamination originates due to the equipment and materials used in the [^{18}F]fluoride production process (e.g., [^{18}O]H$_2$O quality, volume of target, target materials, tubing materials, target loading/unloading process, etc.) [40–42]. While such sources may be out of most radiochemists' control, another significant contribution is the contamination of reaction mixture with extra fluorine-19 fluoride during the synthesis process itself (i.e., all steps upstream of and including the fluorination step). The main sources are the QMA cartridges used in the fluoride drying process, fluorinated materials (e.g.,

Teflon tubing and stirbars) [43], and the reagents used in the synthesis, such as K_2CO_3, Kryptofix, etc.

In preliminary studies, our group observed that microfluidic synthesis on EWOD chips resulted in significantly higher (up to 25–50 times) SA compared to macro-scale synthesis, starting with the same amount of radioactivity [23, 24]. This suggested the potential for microfluidics to significantly reduce fluorine-19 con-tamination in the synthesis process. An in-depth investigation led to the observation that the dependence of SA on reaction parameters was very different for macroscale (100–5000 μL) and microscale (2–8 μL) syntheses. At the macroscale, the SA strongly varied with the reaction volume (amount of reagents) as well as the starting radioactivity (from 10s to 100 s of mCi), whereas the SA was much higher and nearly constant (20–23 Ci/μmol), under all conditions when performed in microdroplets. These results suggest that in the macroscale synthesis, reagents and solvents are the dominant source of fluorine-19, while in microscale volumes, these sources have been nearly eliminated and the fluorine-19 contribution from the cyclotron dominates [44, 45] (Fig. 7.4). The effect of the 120 nm Teflon layer on the chip was also investigated and no impact on SA was seen [43], perhaps due to the radiolysis suppression effect described above.

Small volumes are extremely beneficial for another type of reaction, namely, isotopic exchange (IEX). In IEX reactions, the precursor is identical to the final product, except for the presence of fluorine-19 instead of fluorine-18, and cannot be separated after synthesis. Thus it is desirable to minimize the amount of excess precursor to maintain high SA. In macroscale reactions this is difficult, because the

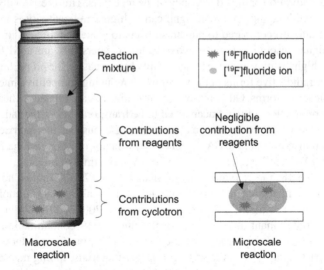

Fig. 7.4 Illustration of specific activity improvement. (*Left*) At the macroscale, reagents are the dominant source of fluorine-19 contamination in the fluorination reaction mixture. (*Right*) At the microscale, the reagents add negligible fluorine-19 contamination to that already present from the cyclotron. After the fluorination reaction, the fluoride (both F-18 and F-19 forms) get incorporated into the precursor and cannot be separated, resulting in [18]F- and ^{19}F-labeled forms of the tracer

concentration of precursor needs to be sufficiently high for efficient reaction. However, Perrin et al. have shown that small volume reactions are an effective way to minimize precursor amount for IEX reactions [46, 47]. It should be noted that the same principles can be applied to other carrier-added situations or to the labeling of proteins or other species where the labeled and unlabeled forms cannot be separated; in all such cases, it is critical to minimize the starting material in order to obtain high SA. The dependence of SA on starting radioactivity for IEX reactions was investigated in simplified EWOD chips using rhodamine clicked to an aryl-BF_3 moiety [44]. Unlike in nucleophilic substitution reactions, SA of microfluidic IEX reactions was found to vary with starting radioactivity, but in a nonlinear manner. This suggests that perhaps the contribution of fluorine-19 from the cyclotron is comparable to other sources and further reduced volume may be beneficial.

For both nucleophilic substitution and IEX reactions, small volume synthesis can achieve high SA even from low starting amounts of radioactivity. This is in contrast to macroscale synthesis, where high SA production typically requires starting with Ci levels of radioactivity. Depending on the amount of tracer radioactivity needed, small volume synthesis could therefore reduce the time/cost of cyclotron bombardment, increase safety, and decrease the required amount of shielding required for production.

7.3 Practical Considerations

7.3.1 Limits of Volume Reduction

Clearly there are enormous advantages to performing radiochemistry in small volumes. The current EWOD chip geometry can reliably handle volumes as small as ~2 μL, which is limited by the size of the electrodes that are used to load and transport reagent droplets. Scaling down the volume of radiochemical reactions below 2 μL could enable further reductions in precursor cost, further improvements in specific activity (for IEX reactions or biomolecule labeling), further simplification of purification and QC testing, or reduction in the size of the EWOD chip, which leads to cost reduction. Even smaller droplets could be manipulated by scaling down the electrode size and/or reducing the gap between the chip plates. In fact, using specialized fabrication techniques, Nelson and Kim have shown that droplets as small as 100 pL can be manipulated in an EWOD chip [48].

As the volume is scaled down, it is important to be mindful of several issues. First, a certain minimum volume will be needed to solvate the desired amount of the radioisotope complexed with phase transfer catalyst along with the precursor. Another limitation will be the droplet lifetime: at extremely small volume scales, droplets quickly evaporate and may not last sufficiently long to carry out the fluorination reaction. The limit of volume reduction for radiochemistry applications remains to be explored.

7.3.2 Radioisotope Concentration

When considering using small reaction volumes, one must also consider how to produce sufficient quantity (radioactivity) of the tracer for the particular application needed. For preclinical imaging, generally a few mCi is sufficient for a study involving several animals, and with modern scanners, <25–50 µCi is sufficient for a single mouse. On the other hand, imaging of a single patient requires on the order of 10 mCi, while producing a large batch in a radiopharmacy for distribution to imaging centers would require 100s–1000s of mCi. Even higher amounts of the radioisotope are needed at the beginning of the synthesis due to nonideal yields and fluid handling, as well as losses due to decay.

Cyclotrons can readily generate multiple Ci levels of $[^{18}F]$fluoride in $[^{18}O]H_2O$ to satisfy any of these applications. However, the output volume is typically in the milliliter range, while the capacity of the current EWOD chip (12 mm diameter reaction zone x 150 µm droplet height) is only ~17 µL, i.e., 1 % of the volume from the cyclotron. From a high-radioactivity bombardment, it would be possible to load as much of tens of mCi of radioisotope into the chip without special measures, but it is not desirable to waste the majority of the radioisotope, and several methods for efficiently concentrating the radioisotope have been developed (Fig. 7.5a).

One approach is to concentrate the $[^{18}F]$fluoride prior to loading it into the chip via a solid-phase extraction (SPE) process. First, the $[^{18}F]$fluoride/$[^{18}O]H_2O$ is flowed through a strong anion exchange cartridge (e.g., quaternary methyl ammonium, QMA) to trap the $[^{18}F]$fluoride. After removing residual water (e.g., with an inert gas flow), an eluent solution (e.g., aqueous K_2CO_3/ $K_{2.2.2}$ or tetrabutylammonium bicarbonate (TBAB), sometimes with MeCN) is passed through the cartridge to release the $[^{18}F]$fluoride. If the cartridge has sufficiently small bed volume, the volume of eluent solution needed to efficiently collect the $[^{18}F]$fluoride can be quite low. For example, using commercial cartridges (OPTI-LYNX, Optimize Technologies), Elizarov et al. concentrated 92 % of 876 mCi starting $[^{18}F]$fluoride into a ~5 µL volume [15], our group demonstrated release into ~12 µL volume [49], and Lebedev et al. [17] and Bejot et al. [50] demonstrated release into 44 µL volume. This approach can be integrated with microfluidics by using packed-tubing cartridges [15], functionalized porous polymer monoliths [51], packed microchannels [52], or resin-filled inserts [12]. Control of trapping and release processes requires the use of valves with small internal volumes to choose which solution is flowed into the cartridge inlet (i.e., $[^{18}F]$fluoride or eluent) and whether the cartridge outlet is direct to an $[^{18}O]H_2O$ collection reservoir or the microfluidic chip. Most commonly, this is accomplished with HPLC injection valves, but can also be achieved with on-chip microvalves if they can be conveniently integrated into the device (Fig. 7.5b, c). Once loaded into the chip, the concentrated $[^{18}F]$fluoride solution is generally evaporated to dryness, and then the subsequent fluorination reaction volume can be controlled by the volume of precursor solution added, provided there is sufficient solvent to dissolve not only the precursor but also the fluoride complex with phase transfer catalyst. Similar trap and release of $[^{18}F]$fluoride can be accomplished with microfluidic electrochemical flow cells

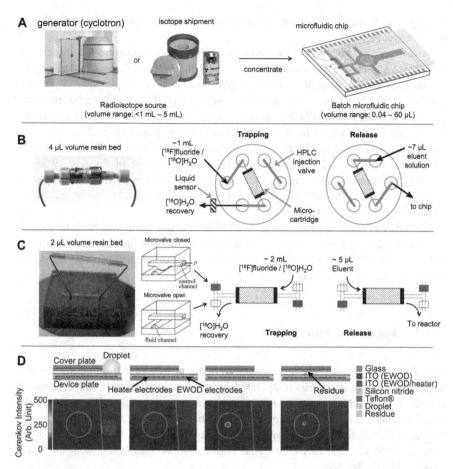

Fig. 7.5 (a) Because the volume of batch microfluidic chips is much smaller than the volume of the radioisotope source, concentration is necessary to ensure sufficient quantity of radioactivity can be loaded onto the chip. (b) Cartridge-based method for concentration described in Ref. [49]. Using an HPLC injection valve with small internal volume, the flow path can be configured in trapping mode, where the [^{18}F]fluoride/[^{18}O]H$_2$O is flowed through a micro-cartridge and the [^{18}F] fluoride trapped, or a release mode, where a small volume of eluent solution is passed through the cartridge to release the [^{18}F]fluoride and deliver it onto the chip. (c) Cartridge-based method using on-chip microvalves implemented in a polydimethylsiloxane (PDMS) chip. Pressure applied to "control channels" can open or close nearby "fluid channels" to configure the flow path into trapping and release modes (Adapted from reference [15] © by the Society of Nuclear Medicine and Molecular Imaging, Inc.). (d) Scheme for evaporative concentration of [^{18}F]fluoride radioisotope. The *top images* show cross-sectional schematics of the concentration process, and the *bottom images* show Cerenkov (radioactivity) images of the *top view* of the chip at corresponding times. *Orange lines* and *circles* were added to depict the cover plate edge and the reaction site, respectively. Initially, a 200 μL droplet of [^{18}F]fluoride solution is loaded to the cover plate edge. By activating a nearby heater, the volume of the droplet is reduced to ~5 μL and then pulled into the chip by electrode actuation. (Reproduced from Ref. [25] with permission from the Royal Society of Chemistry.)

[53, 54] where the [^{18}F]fluoride is trapped at an electrode surface by application of positive voltage.

A different approach is to perform the [^{18}F]fluoride concentration directly on chip [25]. A special chip was fabricated where the bottom plate extended beyond the edge of the cover plate to create a platform. A large droplet of [^{18}F]fluoride solution (with phase transfer catalyst) was loaded onto this platform adjacent to the gap between the two EWOD chip plates and then rapidly evaporated down to a small volume that could be transported between the plates (Fig. 7.5d). Because some groups have reported that the anion exchange resin can contribute fluorine-19 contamination [55], this approach may reduce the amount of fluorine-19 in the reaction mixture and thus enable production of PET tracers with higher specific activity. It also has the advantage of not requiring any valves, but the disadvantage of requiring larger chip real estate.

With any of these approaches, it is possible to concentrate a significant fraction of the radioactivity from a cyclotron bombardment into a volume that can be loaded onto the microfluidic chip, enabling radiochemistry to be performed in microliter volumes with high radioactivity.

7.3.3   Synthesis Automation

As with radiosynthesis in conventional systems at milliliter volume scales, it is important that the apparatus is operated in an automated fashion within radiation shielding to ensure the safety of the operator preparing the PET tracer. Fully automated synthesizers have been developed based on some of the earlier reports of batch microfluidic chips, complete with reagent delivery, radioisotope concentration, synthesis, and cartridge-based purification or interfacing with an HPLC system [15, 17, 50, 56].

For the more recent EWOD microfluidic platform, many aspects of automating the overall system have been demonstrated. Two approaches have been developed for loading reagents from off-chip reservoirs (e.g., standard septum-capped glass reagent vials) into the chip. One simple approach uses an electronically controlled syringe pump to precisely dispense the desired volume of reagent after compensating for evaporation losses at the dispensing tip [57]. Another approach was developed in collaboration with Sofie Biosciences, Inc. to avoid the use of complex, difficult-to-clean components such as syringe pumps and valves, instead of relying on simple disposable fluidic elements such as needles and tubing. Inert gas pressure and gravitational force were used to apply forward and reverse driving forces, respectively, to deliver repeatable volumes to the chip [58]. A multi-reagent loading interface was developed based on this principle and was integrated with a simple cartridge-based method for upstream [^{18}F]fluoride concentration and an automated method for downstream collection of the crude product from the chip and interfacing with miniature solid-phase extraction cartridges or analytical-scale HPLC for purification [34]. Some preliminary progress to develop methods for on-chip purification has also been made including removal of unreacted [^{18}F]fluoride using an alumina surface [35] or beads [36], and more complete separation may be possible by performing on-chip solid-phase extraction. A prototype of a complete EWOD-based PET tracer production system suitable for benchtop operation is under development at Sofie Biosciences in collaboration with our group.

7.4 Conclusions and Outlook

The development of batch microfluidic devices may provide an ideal platform to harness the numerous advantages of performing the synthesis of PET radiotracers in small volumes, including reduced reagent consumption, improved specific activity, reduced radiolysis, and synthesizer miniaturization. In particular, the EWOD platform is compatible with diverse reaction conditions and provides a convenient means to digitally manipulate droplets to perform diverse multistep reactions. By combining these devices with technologies for concentration of radioisotopes into an automated platform, it will become possible to produce not only batches on demand for research use but even large-scale batches in a radiopharmacy for distribution purposes. This microvolume radiochemistry technique could also be a particularly good match for isotopic exchange and biomolecule labeling reactions and could enable novel chemistries by boosting $[^{18}F]$fluoride concentration by orders of magnitude. As a tool for remotely and safely handling small volumes, the EWOD microfluidic platform could open up opportunities for researchers to uncover additional benefits of radiochemistry in extremely small volumes.

Acknowledgments The authors gratefully acknowledge support for writing this review from the National Institute of Biomedical Imaging and Bioengineering (grant R21EB015540), the National Institute on Aging (grant R21AG049918), as well as Sofie Biosciences, Inc., and the National Institute of Mental Health (grant R44MH097271).

References

1. Phelps ME. Positron emission tomography provides molecular imaging of biological processes. PNAS. 2000;97:9226–33.
2. Kelloff GJ, Hoffman JM, Johnson B, et al. Progress and promise of FDG-PET imaging for cancer patient management and oncologic drug development. Clin Cancer Res. 2005;11:2785–808.

3. Lasne M-C, Perrio C, Rouden J, Barré L, Roeda D, Dolle F, Crouzel C. Chemistry of β + −emitting compounds based on fluorine-18. In: Krause W, editor. Contrast agents II. Berlin/Heidelberg: Springer; 2002. p. 201–58.
4. Keng PY, Esterby M, van Dam RM. Emerging technologies for decentralized production of PET tracers. In: Hsieh C-H, editor. Positron emission tomography – current clinical and research aspects. InTech; 2012. p. 153–82.
5. Rensch C, Jackson A, Lindner S, Salvamoser R, Samper V, Riese S, Bartenstein P, Wängler C, Wängler B. Microfluidics: a groundbreaking technology for PET tracer production? Molecules. 2013;18:7930–56.
6. Miller PW, deMello AJ, Gee AD. Application of microfluidics to the ultra-rapid preparation of fluorine-18 labelled compounds. Curr Radiopharm. 2010;3:254–62.
7. Watts P, Pascali G, Salvadori PA. Positron emission tomography radiosynthesis in microreactors. J Flow Chem. 2012;2:37–42.
8. McMullen JP, Jensen KF. Integrated microreactors for reaction automation: new approaches to reaction development. Annu Rev Anal Chem. 2010;3:19–42.
9. Gillies JM, Prenant C, Chimon GN, Smethurst GJ, Perrie W, Hamblett I, Dekker B, Zweit J. Microfluidic reactor for the radiosynthesis of PET radiotracers. Appl Radiat Isot. 2006;64:325–32.
10. Steel CJ, O'Brien AT, Luthra SK, Brady F. Automated PET radiosyntheses using microfluidic devices. J Label Compd Radiopharm. 2007;50:308–11.
11. Wester H-J, Schoultz BW, Hultsch C, Henriksen G. Fast and repetitive in-capillary production of [18F]FDG. Eur J Nucl Med Mol Imaging. 2009;36:653–8.
12. Pascali G, Watts P, Salvadori PA. Microfluidics in radiopharmaceutical chemistry. Nucl Med Biol. 2013;40:776–87.
13. Rensch C, Lindner S, Salvamoser R, et al. A solvent resistant lab-on-chip platform for radiochemistry applications. Lab Chip. 2014;14:2556–64.
14. Arima V, Pascali G, Lade O, et al. Radiochemistry on chip: towards dose-on-demand synthesis of PET radiopharmaceuticals. Lab Chip. 2013;13(12):2328–36.
15. Lee C-C, Sui G, Elizarov A, et al. Multistep synthesis of a radiolabeled imaging probe using integrated microfluidics. Science. 2005;310:1793–6.
16. Elizarov AM, van Dam RM, Shin YS, Kolb HC, Padgett HC, Stout D, Shu J, Huang J, Daridon A, Heath JR. Design and optimization of coin-shaped microreactor chips for PET radiopharmaceutical synthesis. J Nucl Med. 2010;51:282–7.
17. Tseng W-Y, Cho JS, Ma X, Kunihiro A, Chatziioannou A, van Dam RM. Toward reliable synthesis of radiotracers for positron emission tomography in PDMS microfluidic chips: study and optimization of the [18F] fluoride drying process. In: Technical proceedings of the 2010 NSTI nanotechnology conference and trade show, Anaheim, CA. Boca Raton: CRC Press; 2010. p. 472–5.
18. Lebedev A, Miraghaie R, Kotta K, Ball CE, Zhang J, Buchsbaum MS, Kolb HC, Elizarov A. Batch-reactor microfluidic device: first human use of a microfluidically produced PET radiotracer. Lab Chip. 2012;13:136–45.
19. Liu K, Lepin EJ, Wang M-W, et al. Microfluidic-based 18F-labeling of biomolecules for immuno-positron emission tomography. Mol Imaging. 2011;10:168–76.
20. Zeng D, Desai AV, Ranganathan D, Wheeler TD, Kenis PJA, Reichert DE. Microfluidic radiolabeling of biomolecules with PET radiometals. Nucl Med Biol. 2013;40:42–51.
21. Keng PY, Chen S, Ding H, et al. Micro-chemical synthesis of molecular probes on an electronic microfluidic device. PNAS. 2012;109:690–5.
22. Reichert DE. A digital revolution in radiosynthesis. J Nucl Med. 2014;55:181–2.
23. Sadeghi S, Ding H, Shah GJ, Chen S, Keng PY, Kim C-J "CJ", van Dam RM, On chip droplet characterization: a practical, high-sensitivity measurement of droplet impedance in digital microfluidics. Anal Chem. 2012;84:1915–23.
24. Javed MR, Chen S, Kim H-K, Wei L, Czernin J, Kim C-J "CJ," Dam RM van, Keng PY. Efficient radiosynthesis of 3′-deoxy-3′-18F-fluorothymidine using electrowetting-on-dielectric digital microfluidic chip. J Nucl Med. 2014;55:321–8.

25. Javed MR, Chen S, Lei J, Collins J, Sergeev M, Kim H-K, Kim C-J, van Dam RM, Keng PY. High yield and high specific activity synthesis of [18F]fallypride in a batch microfluidic reactor for micro-PET imaging. Chem Commun. 2014;50:1192–4.

26. Chen S, Javed MR, Kim H-K, Lei J, Lazari M, Shah GJ, van Dam M, Keng PY, Kim C-J. Radiolabelling diverse positron emission tomography (PET) tracers using a single digital microfluidic reactor chip. Lab Chip. 2014;14:902–10.

27. Koag MC, Kim H-K, Kim AS. Efficient microscale synthesis of [18F]-2-fluoro-2-deoxy-d-glucose. Chem Eng J. 2014;258:62–8.

28. Koag MC, Kim H-K, Kim AS. Fast and efficient microscale radiosynthesis of 3'-deoxy-3'-[18F]fluorothymidine. J Fluor Chem. 2014;166:104–9.

29. Fawdry RM. Radiolysis of 2-[18F]fluoro-2-deoxy-d-glucose (FDG) and the role of reductant stabilisers. Appl Radiat Isot. 2007;65:1193–201.

30. Búriová E, Macášek F, Melichar F, Kropáček M, Procházka L. Autoradiolysis of the 2-deoxy-2-[18F]fluoro-D-glucose radiopharmaceutical. J Radioanal Nucl Chem. 2005;264:595–602.

31. Jacobson MS, Dankwart HR, Mahoney DW. Radiolysis of 2-[18F]fluoro-2-deoxy-d-glucose ([18F]FDG) and the role of ethanol and radioactive concentration. Appl Radiat Isot. 2009;67:990–5.

32. Levin CS, Hoffman EJ. Calculation of positron range and its effect on the fundamental limit of positron emission tomography system spatial resolution. Phys Med Biol. 1999;44:781.

33. Rensch C, Waengler B, Yaroshenko A, Samper V, Baller M, Heumesser N, Ulin J, Riese S, Reischl G. Microfluidic reactor geometries for radiolysis reduction in radiopharmaceuticals. Appl Radiat Isot. 2012;70:1691–7.

34. Lazari M, Collins J, Shen B, Farhoud M, Yeh D, Maraglia B, Chin FT, Nathanson DA, Moore M, van Dam RM. Fully automated production of diverse 18F-labeled PET tracers on the ELIXYS multireactor radiosynthesizer without hardware modification. J Nucl Med Technol. 2014;42:203–10.

35. Shah GJ, Lei J, Chen S, Kim C-J "CJ," Keng PY, Van Dam RM. Automated injection from EWOD digital microfluidic chip into HPLC purification system. In: Proceedings of the 16th international conference on miniaturized systems for chemistry and life sciences, Okinawa. London: Royal Society of Chemistry; 2012. p. 356–8.

36. Chen S, Lei J, van Dam RM, Keng P-Y, Kim C-J "CJ". Planar alumina purification of 18F-labeled radiotracer synthesis on EWOD chip for positron emission tomography (PET). In: Proceedings of the 16th international conference on miniaturized systems for chemistry and life sciences, Okinawa. London: Royal Society of Chemistry; 2012. p. 1771–3.

37. Chen S, Dooraghi A, Lazari M, van Dam RM, Chatziioannou A, Kim C-J. On-chip product purification for complete microfluidic radiotracer synthesis. In: Proceedings of the 27th IEEE international conference on micro electro mechanical systems (MEMS), San Francisco, CA. Piscataway: IEEE; 2014. p. 284–7.

38. Tarn MD, Pascali G, De Leonardis F, Watts P, Salvadori PA, Pamme N. Purification of 2-[18F] fluoro-2-deoxy-d-glucose by on-chip solid-phase extraction. J Chromatogr A. 2013;1280:117–21.

39. Hume SP, Gunn RN, Jones T. Pharmacological constraints associated with positron emission tomographic scanning of small laboratory animals. Eur J Nucl Med Mol Imaging. 1998;25:173–6.

40. Lapi SE, Welch MJ. A historical perspective on the specific activity of radiopharmaceuticals: What have we learned in the 35 years of the ISRC? Nucl Med Biol. 2013;40:314–20.

41. Satyamurthy N, Amarasekera B, Alvord CW, Barrio JR, Phelps ME. Tantalum [18O]water target for the production of [18F]fluoride with high reactivity for the preparation of 2-deoxy-2-[18F]fluoro-D-glucose. Mol Imaging Biol. 2002;4:65–70.

42. Solin O, Bergman J, Haaparanta M, Reissell A. Production of 18F from water targets. Specific radioactivity and anionic contaminants. Int J Radiat Applications and Instrumentation Part A Applied Radiation and Isotopes. 1988;39:1065–71.

43. Füchtner F, Preusche S, Mäding P, Zessin J, Steinbach J. Factors affecting the specific activity of [18F]fluoride from a [18O]water target. Nuklearmedizin. 2008;47:116–9.
44. Berridge MS, Apana SM, Hersh JM. Teflon radiolysis as the major source of carrier in fluorine-18. J Label Compd Radiopharm. 2009;52:543–8.
45. Lazari M, Sergeev M, Liu Z, Perrin DM, van Dam RM. Study of specific activity in isotopic exchange radiofluorination performed on a microfluidic device. Seoul: World Molecular Imaging Congress; 2014.
46. Sergeev M, Lazari M, Collins J, Morgia F, Javed MR, Keng PY, van Dam RM. Investigation of effect of reaction volume on specific activity in macro- and microscale fluorine-18 radiosynthesis. In: Proceedings of the 6th international symposium on microchemistry and microsystems (ISMM), Singapore; 2014. p. 77–8.
47. Ting R, Lo J, Adam MJ, Ruth TJ, Perrin DM. Capturing aqueous [18F]-fluoride with an arylboronic ester for PET: synthesis and aqueous stability of a fluorescent [18F]-labeled aryltrifluoroborate. J Fluor Chem. 2008;129:349–58.
48. Liu Z, Li Y, Lozada J, Pan J, Lin K-S, Schaffer P, Perrin DM. Rapid, one-step, high yielding 18F-labeling of an aryltrifluoroborate bioconjugate by isotope exchange at very high specific activity. J Label Compd Radiopharm. 2012;55:491–6.
49. Nelson WC, Kim JY. Monolithic fabrication of EWOD chips for picoliter droplets. J Microelectromech Syst. 2011;20:1419–27.
50. Lazari M, Narayanam MK, Murphy JM, Van Dam MR. Automated concentration of 18F-fluoride into microliter volumes. In: 21st international symposium on radiopharmaceutical sciences, Columbia, MO; 2015.
51. Bejot R, Elizarov AM, Ball E, Zhang J, Miraghaie R, Kolb HC, Gouverneur V. Batch-mode microfluidic radiosynthesis of N-succinimidyl-4-[18F]fluorobenzoate for protein labelling. J Label Compd Radiopharm. 2011;54:117–22.
52. Ismail R, Irribarren J, Javed MR, Machness A, van Dam M, Keng PY. Cationic imidazolium polymer monoliths for efficient solvent exchange, activation and fluorination on a continuous flow system. RSC Adv. 2014;4:25348–56.
53. De Leonardis F, Pascali G, Salvadori PA, Watts P, Pamme N. On-chip pre-concentration and complexation of [18F]fluoride ions via regenerable anion exchange particles for radiochemical synthesis of positron emission tomography tracers. J Chromatogr A. 2011;1218:4714–9.
54. Sadeghi S, Liang V, Cheung S, Woo S, Wu C, Ly J, Deng Y, Eddings M, van Dam RM. Reusable electrochemical cell for rapid separation of [18F]fluoride from [18O]water for flow-through synthesis of 18F-labeled tracers. Appl Radiat Isot. 2013;75:85–94.
55. Saiki H, Iwata R, Nakanishi H, Wong R, Ishikawa Y, Furumoto S, Yamahara R, Sakamoto K, Ozeki E. Electrochemical concentration of no-carrier-added [18F]fluoride from [18O]water in a disposable microfluidic cell for radiosynthesis of 18F-labeled radiopharmaceuticals. Appl Radiat Isot. 2010;68:1703–8.
56. Lu S, Giamis AM, Pike VW. Synthesis of [18F]fallypride in a micro-reactor: rapid optimization and multiple-production in small doses for micro-PET studies. Curr Radiopharm. 2009;2:1–13.
57. Van Dam RM, Elizarov AM, Ball CE, et al. Automated microfluidic-chip-based stand-alone instrument for the synthesis of radiopharmaceuticals on human-dose scales. In: Technical proceedings of the 2007 NSTI nanotechnology conference and trade show, Santa Clara, CA. Boca Raton: CRC Press; 2007. p. 300–3.
58. Ding H, Sadeghi S, Shah GJ, Chen S, Keng PY, Kim CJ, van Dam M. Accurate dispensing of volatile reagents on demand for chemical reactions in EWOD chips. Lab Chip. 2012;12:3331–40.
59. Shah GJ, Ding H, Sadeghi S, Chen S, Kim C-J, van Dam RM. Milliliter-to-microliter platform for on-demand loading of aqueous and non-aqueous droplets to digital microfluidics. In: Proceedings of the 16th international solid-state sensors, actuators and microsystems conference (TRANSDUCERS), Beijing. Piscataway: IEEE; 2011. p. 1260–3.

60. Chen Y-C, Liu K, Shen CK-F, van Dam RM. On-demand generation and mixing of liquid-in-gas slugs with digitally programmable composition and size. J Micromech Microeng. 2015;25:084006.
61. Wheeler AR, Moon H, Kim C-J, Loo JA, Garrell RL. Electrowetting-based microfluidics for analysis of peptides and proteins by matrix-assisted laser desorption/ionization mass spectrometry. Anal Chem. 2004;76:4833–8.
62. Cho SK, Moon H, Kim C-J. Creating, transporting, cutting, and merging liquid droplets by electrowetting-based actuation for digital microfluidic circuits. J MEMS. 2003;12:70–80.
63. Barbulovic-Nad I, Yang H, Park P, Wheeler A. Digital microfluidics for cell-based assays. Lab Chip. 2008;8:519.

Chapter 8
Development of a Microreactor for Synthesis of ^{18}F-Labeled Positron Emission Tomography Probe

Norihito Kuno, Naomi Manri, Norifumi Abo, Yukako Asano,
Ken-ichi Nishijima, Nagara Tamaki, and Yuji Kuge

Abstract *Background*: The application of microreactors to positron emission tomography (PET) probe radiosynthesis has attracted a great deal of interest because of its potential to increase specific activity and yields of probes and to reduce reaction time, expensive regent consumption, and the footprint of the device/instrument. To develop a microreactor platform that enables the synthesis of various ^{18}F-labeled PET probes, a prototype microreactor with a novel "split-flow and interflow mixing" (split mixing) was fabricated and applied to ^{18}F-labeling reactions.

Methods: The split mixing microreactor, made of Al_2O_3 resistant to several solvents, had higher mixing performance than that of the conventional batch

N. Kuno (✉)
Center for Exploratory Research, Research and Development Group, Hitachi, Ltd., 1-280, Higashi-koigakubo, Kokubunji, Tokyo 185-8601, Japan
e-mail: norihito.kuno.py@hitachi.com

N. Manri
Center for Technology Innovation – Healthcare, Research and Development Group, Hitachi, Ltd., 1-280, Higashi-koigakubo, Kokubunji, Tokyo 185-8601, Japan
e-mail: naomi.manri.hd@hitachi.com

N. Abo • K. Nishijima
Central Institute of Isotope Science, Hokkaido University, Kita 15 Nishi 7, Kita-ku, Sapporo 060-0815, Japan
e-mail: abo@ric.hokudai.ac.jp; nishijim@ric.hokudai.ac.jp

Y. Asano
Center for Technology Innovation – Mechanical Systems, Research and Development Group, Hitachi, Ltd., 832-2 Horiguchi, Hitachinaka, Ibaraki 312-0034, Tokyo, Japan
e-mail: yukako.asano.dp@hitachi.com

N. Tamaki
Department of Nuclear Medicine, Graduate School of Medicine, Hokkaido University, Sapporo, Japan
e-mail: natamaki@med.hokudai.ac.jp

Y. Kuge
Central Institute of Isotope Science, Hokkaido University Department of Integrated Molecular Imaging, Graduate School of Medicine, Hokkaido University, Sapporo, Japan
e-mail: kuge@ric.hokudai.ac.jp

© The Author(s) 2016
Y. Kuge et al. (eds.), *Perspectives on Nuclear Medicine for Molecular Diagnosis and Integrated Therapy*, DOI 10.1007/978-4-431-55894-1_8

method. Two ^{18}F-labeling reactions (^{18}F labeling of bovine serum albumin (BSA) by N-succinimidyl-4-[^{18}F] fluorobenzoate (SFB) and 1-(2′-nitro-1′-imidazolyl)-2-O-tetrahydropyranyl-3-O-toluenesulfonylpropanediol (NITTP) by ^{18}F) were conducted using the microreactor.

Results: The ^{18}F-labeling yield of BSA obtained by using the microreactor was almost the same as that by using the conventional batch method; however, the reaction time of the microreactor was slightly shorter than that of the batch method. Conversely, the ^{18}F-labeling yield of NITTP obtained by using the microreactor was about half that by using the batch method. The low NITTP-labeling yield was due to adsorption of naked ^{18}F to the surface of micro-mixing channel in the microreactor. The prescreening of candidate materials with lower ^{18}F adsorption for the microreactor was carried out with solvent resistance and solvent absorption as indexes. As a result of this prescreening, cyclo olefin polymer (COP) was selected as a candidate. A prototype COP microreactor has been fabricated and is being evaluated in terms of ^{18}F labeling.

Conclusions: Although the higher mixing performance of the split mixing microreactor did not significantly contribute to increasing ^{18}F-labeling yield, it did contribute to shortening reaction time. Moreover, the material used for the microreactor should be carefully selected from the viewpoint of developing a microreactor platform that enables the synthesis of various ^{18}F-labeled PET probes.

Keywords Positron emission tomography (PET) • Microreactor • ^{18}F-labeled PET probe • Cyclo olefin polymer (COP)

8.1 Introduction

Positron emission tomography (PET) is a noninvasive, nuclear imaging technique that has been widely applied for medical research and clinical diagnosis in the fields of oncology, neurology, and cardiology [1–4]. PET imaging relies on the utilization of a PET probe labeled with short-lived positron-emitting radioisotopes such as [11]C (t1/2 = 20 min) or [18]F (t1/2 = 110 min). Among several PET probes, 2-^{18}F-fluoro-2-deoxy-d-glucose (^{18}F-FDG), an analog of glucose, is most commonly used in the diagnosis and assessment of cancer. Moreover, utilized in clinical oncology, it shows excellent performance as a PET imaging probe [5].

^{18}F-FDG has been extensively utilized as the PET imaging probe in oncologic application. However, in the last few decades, a large number of non-FDG PET probes have been developed to measure and elucidate various biological and physiological processes [6, 7].

With the Increasing variation of PET probes that are applicable to clinical diagnosis, for diagnosis of individual patients, it is necessary to produce a wide variety of PET probes in small quantities. It is therefore also necessary to modify the supply system for PET probe (such as a centralized mass production) and the commercial delivery system that were established for a single PET probe, i.e., ^{18}F-FDG [8].

Meanwhile, decentralized, in-house production of PET probes also has some difficulties in regard to the production of a wide variety of PET probes in small quantities, because of the need for a large investment in infrastructure in accordance with government regulations, an expensive "hot cell" for radiation shielding of PET probe synthesizer, and high personnel and operating costs. Moreover, the number of synthesizer that can be installed in a hot cell is restricted because of the limited workspace in the hot cell; accordingly, it is difficult to accomplish in-house small-scale production of multiple PET probes.

Recently, to solve the abovementioned problems concerning small-scale production of various PET probes, the application of microreactors (or microfluidic devices) to the PET probe radiosynthesis has attracted a great deal of interest because of their potential to increase specific activity and yields of the probes and to reduce reaction time, consumption of expensive reagents, and footprint of the device/instrument [9, 10].

Microreactor can be categorized as flow-through type or batch type. And both a flow-through microreactor and a batch microreactor have been applied to radiosynthesis of PET probes for ^{18}F labeling [11]. Almost all previous studies on applying microreactors for radiosynthesis of PET probes have been limited to preclinical PET imaging; however, a few recent studies attempted to apply microreactors for synthesizing the clinical PET probes such as ^{18}F-fallypride, the dopamine D2/D3 receptors imaging probe [12]; 7-(6-fluoropyridin-3-yl)-5H-pyrido [4,3-b]indole (^{18}F-T807), tau imaging probe [13]; and ^{18}F-labeled 3-fluoro-5-[(pyridin-3-yl)ethynyl]benzonitrile (^{18}F-FPEB), the glutamate receptor subtype type 5 (mGluR5) imaging probe [14].

Moreover, a microreactor for radiosynthesis of a clinical PET probe has not been applied as the routine production method for clinical usage. It is still a great challenge to solve several problems hindering the practical use of microreactors for synthesizing PET imaging probes for clinical applications.

In a previous study, microreactor systems with novel mixing methods were established and applied to achieve large-scale and industrial production of chemicals [15, 16]. In this study, a prototype microreactor with a novel split-flow and interflow mixing (called "split mixing") was fabricated and evaluated in regard to ^{18}F-labeling reactions.

8.2 Materials and Methods

8.2.1 Villermaux-Dushman Method

The mixing performance of the prototype microreactor was evaluated by Villermaux-Dushman method [17]. Solution X (HCl: 0.1374 M) and solution Y (KI, 0.01595 M; CH_3COONa, 1.33 M; KIO_3, 0.003175 M) were separately supplied to the microreactor by Micro Process Server (MPS-α200, Hitachi, Tokyo,

Japan). The solution mixed in the microreactor was collected and left for two minutes. The flow rate of the two solutions was set at 0.2, 0.5, 1.0, 2.0, 4.0, and 6.0 mL/min. Absorbance at 350 nm was measured by a UV-visible spectrometer (U-3010, Hitachi-High Technologies, Tokyo, Japan).

8.2.2 ^{18}F Labeling of BSA by ^{18}F-SFB

Succinimidyl-4-[^{18}F]fluorobenzoate (^{18}F-SFB) was synthesized by a method similar to that reported by Tang et al. [18]. The synthesized ^{18}F-SFB was evaporated at 100 °C under an argon stream and dissolved in 20 % acetonitrile (MeCN) (0.3 MBq/μL). Bovine serum albumin (BSA) dissolved in 125 mM borate buffer (pH8.8) (5 mg/mL) was used as a target protein. By the microreactor method, ^{18}F-SFB and BSA solutions were separately injected into the microreactor by using the MPS-α200. The mixed solution was introduced into a PTFE tube (φ0.17 × 250 mm, GL science, Tokyo, Japan) connected to an outlet of the microreactor. The reaction mixture was collected at times of 2, 10, and 20 min by driving the MPS-α200, and TFA was added to the reaction mixture to terminate the reaction. By the conventional batch method, the ^{18}F-SFB and BSA solutions were mixed in equal amount at room temperature in a 1.5 mL microtube. Trifluoroacetic acid (TFA) was added to the mixture to terminate the reaction at times of 2, 10, and 20 min.

LC analysis was performed using a Nexera X2 UHPLC/HPLC system (Shimadzu, Kyoto, Japan). The reaction mixture (20 μL) was loaded onto a C8 reversed-phase column (CAPCELL PAK C8 SG300, Shiseido, Tokyo, Japan). The LC solvents were (A) 2 % MeCN/0.05 % TFA and (B) 80 % MeCN/0.05 % TFA, and a gradient (40 % B: 0–1.5 min, 100 % B: 1.5–2.5 min, 40 % B: 2.5–9.0 min) was used at a flow rate of 0.3 mL/min. The percentage of ^{18}F-benzoic acid (^{18}F-FBzA), ^{18}F-SFB, and ^{18}F-BSA was calculated from the LC data.

8.2.3 ^{18}F Labeling of NITTP by ^{18}F

An aqueous solution of ^{18}F$^-$, produced by cyclotron using the ^{18}O (p, n) ^{18}F reaction, was passed through a Sep-Pak Light QMA cartridge (Waters Corporation, MA, USA). The ^{18}F activity was eluted with a 0.9 mL (0.7 mL MeCN/0.2 mL water) solution containing 14 mg Kryptofix222 (K222) and 1.4 mg K$_2$CO$_3$. The eluent was then evaporated at 100 °C under an argon stream. The residue, containing [K/K222]$^{+18}$F$^-$, was dissolved in dimethyl sulfoxide (DMSO) (0.22 MBq/μL).

1-(2'-Nitro-1'-imidazolyl)-2-O-tetrahydropyranyl-3-O-toluenesulfonyl-propanediol (NITTP, ABX GmbH, Radeberg, Germany) was dissolved in DMSO (1.3 mg/mL). By the microreactor method, [K/K222]$^{+18}$F$^-$ and NITTP solutions were separately sent to the microreactor by using a dual syringe pump (TSP-202, YMC, Kyoto, Japan). The solution mixed in the microreactor was then sent to a PTFE tube ($\varphi 0.5 \times 510$ mm, GL science) connected to an outlet of the microreactor, and the reaction in the PTFE tube was allowed to proceed for 3 or 10 min at 80 °C. By the batch method, [K/K222]$^{+18}$F$^-$ and NITTP solutions were mixed in equal amount in a 1.5 mL microtube. The reaction was allowed to proceed for 3 or 10 min at 80 °C. LC analysis was performed using a Nexera X2 (Shimadzu). The reaction mixture (10 μL) was loaded onto a C18 reversed-phase column (XBridge C18, 5 μm, 4.6 mm × 150 mm, Waters Corporation). The LC solvents were (A) 50 mM (NH$_4$)$_2$HPO$_4$ and (B) MeCN, and isocratic elution (45 % B) was used at a flow rate of 1 mL/min. Percentage of ^{18}F-NITTP was calculated from the LC data.

8.2.4   Solvent Resistance Test

The chemical resistance of seven materials (polyvinyl chloride [PVC], polystyrene [PS], acrylonitrile-butadiene-styrene resin [ABS], methacrylate resin [PMMA], polycarbonate [PC], polypropylene [PP], and cyclo olefin polymer [COP]) against five chemicals (acetonitrile [MeCN], dimethyl sulfoxide [DMSO], hydrochlonic [HCl], sodium hydroxide [NaOH], and ethanol [EtOH]) was tested. A test piece (size: $10 \times 10 \times t2$ mm) was dropped into each of the chemicals set at 25, 50, 80, or 120 °C, and the reaction was allowed to proceed for 30 min. The condition of the test piece was observed, and the weight of the test piece was measured (W1) after the reaction was completed. After the test piece was washed with water, it was dehydrated for 24 h at 50 °C. The weight of the test piece was measured again (W2). The volume of the chemical absorbed in the test piece was calculated from the difference between W1 and W2.

8.3   Results and Discussion

8.3.1   Microreactor with Novel Mixing System

Two microreactors with different types of mixing, i.e., split-flow and interflow ("split mixing") and multilayer channels contracting toward the downstream ("multimixing"), were fabricated (Fig. 8.1a, b). The split mixing microreactor was made of Al$_2$O$_3$, and the multimixing one was made of PEEK. Both materials, Al$_2$O$_3$ and PEEK, were selected from the viewpoint of resistance to several solvents and fabricability of micro channel structure for mixing.

On the split mixing microreactor, the first liquid (solution A) and the second liquid (solution B) were injected into the micro channels of the microreactor. The

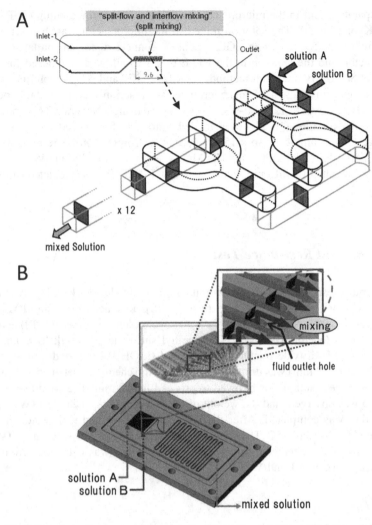

Fig. 8.1 Schematics of microreactors used in this study. (**a**) The split-flow and interflow microreactor. The flow of fluids in the micro channel for mixing is shown in the cross section of the micro channel. (**b**) The multilayer channels contracting toward the downstream microreactor

parallel flow of two fluids (solutions A and B) was split, rotated 90° (inversion), and interflowed repeatedly (12 times) as the fluids pass through the repeated split mixing structures of the microreactor. Finally, the flow of two fluids formed an alternately multilayered thin flow of fluids (Fig. 8.1a). As the thickness of each fluid became small, the diffusion time of the reactants of fluids (solutions A and B) was reduced, causing faster mixing of the solutions.

On the multimixing microreactor, the first liquid (solution A) flows from each nozzle in layer form on top of the chip. In the center of the chip, the second liquid (solution B) supplied from multi-outlet holes flows into the layered first liquid. Then, both fluids form a multilayered flow at a contraction flow part on the bottom of the chip to produce the thin flow of fluids (Fig. 8.1b).

8.3.2 Evaluation of Mixing Performance of Prototype Microreactors

Mixing performance of the prototype microreactors was evaluated by using the Villermaux-Dushman method [17], shown in Fig. 8.2a. By this method, the side reaction product, I_3^-, was spectroscopically measured by using the mean of UV absorbance at 350 nm. Therefore, lower UV absorbance indicates higher mixing performance. The mixing performance of the split mixing microreactor was higher than that of the multimixing microreactor and that of a conventional batch method (Fig. 8.2b). From this result, the split mixing microreactor was selected for further analysis of ^{18}F-labeling reaction.

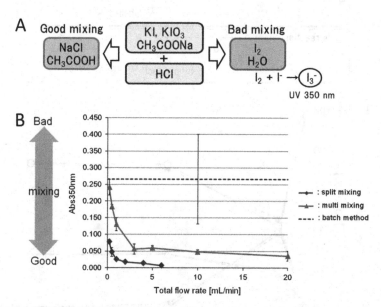

Fig. 8.2 (a) Schematic of the Villermaux-Dushman method. (b) Mixing performance of the split-flow and interflow ("split mixing") microreactor (◇) and the multilayer channels contracting toward the downstream ("multimixing") microreactor (△)

8.3.3 ^{18}F Labeling of Bovine Serum Albumin (BSA) by N-succinimidyl-4-^{18}F Fluorobenzoate (^{18}F-SFB)

The ^{18}F-labeling reaction of BSA by ^{18}F-SFB was examined to evaluate the ^{18}F-labeling performance of the split mixing microreactor. This reaction consists of a main reaction (^{18}F labeling of BSA) and a side reaction which produce ^{18}F-fluorobenzoic acid (^{18}F-FBzA) as a by-product (Fig. 8.3a).

As shown in Fig. 8.3b, the ^{18}F-labeling yield of BSA obtained by using the split mixing microreactor was almost the same as that by using the conventional batch method (Fig. 8.3b). A by-product, ^{18}F-FBzA, was synthesized in the same manner as that of batch method. These results suggest that as well as the main reaction, the side reaction is likely to proceed due to the higher mixing performance of the split mixing-type microreactor; therefore, the higher mixing performance might not be effective for increasing the ^{18}F-labeling yield of BSA.

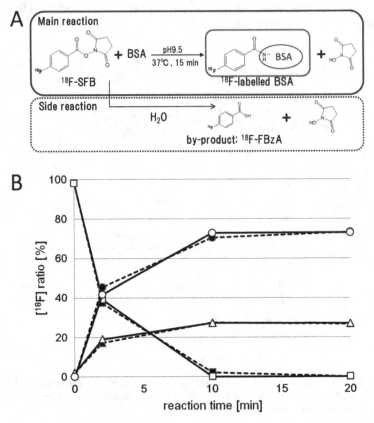

Fig. 8.3 (a) Synthesis of ^{18}F-labeled BSA by N-succinimidyl-4-^{18}F fluorobenzoate (^{18}F-SFB). (b) Time courses of ^{18}F-BSA (○, ●), ^{18}F-FBzA (△, ▲), and ^{18}F-SFB (◇, ◆) synthesis of the split mixing microreactor (*solid line*) and the conventional batch method (*broken line*)

The reaction time of ^{18}F labeling of BSA was estimated from a reaction rate constant calculated from the HPLC data. The estimated reaction time (10 min) for the ^{18}F labeling of BSA by the microreactor method was shorter than that by the batch method (12 min). This result suggests that high mixing performance contributes to shortening the reaction time.

8.3.4   [18]F Labeling of 1-(2′-nitro-1′-imidazolyl)-2-O-tetrahydropyranyl-3-O-toluenesulfonylpropanediol (NITTP) by [18]F

To further evaluate the ^{18}F-labeling performance of the split mixing microreactor, the ^{18}F-labeling reaction of NITTP was investigated (Fig. 8.4a). NITTP is a precursor for the synthesis of ^{18}F-fluoromisonidazole (^{18}F-FMISO), which is a PET imaging probe for determining the tumor hypoxia in vivo [19].

The ^{18}F-labeling yield of NITTP (at reaction time of 10 min) obtained by using the microreactor was 26 %, which is about half of that by using the batch method (59 %) (Fig. 8.4b). By measuring the total ^{18}F activity of all solutions applied for the microreactor reaction, only 65 % of the initial ^{18}F activity was recovered, and about 20 % of that was remained in the micro channels of microreactor. This result suggests that the low NITTP-labeling yield is due to adsorption of naked ^{18}F to the

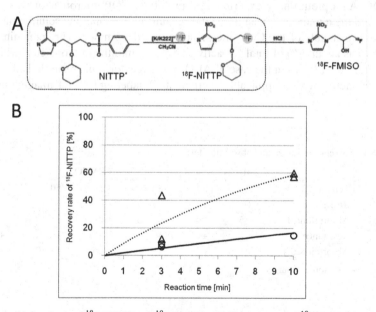

Fig. 8.4   (a) Synthesis of ^{18}F-NITTP and ^{18}F-FMISO. (b) Time courses of ^{18}F-NITTP synthesis of the split mixing microreactor (○, *solid line*) and the conventional batch method (△, *broken line*)

surface of micro channels. To improve the ^{18}F-labeling yield of NITTP attained by naked ^{18}F, the material used for the microreactor should be reexamined.

8.3.5 Screening of Material for the Split Mixing Microreactor

As a first step of selecting the material for the microreactor, prescreening of candidate materials was carried out with solvent resistance and solvent absorption as indexes. The solvent resistance and absorption of seven kinds of materials, namely, polyvinyl chloride (PVC), polystyrene (PS), acrylonitrile-butadiene-styrene resin (ABS), methacrylate resin (PMMA), polycarbonate (PC), polypropylene (PP), and cyclo olefin polymer (COP), were tested for acetonitrile (MeCN), dimethyl sulfoxide (DMSO), hydrochloric acid (HCl), sodium hydroxide (NaOH), and ethanol (EtOH) at 25, 50, and 80 °C. Among these materials, PP and COP exhibited relatively better solvent resistant and lower solvent absorption than other materials. PP and COP exhibited excellent solvent resistant and lower absorption for HCl, NaOH, and EtOH; however, at the higher temperature, PP showed a decrease of solvent resistant and COP showed little absorption of solvent (Table 8.1).

As a candidate material for the microreactor, COP was selected for the microreactor because of the higher solvent resistance at high temperature (80 °C) of COP. As a preliminary experiment, a prototype COP microreactor was fabricated, and the remaining ^{18}F activity after passing a ^{18}F containing solution through the micro channels of the COP microreactor was determined. The remaining ^{18}F activity was about 5 % of total ^{18}F activity injected into the microreactor, which is lower than that (35 %) in the case of Al$_2$O$_3$ microreactor. This result indicates that the COP microreactor is applicable to efficient ^{18}F labeling for PET imaging probe.

Table 8.1 Solvent resistance and absorption test

		MeCN			DMSO		
	Temp (°C)	25	50	80	25	50	80
PP	Resistance	+	+	−	+	+	+
	Absorption(µl)	<5	<5	5 ~ 10	<5	<5	<5
COP	Resistance	+	+	+	+	+	+
	Absorption(µl)	<5	<5	<5	<5	5 ~ 10	5 ~ 10

+, resistance; −, nonresistance

8.4   Conclusion

Although the higher mixing performance of the microreactor did not significantly contribute to increasing the ^{18}F-labeling yield, it did contribute to shortening the reaction time. Moreover, selecting the appropriate material for the microreactor is crucial from the viewpoint of developing a microreactor platform that enables the synthesis of various ^{18}F-labeled PET probes.

Acknowledgment   This work was supported in part by the Creation of Innovation Centers for Advanced Interdisciplinary Research Areas Program, Ministry of Education, Culture, Sports, Science and Technology, Japan.

References

1. Phelps ME. Positron emission tomography provides molecular imaging of biological processes. Proc Natl Acad Sci U S A. 2000;97:9226–33.
2. Gambhir SS. Molecular imaging of cancer with positron emission tomography. Nat Rev Cancer. 2002;2:683–93.
3. Politis M, Piccini P. Positron emission tomography imaging in neurological disorders. J Neurol. 2012;259:1769–80.
4. Schindler TH, Schelbert HR, Quercioli A, Dilsizian V. Cardiac PET imaging for the detection and monitoring of coronary artery disease and microvascular health. JACC Cardiovasc Imaging. 2010;3:623–40.
5. Otsuka H, Graham M, Kubo A, Nishitani H. Clinical utility of FDG PET. J Med Invest. 2004;51:14–9.
6. Brower V. Beyond FDG: many molecular imaging agents are in development. J Natl Cancer Inst. 2011;103:13–5.
7. The Radiosynthesis Database of PET Probes (RaDaP). National Institute of Radiological Sciences, Japan. 2013. http://www.nirs.go.jp/research/division/mic/db2/
8. Keng PY, Esterby M, van Dam RM. Emerging technologies for decentralized production of PET tracers. In: Hsieh CH, editor. Positron emission tomography – current clinical and research aspects. Rijeka: InTech; 2012. p. 53–182.
9. Lu SY, Pike VW. Micro-reactors for PET tracer labeling. In: Schubiger PA, Lehmann L, Friebe M, editors. PET chemistry. Berlin: Springer; 2007. p. 271–87.
10. Pascali G, Watts P, Salvadori PA. Microfluidics in radiopharmaceutical chemistry. Nucl Med Biol. 2013;40:776–87.
11. Elizarov AM. Microreactors for radiopharmaceutical synthesis. Lab Chip. 2009;9:1326–33.

12. Lebedev A, Miraghaie R, Kotta K, Ball CE, Zhang J, Buchsbaum MS, Kolb HC, Elizarov A. Batch-reactor microfluidic device: first human use of a microfluidically produced PET radiotracer. Lab Chip. 2013;13:136–45.
13. Liang SH, Yokell DL, Normandin MD, Rice PA, Jackson RN, Shoup TM, Brady TJ, El Fakhri G, Collier TL, Vasdev N. First human use of a radiopharmaceutical prepared by continuous-flow microfluidic radiofluorination: proof of concept with the tau imaging agent [^{18}F]T807. Mol Imaging 2014;13. doi:10.2310/7290.2014.00025.
14. Liang SH, Yokell DL, Jackson RN, Rice PA, Callahan R, Johnson KA, Alagille D, Tamagnan G, Collier TL, Vasdev N. Microfluidic continuous-flow radiosynthesis of [^{18}F] FPEB suitable for human PET imaging. Medchemcomm. 2014;5:432–5.
15. Asano Y, Togashi S, Tsudome H, Murakami S. Microreactor technology: innovations in production processes. Pharm Eng. 2010;8:32–42.
16. Asano Y, Miyamoto T, Togashi S, Endo Y. Study on the sandmeyer reaction via an unstable diazonium ion in microreactors with reaction rate analyses. J Chem Eng Jpn. 2014;47:287–95.
17. Ehrfeld W, Golbig K, Hessel V, Löwe H, Richter T. Characterization of mixing in micromixers by a test reaction: single mixing units and mixer arrays. Ind Eng Chem Res. 1999;38:1075–82.
18. Tang G, Zeng W, Yu M, Kabalka G. Facile synthesis of N-succinimidyl 4-[^{18}F]fluorobenzoate ([^{18}F]SFB) for protein labeling. J Label Compd Radiopharm. 2008;51:68–71.
19. Dubois L, Landuyt W, Haustermans K, Dupont P, Bormans G, Vermaelen P, Flamen P, Verbeken E, Mortelmans L. Evaluation of hypoxia in an experimental rat tumour model by [(18)F] fluoromisonidazole PET and immunohistochemistry. Br J Cancer. 2004;91:1947–54.

Chapter 9
Preclinical Evaluation of a Thymidine Phosphorylase Imaging Probe, [^{123}I]IIMU, for Translational Research

Ken-ichi Nishijima, Songji Zhao, Fei Feng, Yoichi Shimizu, Hiromichi Akizawa, Kazue Ohkura, Nagara Tamaki, and Yuji Kuge

Abstract The expression of thymidine phosphorylase (TP) is closely associated with angiogenesis, tumor invasiveness, and activation of antitumor agents. We developed a radiolabeled uracil derivative, I-123-labeled 5-iodo-6-[(2-iminoimidazolidinyl)methyl]uracil ([^{123}I]IIMU), as a novel SPECT probe for TP. A clinical study to verify the safety of [^{123}I]IIMU injection was approved by the Institutional Review Board of Hokkaido University Hospital for Clinical Research, and first-in-human (FIH) clinical studies of healthy adults were started.

Here, we will introduce our research, including the synthesis of [^{123}I]IIMU and its efficacy and safety evaluation, toward its FIH clinical study.

Radiosynthesis of [^{123}I]IIMU: [^{123}I]IIMU synthesis was achieved by radioiodination of the precursor, 6-(2-iminoimidazolidinyl)methyluracil at the

K. Nishijima
Central Institute of Isotope Science, Hokkaido University, Sapporo, Japan

Graduate School of Medicine, Hokkaido University, Sapporo, Japan

S. Zhao • F. Feng
Graduate School of Medicine, Hokkaido University, Sapporo, Japan

Y. Shimizu
Faculty of Pharmaceutical Sciences, Hokkaido University, Sapporo, Japan

H. Akizawa
Showa Pharmaceutical University, Machida, Japan

K. Ohkura
Faculty of Pharmaceutical Sciences, Health Sciences University of Hokkaido, Sapporo, Japan

N. Tamaki
Department of Nuclear Medicine, Graduate School of Medicine, Hokkaido University, Sapporo, Japan

Y. Kuge (✉)
Central Institute of Isotope Science, Hokkaido University Department of Integrated Molecular Imaging, Graduate School of Medicine, Hokkaido University, Sapporo, Japan
e-mail: kuge@ric.hokudai.ac.jp

© The Author(s) 2016
Y. Kuge et al. (eds.), *Perspectives on Nuclear Medicine for Molecular Diagnosis and Integrated Therapy*, DOI 10.1007/978-4-431-55894-1_9

C-5 position with *N*-chlorosuccinimide/[^{123}I]NaI. After purification by HPLC, [^{123}I]IIMU was obtained in high radiochemical yields.

In vitro and in vivo *studies*: The in vitro and in vivo uptake of [^{125}I]IIMU by the A431 tumor was attributable to the binding of the radiotracer to its target enzyme, i.e., TP. SPECT/CT imaging with [^{123}I]IIMU clearly visualized the A431 tumor 3 h after the injection of n.c.a. [^{123}I]IIMU.

Safety *assessment*: The human radiation absorbed dose was estimated as 17 μSv/ MBq on the basis of the biodistribution data of [I]IIMU in normal mice. The no observed adverse effect level (NOAEL) for intravenous administration of non-radiolabeled IIMU to mice was higher than 1.8 mg/kg. The bacterial reverse mutation assay showed negative results.

Keywords Thymidine • Phosphorylase • SPECT

9.1 Introduction

Thymidine phosphorylase (TP) catalyzes the reversible phosphorolysis of thymidine to thymine and 2-deoxyribose-1-phosphate. The expression of TP is highly associated with angiogenesis, infiltration, and metastasis of tumors. The activity and expression level of TP in many tumors are higher than those in the adjacent nonneoplastic tissues [1].

We developed a radiolabeled uracil derivative, I-123-labeled 5-iodo-6-[(2-iminoimidazolidinyl)methyl]uracil ([^{123}I]IIMU, Fig. 9.1), as a novel SPECT probe for TP. A clinical study to verify the safety of [^{123}I]IIMU injection was approved by the Institutional Review Board of Hokkaido University Hospital for Clinical Research, and first-in-human (FIH) clinical studies on healthy adults were started.

Here, we will introduce our research, including the synthesis of [^{123}I]IIMU [2, 3] and its efficacy [4–6] and safety evaluation, toward its FIH clinical study.

9.2 Radiosynthesis of [^{123}I]IIMU [2]

[^{123}I]IIMU was synthesized according to a method previously reported [3]. Briefly, dry acetone containing *N*-chlorosuccinimide/AcOH was added to [^{123}I]NaI (370 MBq) in a reaction vial, and the mixture was allowed to stand for 10 min at room temperature. Acetone was then removed completely under a stream of N$_2$. A

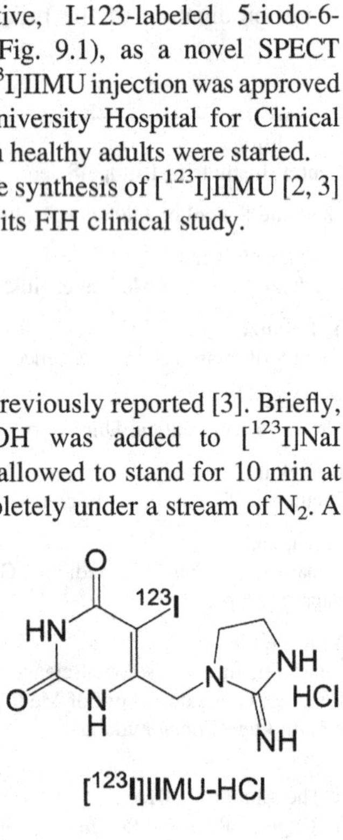

Fig. 9.1 Structure of [^{123}I] IIMU hydrochloride

[^{123}I]IIMU-HCl

Table 9.1 Production data for three consecutive syntheses of $[^{123}I]IIMU$

Parameter	Run number			Mean ± SD
	1	2	3	
Yield at the end of preparation (MBq)	232	189	193	205 ± 24
Radiochemical yield (%)	62	51	52	55 ± 6
Radiochemical purity (%)	>99	>99	>99	>99

Table 9.2 Results of quality control tests for three consecutive syntheses of $[^{123}I]IIMU$

Parameter		Run number			Mean ± SD
		1	2	3	
pH		7	7	7	7 ± 0
Residual organic solvent (ppm)	EtOH	46.8	232.6	33.4	104 ± 111
	MeCN	2.2	ND	2.3	1.5 ± 1.3
	Acetone	ND	ND	ND	–
Tests for bacterial endotoxins		Negative	Negative	Negative	–
Sterility test		Negative	Negative	Negative	–
ND: Not detected (<1.0)					

solution of 6-[(2-iminoimidazolidinyl)methyl]uracil (HIMU-TFA) in aqueous acetonitrile ($CH_3CN/H_2O = 2:1$) was added to the residue, and the capped vial was heated for 35 min at 50 °C. After removal of the solvent, the crude product was converted to $[^{123}I]IIMU$-HCl and purified simultaneously by reversed-phase HPLC using a solvent system containing HCl. The radioactive fraction was sterilized through a 0.22 µm membrane filter. The radiochemical purity of $[^{123}I]IIMU$ was determined with HPLC. Residual organic solvents were determined with GC. Sterility tests and bacterial endotoxin tests were also performed.

$[^{123}I]IIMU$ for intravenous injection was prepared in 2.5 h with a yield of 205 ± 24 MBq ($n = 3$). The radiochemical purity of $[^{123}I]IIMU$ was found to be more than 99 % (Table 9.1). The results of the quality control tests are summarized in Table 9.2. Acetone was not detected in the solution. The ethanol concentration was 104 ± 111 ppm. Sterility tests and bacterial endotoxin tests showed negative results (Table 9.2). We successfully prepared $[^{123}I]IIMU$ for intravenous injection with high purity. Results of quality control tests demonstrate that the $[^{123}I]IIMU$ preparation is suitable for clinical studies.

9.3   In Vitro *Study*: Uptake of $[^{125}I]IIMU$ in Cultured A431 and AZ521 Cells [4]

Immunoblotting for the detection of TP demonstrated high enzyme expression in A431 human epithelial carcinoma cells and very low expression in AZ521 human gastric cancer cells. A431 or AZ521 cells in 24-well plates were incubated at 37 °C in 1 mL of PBS(−) containing 37 kBq of $[^{125}I]IIMU$ for 10, 30, 60, or 120 min. The incubation solution was removed, and cells were washed and solubilized in 0.7 mL of 0.2 M NaOH. The radioactivity and protein content of the cell lysate were evaluated. When the radiotracer was incubated with A431 cells, the uptake level of the radiotracer increased with an increase in the incubation time, with 5.3 % dose/mg protein at 2 h of incubation. In the case of AZ521 cells, uptake of radioactivity was extremely low, 0.68 % dose/mg protein at most, regardless of incubation time. To confirm whether the observed uptake is due to the binding of the tracer to TP, similar experiments with A431 tumors were conducted in the presence of various concentrations of nonlabeled IIMU. The uptake level of [^{125}I] IIMU in A431 cells was reduced depending on the concentration of nonlabeled IIMU.

9.4 In Vivo *Study*: Biodistribution of [^{125}I]IIMU in A431 and AZ521 Tumor-Bearing Nude Mice [4]

The entire experimental protocol was approved by the Laboratory Animal Care and Use Committee of Hokkaido University. A saline solution of [^{125}I]IIMU (37 kBq, 0.1 mL) was injected into the tail vein of A431 or AZ521 tumor-bearing female Balb/cAJc1-nu/nu mice (8 weeks old; about 20 g). At 0.5, 1, 3, and 24 h after administration, animals were euthanized and the organs of interest and blood were collected. Radioactivity levels in the blood and muscle were similar in A431 and AZ521 tumor-bearing mice. However, tumor accumulation levels were markedly different between the two; the A431 tumor with high TP expression showed high accumulation, while AZ521 tumor with low TP expression showed low accumulation. To hamper the binding of the tracer to TP, an excess amount of non-radiolabeled IIMU was administered to A431 tumor-bearing mice and the biodistribution was evaluated at 0.5 h postinjection. The radioactivity in A431 tumor was reduced by co-injection of nonlabeled IIMU.

The in vitro and in vivo uptake of [^{125}I]IIMU by the A431 tumor was attributable to the binding of the radiotracer to its target enzyme, i.e., TP.

9.5 SPECT/CT Imaging Study [2]

Small-animal SPECT imaging studies were performed in mice bearing A431 xenografts after intravenous injection of non-carrier-added (n.c.a.) [^{123}I]IIMU or [^{123}I]IIMU with an excessively large amount of nonlabeled IIMU (n = 3 per group) by using a small-animal PET/SPECT/CT. SPECT/CT imaging with [^{123}I]IIMU clearly visualized A431 tumor 3 h after the injection of n.c.a. [^{123}I]IIMU (Fig. 9.2a). The accumulation of [^{123}I]IIMU in the tumor and liver was inhibited by the co-injection of non-radiolabeled IIMU (Fig. 9.2b).

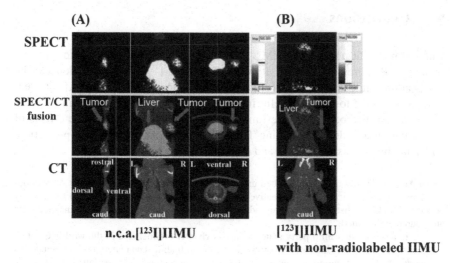

(A)   **(B)**

SPECT

SPECT/CT
fusion

CT

n.c.a.[^{123}I]IIMU   [^{123}I]IIMU
with non-radiolabeled IIMU

Fig. 9.2 SPECT/CT images of mice bearing A431 tumors. Mice were injected with 25 MBq of n.c.a. [^{123}I]IIMU (**a**) or [^{123}I]IIMU with non-radiolabeled IIMU (**b**)

9.6   Safety Assessment

To realize the application of [^{123}I]IIMU to clinical studies, we performed safety assessment of [^{123}I]IIMU. Evaluation of radiation absorbed dose is important for the safety assessment of radiopharmaceuticals. The human radiation absorbed dose was estimated as 17 µSv/MBq on the basis of the biodistribution data of [^{125}I]IIMU in normal mice. The highest radiation dose was of the urinary bladder (130 µGy/MBq), followed by the liver (75.1 µGy/MBq), thyroid (47.3 µGy/MBq), and gallbladder (20.4 µGy/MBq). The human radiation absorbed dose of [^{123}I]IIMU was considered to be within the allowable range and is equal to or less than the human radiation absorbed dose of [^{18}F]FDG (21 µSv/MBq; ICPR 60).

Also, based on the "guidance for conducting microdose clinical trials," we performed an extended single-dose toxicity study and the bacterial reverse mutation assay (Ames test). In the extended single-dose toxicity study, SD rats were given a single intravenous dose (0, 0.18, and 1.8 mg/kg) on Day 1, followed by observations until termination on Day 14. There were no deaths or in-life clinical signs and there were no microscopic effects. The no observed adverse effect level (NOAEL) for intravenous administration of nonlabeled IIMU to mice was greater than 1.8 mg/kg. The bacterial reverse mutation assay showed negative results.

9.7 Conclusions

Our findings indicate that [^{123}I]IIMU should be developed as a diagnostic agent for imaging TP-expressing tumors. It was shown that [^{123}I]IIMU injection can be safely administered in preclinical studies. Examinations using [^{123}I]IIMU for injection are expected to provide useful information that is difficult to obtain by other conventional methods, such as estimation/determination of therapeutic effects of anticancer drugs, decision-making for a treatment plan, prognostic prediction, understanding of disease stages, and malignancy assessment.

References

1. Takebayashi Y, Yamada K, Miyadera K, et al. The activity and expression of thymidine phosphorylase in human solid tumors. Eur J Cancer. 1996;32A:1227–32.
2. Nishijima K, Zhao S, Zhao Y, et al. Preparation and evaluation of [^{123}I]IIMU for SPECT imaging of thymidine phosphorylase expression in tumors. J Label Compd Radiopharm. 2013;56:S1–S349.
3. Takahashi M, Seki K, Nishijima K, et al. Synthesis of a radioiodinated thymidine phosphorylase inhibitor and its preliminary evaluation as a potential SPECT tracer for angiogenic enzyme expression. J Label Compd Radiopharm. 2008;51:384–7.
4. Akizawa H, Zhao S, Takahashi M, et al. In vitro and in vivo evaluations of a radioiodinated thymidine phosphorylase inhibitor as a tumor diagnostic agent for angiogenic enzyme imaging. Nucl Med Biol. 2010;37:427–32.
5. Li H, Zhao S, Jin Y, et al. Radiolabeled uracil derivative as a novel SPECT probe for thymidine phosphorylase: suppressed accumulation into tumor cells by target gene knockdown. Nucl Med Commun. 2011;32:1211–5.
6. Zhao S, Li H, Nishijima K et al. Relationship between biodistribution of a novel thymidine phosphorylase (TP) imaging probe and TP expression levels in normal mice. Ann Nucl Med. 2015;29:582-7.

Chapter 10
Discovery and Evaluation of Biomarkers for Atherosclerosis

Differential Proteomics of Plasma and Tissues

Takeshi Sakamoto, Hiroko Hanzawa, Naomi Manri, Mamoru Sakakibara, Yoichi Shimizu, Yan Zhao, Songji Zhao, Shiro Yamada, Kiwamu Kamiya, Yutaka Eki, Akihiro Suzuki, Haruhiko Higuchi, Chiaki Sugano, Hiroyuki Tsutsui, Nagara Tamaki, and Yuji Kuge

Abstract The usage of biomarkers reflecting atherosclerosis progression is important for preventing serious incidence of cardiovascular events. To elucidate clinically relevant molecular determinants in atherosclerosis, we have taken a comprehensive approach to combine mass spectrometry-based differential proteomics using both clinical and animal model specimens. Clinical plasma samples were collected from patients with acute myocardial infarction (AMI), stable angina (SA), and healthy/low-risk individuals (H-LR). We also obtained plasma and arterial tissue samples from apolipoprotein E-deficient and wild-type mice at various pathognomonic points of age. Cleavable isotope-coded affinity tags were

T. Sakamoto (✉)
Research & Development Group, Hitachi, Ltd., 1-280, Higashi-koigakubo, Kokubunji, Tokyo 185-8601, Japan

Department of Nuclear Medicine, Graduate School of Medicine, Hokkaido University, Sapporo 060-8638, Japan
e-mail: takeshi.sakamoto.yg@hitachi.com

H. Hanzawa • N. Manri
Research & Development Group, Hitachi, Ltd., 1-280, Higashi-koigakubo, Kokubunji, Tokyo 185-8601, Japan

Central Institute of Isotope Science, Hokkaido University, Sapporo 060-0814, Japan

M. Sakakibara • S. Yamada • K. Kamiya • H. Tsutsui
Department of Cardiovascular Medicine, Graduate School of Medicine, Hokkaido University, Sapporo 060-8638, Japan

Y. Shimizu
Laboratory of Bioanalysis and Molecular Imaging, Faculty of Pharmaceutical Sciences, Hokkaido University, Sapporo 060-0812, Japan

Y. Zhao • N. Tamaki
Department of Nuclear Medicine, Graduate School of Medicine, Hokkaido University, Sapporo 060-8638, Japan

© The Author(s) 2016   131
Y. Kuge et al. (eds.), *Perspectives on Nuclear Medicine for Molecular Diagnosis and Integrated Therapy*, DOI 10.1007/978-4-431-55894-1_10

used for differential mass spectrometry. Differential proteomics of clinical plasma samples revealed that more than 10 proteins appeared to be upregulated (relative abundance AMI/H-LR or SA/H-LR >1.5) and 5 proteins downregulated (AMI/H-LR or SA/H-LR <1/1.5). These trends associated with the disease progression are not always coincident with those of mouse ortholog proteins, suggesting a pathophysiological difference between humans and the mouse model. Among the downregulated proteins, the complement factor D (CFD) showed monotonic decrease that was in good agreement with the enzyme-linked immunosorbent assay. These results suggest that the comprehensive and systematic proteomic approach may be promising in terms of the selection and evaluation of biomarker candidates.

Keywords Proteomic study • Atherosclerosis • Inflammation • apoE-deficient mouse

10.1 Introduction

Atherosclerosis is a chronic inflammatory disease and often causes subsequent thrombotic complication. It is well known as a main etiology of critical diseases such as acute coronary syndrome including myocardial infarction, sudden cardiac death, and stroke [1]. To detect the signs of severe incidences, it is important to accurately evaluate the progression stages of atherosclerosis, vulnerability, and rupture risk of atherosclerotic plaques. Therefore, a variety of approaches to establish novel biomarkers directly reflecting the status of atherosclerosis have been conducted to date [2]. However, due to the complexity of the disease, discovery and clinical validation of such biomarkers are still underway in many institutions.

S. Zhao
Department of Tracer Kinetics & Bioanalysis, Graduate School of Medicine, Hokkaido University, Sapporo 060-8638, Japan

Y. Eki • A. Suzuki • H. Higuchi
Hitachi General Hospital, Hitachi, Ltd., Hitachi 317-0077, Japan

C. Sugano
Hitachinaka General Hospital, Hitachi, Ltd., Hitachinaka 312-0057, Japan

Y. Kuge
Central Institute of Isotope Science, Hokkaido University Department of Integrated Molecular Imaging, Graduate School of Medicine, Hokkaido University, Sapporo, Japan

Disease proteomics is a profiling technology using mass spectrometry that makes it possible to identify disease-related alteration of protein expression comprehensively in a wide variety of biological specimens including serum or plasma or extracts from tissues of interests [3]. Numerous studies have been conducted to develop biomarkers for early diagnosis, selection of appropriate therapy, and prognosis assessment. A decade of progress to determine changes in disease-related protein expression has achieved accurate and high-throughput quantification of the individual proteins within mixtures by using differential stable isotopic labeling, such as cleavable isotope-coded affinity tags (cICATs) [4]. Either light or heavy cICATs are labeled at the free thiol groups of cysteine residues of which proteins are isolated from two distinct samples (i.e., disease and healthy states). The ratio of protein amount between these states is estimated by comparing MS signal intensity of the corresponding proteolytic peptide fragments [4].

To elucidate clinically relevant molecular determinants in atherosclerotic development, we have taken a comprehensive approach by using mass spectrometry-based differential proteomics. First, we conducted differential human plasma proteomic studies using clinical samples of patients with atherosclerosis-related cardiovascular disease and healthy (or low-risk) volunteers. Second, to validate the results we obtained in the studies, a biomarker candidate, the complement factor D (CFD) level of patients with atherosclerosis-related cardiovascular disease, was determined by carrying out an enzyme-linked immunosorbent assay (ELISA). Then, we tried combining differential proteome of plasma and arterial tissue obtained from both wild-type (WT) and apoED mice at four pathognomonic time points of age. Finally, we compared identified proteins in humans with mouse plasma proteome.

10.2   Materials and Methods

This study was approved by the Ethics Committee of Hokkaido University Hospital (no. 010–0118) and the institutional ethics committees of Hitachi, Ltd. Clinical plasma samples were collected prospectively for 48 acute myocardial infarction (AMI) patients, 73 stable angina (SA) patients, and 69 healthy/low-risk (H-LR) individuals.

Animal care and animal experiments were conducted at Japan SLC, Inc. (Hamamatsu, Japan), under the approval of the company's animal care committee. The apoED (C57BL/6.KOR/StmSlc-Apoeshl) and WT (C57BL/6) mice were fed a high-fat diet from 8 weeks of age. Plasma and arterial tissues were collected from each group of male or female mice at ages of 12, 18, 25, and 35 weeks.

Proteins prepared from plasma or arterial tissue as described above were labeled with isotope-coded affinity tags using the Cleavable ICAT® Reagent Kit (Applied Biosystems, Foster City, USA) according to the manufacturer's instructions with minor modifications. Tryptic peptides were applied to the strong cation exchange (SCX) column, and the eluted solution was fractionated into 25 fractions. The SCX separated fractions were analyzed using NanoFrontier LD, a liquid chromatograph mass spectrometry (LC-MS) system (Hitachi High-Technologies Corporation, Tokyo, Japan). Original MS/MS peak lists (PLs) were generated using built-in PL generation software in the mass spectrometer, and further protein/peptide identification and cICAT quantitative analyses were conducted using a custom developed software platform with a relational database.

Plasma CFD levels were measured with the use of ELISA kits according to the manufacturer's instructions (Quantikine, DFD00, R&D Systems, Inc., Minneapolis, USA). Plasma levels of known markers including high-sensitive C-reactive protein (hsCRP), amino-terminal pro-brain natriuretic peptide (NT-pro BNP), and adiponectin were also determined (SRL, Inc., Tokyo, Japan).

10.3 Results and Discussion

Atherosclerosis is a chronic inflammatory disease, in which atherosclerotic lesions are formed in blood vessels through complicated molecular processes occurring between the circulating blood stream and lesions. To identify proteins showing changes in expression levels associated with atherosclerotic plaque progression, we

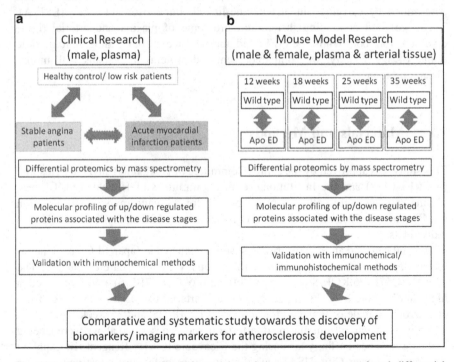

Fig. 10.1 Entire research workflow of stage-dependent, mass spectrometry-based differential proteomics. (**a**) Clinical proteomic study using human plasma samples. (**b**) Animal model proteomic study using plasma and arterial tissue samples from WT and atherosclerotic model mice

conducted mass spectrometry-based proteomic analyses. Figure 10.1 shows an overall picture of the proteomic experiments we have done. Most previous proteomic studies have focused on only one point of the disease. However, these strategies would not be adequate to indentify proteins showing serial quantitative change in accordance with progression of atherosclerosis. In this study, we conducted a differential proteome study at several characteristic points of disease stage and compared the results of identified proteins. The proteins we identified that showed changes in plasma level according to the severity of the atherosclerosis-related disease (e.g., ischemic heart disease) or atherosclerosis progression of the mouse model might be diagnostic or predictive biomarker candidates for blood testing. On the other hand, the proteins that showed changes, especially an increase tendency, in arterial tissues might be biomarkers for diagnostic imaging.

10.3.1 Disease Stage-Dependent Differential Proteome in Human Plasma

As shown in Fig. 10.1, we conducted disease stage-dependent differential human plasma proteomic experiments using clinical samples. We selected three clinical conditions, H-LR, SA, and AMI (Table 10.1). Two independent age-matched plasma pools from each group ($n = 7$) were used for the experiments with combinations of H-LR vs. SA, H-LR vs. AMI, and SA vs. AMI. Table 10.2 shows the summary of identified proteins by differential proteomics of clinical plasma samples. We identified about 110 proteins in each trial of differential proteome and found that 8–13 proteins appeared to be upregulated (relative abundance AMI/H-LR or SA/H-LR >1.5), and 2–8 proteins were downregulated (AMI/H-LR or SA/H-LR <1/1.5). Finally, five identical proteins were identified in common between trials 1 and 2. Three were blood coagulation related, such as von Willebrand factor, and the other two were categorized as structural-integrity-related or immuno-response (immunoglobulin)-related proteins. The downregulated proteins identified in common between trials were found to be apolipoproteins involving cholesterol homeostasis, blood coagulation, and CFD.

To validate the results we obtained in the differential proteome experiments as described above, we determined the CFD level of plasma of clinical samples by ELISA as a representative example. We found that CFD levels in plasma of the AMI group were the lowest among the three clinical groups. The statistical

Table 10.1 Description of three clinical groups in human plasma proteome

Description	H-LR	SA	AMI
Group	Healthy and low-risk volunteers	Patients with stable angina	Patients with acute myocardial infarction
Risk and progression stage of atherosclerosis	Low	Moderate/early	High/advanced

Table 10.2 Up- or downregulated proteins detected by differential proteomic analysis in clinical pooled plasma samples

Group		SA/H-LR	AMI/H-LR	AMI/SA
Total number of identified proteins	Trial 1	116	115	110
	Trial 2	106	112	114
Upregulated	Trial 1	8	8	5
	Trial 2	7	8	13
	Common	1	5	2
Downregulated	Trial 1	4	6	8
	Trial 2	7	2	5
	Common	2	1	1

H-LR group of healthy control and low-risk volunteers, *SA* group of patients with stable angina, *AMI* group of patients with acute myocardial infarction, *Upregulated* proteins showed expression ratio >1.5, *Downregulated* proteins showed expression ratio <1/1.5

difference of AMI to H-LR was the most pronounced (H/LR vs. AMI, $p = 2.4 \times 10^{-10}$; H/LR vs. SA, $p = 0.54$). The diminished plasma levels of CFD in AMI patients showed that the results we obtained in our proteomic study were basically verified. Furthermore, the plasma CFD levels showed no correlation with body mass index (BMI) ($r = 0.03$, $P < 0.05$), hsCRP ($r = -0.09$, $P < 0.05$), NT-proBNP ($r = -0.03$, $P < 0.05$), and adiponectin ($r = 0.11$, $P < 0.05$). In recent years, it has been suggested that the activation of the complement system plays a role in atherosclerosis progression [5]. Among the components of the complement pathway, CFD is known as a key regulatory serine protease of the alternative complement pathway. CFD mRNA and protein are abundantly expressed in adipose tissue, and the protein is found at high levels in serum [6]. CFD expression levels in rodent models of obesity are reduced [7]. Our results may suggest some kind of CFD implication in atherosclerosis.

10.3.2 Disease Stage-Dependent Differential Proteome in Atherosclerosis Mouse Model

As shown in Fig. 10.1, we conducted differential proteome experiments using plasma and arterial tissues of WT and apolipoprotein E-deficient (apoED) mice. Table 10.3 shows phenotypic characteristics of atherosclerotic lesions of WT and apoED at each point of age. As we previously demonstrated, on a high-fat diet, early lesions were observed in apoED at 12–18 weeks of age, and advanced lesions were prominent at 25–35 weeks. No atherosclerotic lesions were found in WT mice throughout four points of age [8]. At 25 weeks of age, vulnerable atheromatous lesions were more abundant, but fibroatheromatous lesions were less at 25 weeks than those at 35 weeks [8]. Table 10.4 shows a summary of identified proteins. In plasma, the total number of identified proteins and the ratio of their upregulated

Table 10.3 Description of possible progression stages of atherosclerotic lesion of atherosclerosis mouse model

Age (weeks)		12	18	25	35
Risk and progression stage of atherosclerosis	WT	None	None	None	None
	apoED	Low/early	Low/early	High/advanced	Moderate/advanced
Lesion phenotype	WT	None	None	None	None
	apoED	Monocyte adhesion	Foam cell formation	Vulnerable plaque	Stable plaque

Table 10.4 Summary of up- or downregulated proteins detected in plasma and arterial tissues by differential proteome of mouse model

	Plasma				Arterial tissue			
Age (weeks)	12	18	25	35	12	18	25	35
Total number of identified proteins	146	133	119	124	446	616	659	693
Upregulated (%)	7	14	15	11	8	6	16	16
Downregulated (%)	5	5	11	15	2	5	8	9
No change (%)	88	81	74	74	90	89	76	75

Upregulated expression ratio (apoED/WT) >1.5, *Downregulated* expression ratio (apoED/WT) $<1/1.5$, *No change* $1/1.5 <$ expression ratio (apoED/WT) < 1.5. This table is modified from reference [9]

proteins (expression ratio, apoED/WT; > 1.5) did not significantly change throughout the time course (Table 10.4). However, the ratio of downregulated proteins (apoED/WT; $<1/1.5$) increased on and after 25 weeks of age (Table 10.4). We finally found 100 proteins in the plasma, and 390 proteins in the arterial tissues were detected throughout all four time points: 29 were identified in common between plasma and arterial tissues [data not shown, 9]. Interestingly, we found that disease stage-dependent quantitative variation patterns did not always correspond between plasma and arterial tissues. Furthermore, proteins showed characteristic change in abundance in plasma, and/or arterial tissues were found to be components of inflammation, thrombus formation, and vascular remodeling [9].

10.3.3 Comparison Between Human and Mouse Plasma Proteome

In this study, we conducted disease stage-dependent differential proteome experiments in two identical studies: one for human plasma proteome using clinical samples and one for plasma/arterial tissue proteome using an atherosclerotic mouse model, apoED. Importantly, we found that the changes associated with the disease progression in the amount of identified proteins were not always coincident with those of mouse ortholog proteins in plasma or arterial tissues determined by proteomic studies (data not shown). In case of CFD, the plasma level of CFD in humans determined in the proteomic study or ELISA decreased in accordance with the severity of the clinical conditions. On the other hand, the plasma level of CFD in mice showed a slight but not significant decreasing tendency determined in differential proteome between WT mice and the apoED mouse model. We preliminarily determined the plasma level of CFD in mice by ELISA and detected no statistical significance between WT mice and apoED throughout all four time points. CD5L, a soluble member of the scavenger receptor cysteine-rich domain superfamily protein, did not show any significant change in abundance as determined by human plasma differential analyses. However, the expression ratios (apoED/WT) of CD5L in mouse plasma were high throughout the four time points [9]. In addition, we found that CD5L accumulated in advanced lesions of apoED in accordance with macrophage infiltration by immunohistochemistry. These results suggest that fundamental mechanisms of atherosclerosis development are similar to each other; however, there would be a pathophysiological difference between humans and the mouse model.

10.3.4 Limitation

We failed to detect several known atherosclerotic plaque-related proteins such as cytokines, monocyte chemoattractant protein-1 (MCP-1), and intercellular adhesion molecule-1(ICAM-1). We assume that there were several technical reasons for this. For example, the practical detection limit in our mass spectrometry system was assumed to be 1–10 ng/mL, which is much higher than the normal concentration of cytokines. We used cICAT labeling reagents, which covalently bind only to cysteine residues of targeted proteins. Therefore, it becomes difficult to detect proteins with trypsin-digested peptides with few or no cysteine residues.

10.4 Conclusion

To identify proteins showing changes in expression levels associated with atherosclerotic plaque progression, we conducted mass spectrometry-based proteomic analyses. We adopted two separate study designs: one for human plasma differential proteome using clinical samples and one for mouse plasma/arterial tissue differential proteome using samples obtained from wild-type mice and an atherosclerotic mouse model apoED. Then several proteins showing quantitative changes in accordance with disease were found, including the complement factor D (CFD). The diminished plasma levels of CFD in acute myocardial infarction patients were verified in an enzyme-linked immunosorbent assay. These results suggest that CFD might be a potential biomarker for atherosclerosis. The comprehensive and systematic proteomic approach using different states of samples is promising in terms of the selection of biomarker candidates.

Acknowledgments This study was supported in part by the grant "The matching program for innovations in future drug discovery and medical care" from the Ministry of Education, Culture, Sports, Science, and Technology, Japan (to Tamaki, N.). The authors thank Megumi Hikichi, Yuko Komori, and Yumi Yanagiya for their technical assistance. Without their help and support, we could never have done this study.

References

1. Ross R. Atherosclerosis – an inflammatory disease. N Engl J Med. 1999;340:115–26.
2. Wang X, Connolly TM. Biomarkers of vulnerable atheromatous plaques: translational medicine perspectives. Adv Clin Chem. 2010;50:1–22.
3. Hanash S. Disease proteomics. Nature. 2003;422:226–32.
4. Gygi SP, Rist B, Gerber SA, et al. Quantitative analysis of complex protein mixtures using isotope-coded affinity tags. Nat Biotechnol. 1999;17:994–9.
5. Torzewski M, Bhakdi S. Complement and atherosclerosis-united to the point of no return? Clin Biochem. 2013;46:20–5.
6. Cook KS, Min HY, Jonson D, et al. Adipsin: a circulating serine protease homolog secreted by adipose tissue and sciatic nerve. Science. 1987;237:402–5.
7. Flier JS, Cook KS, Usher P, et al. Severely impaired adipsin expression in genetic and acquired obesity. Science. 1987;237:405–8.
8. Zhao Y, Kuge Y, Zhao S, et al. Prolonged high-fat feeding enhances aortic ^{18}F-FDG and ^{99m}Tc-Annexin A5 uptake in apolipoprotein E-deficient and wild-type C57BL/6J Mice. J Nucl Med. 2008;49:1707–14.
9. Hanzawa H, Sakamoto T, Kaneko A, et al. Combined plasma and tissue proteomic study of atherogenic model mouse: Approach to elucidate molecular determinants in atherosclerosis development. J Proteome Res. 2015;14:4257–69.

Chapter 11
Radioimmunodetection of Atherosclerotic Lesions Focusing on the Accumulation Mechanism of Immunoglobulin G

Yoichi Shimizu, Hiroko Hanzawa, Yan Zhao, Ken-ichi Nishijima, Sagiri Fukura, Takeshi Sakamoto, Songji Zhao, Nagara Tamaki, and Yuji Kuge

Abstract In the diagnosis of atherosclerosis, detailed evaluation of biomarkers related to its lesion formation is desired for estimation of its progression rate. In our previous proteomic studies of atherosclerosis mice, the protein level of thrombospondin-4 (TSP4) in the aorta, but not in plasma, elevated relatively with atherosclerotic plaque formation. Therefore, we supposed that TSP4 would be a potential biomarker for diagnostic imaging of atherosclerotic progression. Immunoglobulin G (IgG) has been widely used as a basic molecule of imaging probes providing images specific to their target biomolecules, owing to the antigen-antibody reaction. Therefore, we first developed anti-TSP4 monoclonal IgG radiolabeled with ^{99m}Tc (^{99m}Tc-TSP4-mAb). ^{99m}Tc-TSP4-mAb showed higher accumulation in atherosclerotic aortas of apoE$^{-/-}$ mice (atherosclerotic model

Y. Shimizu (✉)
Faculty of Pharmaceutical Sciences, Hokkaido University, Sapporo, Japan

Central Institute of Isotope Science, Hokkaido University, Sapporo, Japan

Graduate School of Medicine, Hokkaido University, Sapporo, Japan
e-mail: yshimizu@pharm.hokudai.ac.jp

H. Hanzawa • T. Sakamoto
Research & Development Group, Hitachi, Ltd., Kokubunji, Tokyo, Japan

Y. Zhao • S. Fukura • S. Zhao
Graduate School of Medicine, Hokkaido University, Sapporo, Japan

K. Nishijima
Central Institute of Isotope Science, Hokkaido University, Sapporo, Japan

Graduate School of Medicine, Hokkaido University, Sapporo, Japan

N. Tamaki
Department of Nuclear Medicine, Graduate School of Medicine, Hokkaido University, Sapporo, Japan

Y. Kuge
Central Institute of Isotope Science, Hokkaido University Department of Integrated Molecular Imaging, Graduate School of Medicine, Hokkaido University, Sapporo, Japan

© The Author(s) 2016
Y. Kuge et al. (eds.), *Perspectives on Nuclear Medicine for Molecular Diagnosis and Integrated Therapy*, DOI 10.1007/978-4-431-55894-1_11

141

mice); however, we found that the non-targeted monoclonal IgG radiolabeled with ^{99m}Tc also showed similar distribution in atherosclerotic aortas of apoE$^{-/-}$ mice. IgG has also known to accumulate nonspecifically in the immunological disease such as inflammatory arthritis. However, the accumulation mechanism of IgG has still been unclear in detail. In this chapter, we would like to introduce recent topics on atherosclerotic imaging, focused on our work exploring the accumulation mechanisms of IgG in atherosclerotic lesions, and elucidating the usefulness of radiolabeled IgG images in the diagnosis of atherosclerosis.

Keywords Atherosclerosis • Immunoglobulin G • Polarized macrophage

11.1 Introduction

Rupture of vulnerable plaques and the subsequent thrombogenesis induce ischemic diseases such as cerebral and myocardial infarction [1]. Therefore, it is necessary to detect vulnerable lesions precisely for the diagnosis of such diseases. Various biomolecules are expressed or activated as atherosclerosis progresses. Thus, the detection and imaging of such biomolecules would make possible the determination of the progression of atherosclerosis in detail. In our previous proteomic studies of atherosclerotic model mice [2], the relative thrombospondin-4 (TSP4) levels of atherosclerotic model mice/normal mice in the aorta, but not in plasma, increased with the atherosclerotic plaque formation. TSP4 belongs to the thrombospondin families and has been reported to play some roles such as promotion of proliferation of smooth muscle cells and adhesion and migration of neutrophils [3]. It has also been reported that apoE and TSP4 double knockout mice showed fewer atherosclerotic lesions than the atherosclerosis apoE knockout mice, which suggests that TSP4 has a crucial role in the progression of atherosclerotic lesions [4]. Therefore, we supposed that TSP4 would be a potential biomarker for diagnostic imaging of atherosclerotic progression. Immunoglobulin G (IgG) is widely used particularly for the target-specific imaging of cancer, because it provides images specific to their target biomolecules owing to the antigen-antibody reaction [5]. Thus, we first developed an IgG-based TSP4 targeting SPECT imaging probe (^{99m}Tc-TSP4-mAb). ^{99m}Tc-TSP4-mAb accumulated in the atherosclerotic lesions of apoE$^{-/-}$ mouse aortas. However, ^{99m}Tc-NC-mAb, which was composed of non-targeting IgG, also accumulated highly in the atherosclerotic lesions similar to ^{99m}Tc-TSP4-mAb. IgG itself is known to be delivered to atherosclerotic lesions nonspecifically, but the detailed mechanism of the accumulation is still unknown [6].

In this report, we would like to introduce our above-mentioned work in which we explored the accumulation mechanisms of IgG in atherosclerotic lesions and elucidated the usefulness of radiolabeled IgG imaging in the diagnosis of atherosclerosis.

11.2 Materials and Methods

11.2.1 Materials

All chemicals used in this study were commercially available and of the highest purity. HYNIC-N-hydroxysuccinimide was prepared as previously reported [7]. ^{99m}Tc-pertechnetate was purchased from Nihon Medi-Physics Co., Ltd. (Tokyo, Japan). As a TSP4-targeting monoclonal antibody, we used anti-thrombospondin-4 mouse IgG$_{2b}$ (Clone #276523, R&D Systems, Abingdon, UK). As for the negative control non-targeted mouse IgG, we chose mouse IgG$_{2b}$, a kappa monoclonal [MG2b-57] isotype control (Abcam, Cambridge, UK) whose immunogen is trinitrophenol + keyhole-limpet hemocyanin (KLH).

11.2.2 Preparation of Radiolabeled IgG

Anti-TSP4 monoclonal IgG (TSP4-mAb) or non-targeting IgG (NC-mAb) was radiolabeled with ^{99m}Tc after derivatization with 6-hydrazinonicotinic acid (HYNIC), as previously reported (Fig. 11.1) [8]. In brief, to HYNIC-N-hydroxysuccinimide (8.25 μg) in N,N-dimethylformamide (8.25 μl), TSP4-mAb or NC-mAb solution in 0.16 M borate buffer (pH 8.0) (250 μl, 2 mg/ml) was added, and the

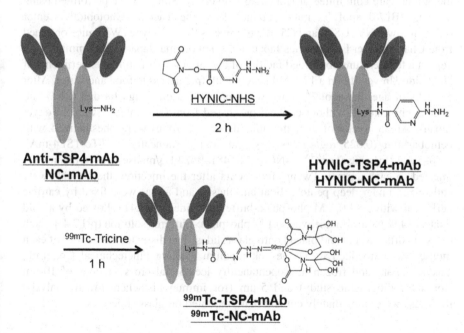

Fig. 11.1 Scheme of ^{99m}Tc-TSP4-mAb or ^{99m}Tc-NC-mAb preparation

mixture was incubated at room temperature for 2 h. The mixture was purified by size-exclusion filtration using a diafiltration membrane (Amicon Ultra 4 [cutoff molecular weight, 30,000]; Millipore Co., Billerica, MA). ^{99m}Tc-(tricine)$_2$(740 MBq/ml, 300 μl) was prepared by the method of Larsen et al. [9]. It was added to the purified solution of HYNIC-TSP4-mAb or NC-mAb solution in 10 mM citrate buffer (pH 5.2) (30 μl, 1 mg/ml), and the mixture was incubated at room temperature for 1 h. The mixture was then purified on a Sephadex G-25 column (PD-10, GE Healthcare, Buckinghamshire, UK) equilibrated with 0.1 M PBS (pH7.4) to obtain ^{99m}Tc-TSP4-mAb or ^{99m}Tc-NC-mAb. The radio-chemical purity of ^{99m}Tc-TSP4-mAb or ^{99m}Tc-NC-mAb was measured by size-exclusion filtration of the PD-10 column and size-exclusion high-performance liquid chromatography (HPLC). The stability of ^{99m}Tc-TSP4-mAb or ^{99m}Tc-NC-mAb in plasma was evaluated by the method described below. First, the probes (^{99m}Tc-TSP4-mAb, 27.7 MBq/ml; ^{99m}Tc-NC-mAb, 34.9 MBq/ml; 50 μl) were incubated with the plasma derived from C57BL/6 (male, 30 weeks) for 24 h, and then the mixture was analyzed by size-exclusion filtration of the PD-10 column.

11.2.3 Animal Study

Animal care and all experimental procedures were performed with the approval of the animal care committee of Hokkaido University. Studies were performed using male C57BL/6J apoE$^{-/-}$ mice obtained from the Taconic Gnotobiotic Center (Germantown, NY, USA) and C57BL/6J mice as the wild-type (WT) mice obtained from Charles River Laboratories Japan, Inc. (Yokohama, Japan). The animals were kept in a temperature-controlled facility of the laboratory of animal experiments of Hokkaido University on a 12-h light cycle with free access to food and water. After 5 weeks of age, the apoE$^{-/-}$ mice were maintained on a high-fat diet (21 % fat, 0.15 % cholesterol, without cholate; purchased from Oriental Yeast Ltd., Tokyo, Japan). At 35 weeks of age, the animals ($n = 4$/group) were anesthetized with pentobarbital (0.025 mg/kg body weight, intraperitoneally). ^{99m}Tc-TSP4-mAb (200–592 kBq/mouse) or ^{99m}Tc-NC-mAb (481–962 kBq/mouse) was intravenously injected to each animal. Twenty-four hours after the injection, the animals were euthanized under deep pentobarbital anesthesia, and aortas were fixed by cardiac perfusion with cold 0.1 M phosphate-buffered saline (pH 7.4) followed by a cold fixative [4 % paraformaldehyde, 0.1 M phosphate-buffered solution (pH 7.4)]. Each excised aorta was cut and placed onto glass slides. The dissected aortic root of each mouse was embedded in Tissue-Tek medium (Sakura Finetechnical Co., Ltd., Tokyo, Japan) and frozen in isopentane/dry ice. Serial cross sections of 10-μm (for autoradiographic study) and 5-μm (for immunohistochemistrical analysis) thickness were immediately cut and thaw-mounted on glass slides.

11.2.3.1 Autoradiography (ARG) Study

The excised and cut aortas on glass slides were exposed to phosphor imaging plates (Fuji Imaging Plate BAS-UR, Fujifilm, Tokyo, Japan) for 12 h, together with a set of calibrated standards. The autoradiographic images were acquired using a computerized imaging analysis system (Fuji bio-imaging analyzer FLA7000). The acquired data was analyzed using MultiGauge version 3.2 (Fujifilm).

11.2.4 Histochemical Study

Movat's pentachrome staining of serial aortic root sections was performed [10]. Immunohistochemical staining of the serial sections with a mouse macrophage-specific antibody (Mac-2, clone m3/38, Cedarlane, Ontario, Canada) was performed in accordance with a previously reported immunohistochemical procedure [11]. The TSP4 immunohistochemical staining of the serial sections was performed as shown below. At first, endogenous peroxidase activity was blocked for 10 min with 3 % hydrogen peroxide after rehydration. Slides were then incubated with anti-thrombospondin-4 mouse IgG_{2b} (Clone #276523, R&D Systems) overnight at 4 °C, followed by incubation with a peroxidase-labeled amino acid polymer-conjugated goat anti-mouse F(ab')2 fragment of IgG (Histofine Mouse Stain kit, Nichirei, Tokyo, Japan) for 30 min at room temperature. The bound antibody complex was then visualized by incubation with 3,3-'-diaminobenzidine tetrahydrochloride. The images of the staining shown above were captured under a microscope (Biozero BZ-8000; Keyence Co., Osaka, Japan).

11.3 Results

11.3.1 Probe Preparation

^{99m}Tc-TSP4-mAb or ^{99m}Tc-NC-mAb was obtained with a radiochemical yield of 17.6 ± 3.8 % or 31.8 ± 6.8 % (n = 3) and with the radiochemical purity of 99.5 ± 0.1 % or 99.2 ± 0.5 % (n = 3). The stability of ^{99m}Tc-TSP4-mAb or ^{99m}Tc-NC-mAb in the mouse plasma was over 90 % for 24-hour incubation.

11.3.2 In Vivo Study

The distributions of ^{99m}Tc-TSP4-mAb in apoE$^{-/-}$ mice and wild-type (WT) mice at 24 h after administration are shown in Table 11.1. The ^{99m}Tc-TSP4-mAb

Table 11.1 Biodistribution of ^{99m}Tc-TSP4-mAb in apoE$^{-/-}$ or wild-type (WT) mice 24 h after administration

	apoE$^{-/-}$	WT
Aorta	5.3 ± 1.1	2.4 ± 0.3
Heart	1.8 ± 0.3	1.5 ± 0.2
Lung	1.7 ± 1.4	1.9 ± 1.6
Liver	5.5 ± 1.8	5.9 ± 1.3
Kidney	2.5 ± 0.2	2.3 ± 0.3
Stomach	1.8 ± 0.5	1.1 ± 0.2
Small intestine	1.3 ± 0.2	1.5 ± 0.2
Large intestine	3.8 ± 1.9	2.5 ± 0.3
Pancreas	0.8 ± 0.2	0.7 ± 0.1
Spleen	7.5 ± 1.2	6.7 ± 0.8
Brain	0.1 ± 0.1	0.1 ± 0.0
Muscle	0.5 ± 0.2	0.6 ± 0.1
Blood	17.2 ± 2.1	17.2 ± 1.5

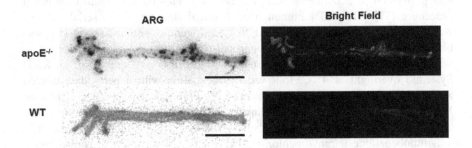

Fig. 11.2 ARG images (*left*) and bright field images (*right*) of the excised aortas of apoE$^{-/-}$ mouse (*upper*) and of wild-type (WT) mouse (*lower*) 24 h after administration of ^{99m}Tc-TSP-mAb

accumulation levels in the aortas of apoE$^{-/-}$ mice were significantly higher than those in WT mice (5.3 ± 1.1 vs. 2.4 ± 0.3 %ID/g, $p < 0.05$), whereas the radioactivities in other organs were not significantly different between apoE$^{-/-}$ mice and wild mice. On the other hand, the ^{99m}Tc-NC-mAb accumulation levels in the aortas of apoE$^{-/-}$ mice were also significantly higher than those of WT mice (5.1 ± 1.4 vs. 2.8 ± 0.5 %ID/g, $p < 0.05$), whereas the radioactivities in other organs were not different between apoE$^{-/-}$ mice and wild-type mice.

The ARG images of the apoE$^{-/-}$ aortas injected with ^{99m}Tc-TSP4-mAb showed heterogeneous distribution of the radioactivity where the plaque formation was observed in the bright field (Fig. 11.2). The radioactive distribution in the aortic roots of apoE$^{-/-}$ mice injected with ^{99m}Tc-TSP4-mAb measured by ARG was inside of the atherosclerotic plaque lesions and coincided with the Mac-2-positive areas (Fig. 11.3). These results suggest that ^{99m}Tc-TSP4-mAb accumulated in the macrophage-infiltrated area of the plaque lesions.

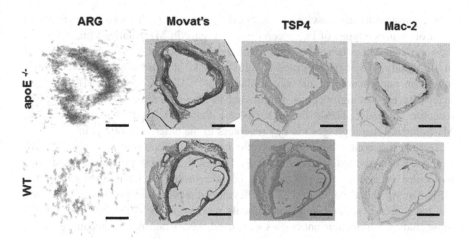

Fig. 11.3 ARG images, Movat's pentachrome staining, TSP4 immunohistochemical staining, and Mac-2 immunohistochemical staining of the aortic roots of apoE$^{-/-}$ mouse (*upper*) and wild-type (WT) (*lower*) mouse 24 h after administration of ^{99m}Tc-TSP4-mAb

11.3.3 Discussion

In this study, we observed that ^{99m}Tc-TSP4-mAb accumulated in the atherosclerotic lesions of apoE$^{-/-}$ mouse aortas. However, ^{99m}Tc-NC-mAb, which was composed of non-targeting IgG, also accumulated highly in the atherosclerotic lesions similar to ^{99m}Tc-TSP4-mAb (Fig. 11.2). Moreover, the ^{99m}Tc-TSP4-mAb accumulation area coincided with the Mac-2-positive areas in the plaques in aortic root (Fig. 11.3), which suggests that IgG itself was delivered and accumulated in atherosclerotic lesions, especially macrophage infiltration areas.

Previously, various types of polarized macrophage were identified and reported [12]. Among the polarized macrophages, pro-inflammatory M1-polarized macrophages were reported to be abundant in lipids and to localize in areas that are distinct from those in which anti-inflammatory M2-polarized macrophages (which are also called alternatively activated macrophages) localize in human plaques [13]. Although the origin of M1 and polarized macrophages and how polarized macrophages are involved in the progression of atherosclerotic plaques are still being unclarified, polarized macrophages would have a critical role in the development of atherosclerotic plaques [14]. Therefore, we examined the correlation of the macrophages, especially polarized macrophages, with IgG accumulation. In our preliminary in vitro study, M1-polarized macrophages showed a higher uptake of ^{99m}Tc-NC-mAb than M2-polarized and non-polarized M0 macrophages [15]. To clarify the mechanism of ^{99m}Tc-NC-mAb accumulation in M1-polarized macrophages, we next focus on the expression levels of Fcγ receptors. Fcγ receptors recognize the Fc region of IgG and play a role in the activation of immune systems [16]. Furthermore, it has been reported that deficiency of Fcγ receptors induces protection against atherosclerosis in apoE$^{-/-}$ mice [17]. Indeed, the expression level of some subtypes of Fcγ receptors was higher in M1-polarized macrophages than those in M2-polarized or non-polarized M0 macrophages in our unreported in vitro study. We also performed a cellular uptake study under the Fcγ receptor's inhibition and found that the accumulation of ^{99m}Tc-NC-mAb in M1-polarized macrophages was significantly suppressed by the pretreatment with an anti-Fcγ receptor antibody. These findings suggest that IgG itself is accumulated in M1-polarized macrophages via Fcγ receptors in the atherosclerotic plaques.

During the course of atherosclerotic progression, various biomolecules are expressed or activated. Thus, various PET/SPECT imaging probes targeting bio-molecules related to the progression of atherosclerosis have been developed [18]. Among them, some probes are developed with based on monoclonal IgG and have been evaluated in animal models such as mouse and rabbit [19, 20]. In those studies, xenogeneic antibodies were used, whose nonspecific accumulation in atherosclerotic lesions was not taken into consideration. However, considering that the probes will be used clinically, the IgG used as a basic component of probes should be humanized, and it would be necessary to note its nonspecific accumulation as we have seen in this study.

Radiolabeled IgG has been widely applied to the diagnosis of inflammatory diseases such as rheumatoid arthritis and infections, although the mechanism of its accumulation is still unclarified [21]. Our preliminary study is the first to show that pro-inflammatory M1-polarized macrophages contribute to the accumulation of radiolabeled IgG, which is in agreement with the conventional use of such IgG as mentioned above.

In the nuclear imaging for diagnosis of atherosclerosis, 18-fluoro-deoxyglucose (^{18}F-FDG) has been widely used [22]. ^{18}F-FDG is reported to accumulate in macrophages, particularly M1-polarized macrophages in atherosclerotic lesions [23], which is similar to radiolabeled IgG behavior. Therefore, radiolabeled IgG would provide information similarly to ^{18}F-FDG in the diagnosis of atherosclerosis.

In this study, we found that IgG itself can be potentially used for the visualization of atherosclerotic plaques, especially atherosclerotic lesions in active inflammation independent of its target biomolecules. However, we also observed the high retention of radioactivities in blood 24 h after administration of ^{99m}Tc-TSP4-mAb (apoE$^{-/-}$, 17.2 ± 2.1 %ID/g; WT, 17.2 ± 1.5 %ID/g), which were about three times higher than those in aortas. This may be because that IgG has a high molecular weight (about 150 kDa), which leads to a low rate of clearance from blood. To overcome this problem, the molecular weight of IgG should be decreased with its affinity to Fcγ receptors maintained. That is, an Fc fragment (about 50 kDa) obtained from IgG would be a suitable basic compound for atherosclerotic imaging. We are now developing an Fc fragment-based probe and evaluating to determine whether this probe can be used to visualize the inflammatory active areas of atherosclerotic lesions.

Acknowledgments This study was supported in part by MEXT KAKENHI (Grant Numbers: 24890003 and 26860961) and the Creation of Innovation Centers for Advanced Interdisciplinary Research Areas Program, Ministry of Education, Culture, Sports, Science and Technology, Japan.

References

1. Ruberg FL, Leopold JA, Loscalzo J. Atherothrombosis: plaque instability and thrombogenesis. Prog Cardiovasc Dis. 2002;44:381–94.
2. Hanzawa H, Sakamoto T, Kaneko A, Manri N, Zhao Y, et al. Combined plasma and tissue proteomic study of atherogenic model mouse: approach to elucidate molecular determinants in atherosclerosis development. J Proteome Res. 2015;14:4257–69.
3. Stenina OI, Desai SY, Krukovets I, Kight K, Janigro D, Topol EJ, et al. Thrombospondin-4 and its variants: expression and differential effects on endothelial cells. Circulation. 2003;108:1514–9.
4. Frolova EG, Pluskota E, Krukovets I, Burke T, Drumm C, Smith JD, et al. Thrombospondin-4 regulates vascular inflammation and atherogenesis. Circ Res. 2010;107:1313–25.
5. Larson SM. Radiolabeled monoclonal anti-tumor antibodies in diagnosis and therapy. J Nucl Med. 1985;26:538–45.
6. Fischman AJ, Rubin RH, Khaw BA, Kramer PB, Wilkinson R, Ahmad M, et al. Radionuclide imaging of experimental atherosclerosis with nonspecific polyclonal immunoglobulin G. J Nucl Med. 1989;30:1095–100.
7. Abrams MJ, Juweid M, TenKate CI, Schwartz DA, Hauser MM, Gaul FE, et al. Technetium-99m-human polyclonal IgG radiolabeled via the hydrazino nicotinamide derivative for imaging focal sites of infection in rats. J Nucl Med. 1990;31:2022–8.
8. Ono M, Arano Y, Mukai T, Uehara T, Fujioka Y, Ogawa K, et al. Plasma protein binding of (99m)Tc-labeled hydrazino nicotinamide derivatized polypeptides and peptides. Nucl Med Biol. 2001;28:155–64.
9. Larsen SK, Solomon HF, Caldwell G, Abrams MJ. [99mTc]tricine: a useful precursor complex for the radiolabeling of hydrazinonicotinate protein conjugates. Bioconjug Chem. 1995;6:635–8.
10. Vucic E, Dickson SD, Calcagno C, Rudd JH, Moshier E, Hayashi K, et al. Pioglitazone modulates vascular inflammation in atherosclerotic rabbits noninvasive assessment with FDG-PET-CT and dynamic contrast-enhanced MR imaging. JACC Cardiovasc Imaging. 2011;4:1100–9.
11. Zhao Y, Kuge Y, Zhao S, Morita K, Inubushi M, Strauss HW, et al. Comparison of 99mTc-annexin A5 with 18F-FDG for the detection of atherosclerosis in ApoE−/− mice. Eur J Nucl Med Mol Imaging. 2007;34:1747–55.
12. Mantovani A, Sica A, Sozzani S, Allavena P, Vecchi A, Locati M. The chemokine system in diverse forms of macrophage activation and polarization. Trends Immunol. 2004;25:677–86.

13. Chinetti-Gbaguidi G, Baron M, Bouhlel MA, Vanhoutte J, Copin C, Sebti Y, et al. Human atherosclerotic plaque alternative macrophages display low cholesterol handling but high phagocytosis because of distinct activities of the PPARgamma and LXRalpha pathways. Circ Res. 2011;108:985–95.

14. Moore KJ, Sheedy FJ, Fisher EA. Macrophages in atherosclerosis: a dynamic balance. Nat Rev Immunol. 2013;13:709–21.

15. Shimizu Y, Hanzawa H, Zhao Y, Fukura S, Nishijima K, Sakamoto T, et al. Accumulation mechanism of non-targeted immunoglobulin G in atherosclerotic lesions. J Nucl Med. 2015;56 Suppl 3:462.

16. Ravetch JV, Bolland S. IgG Fc receptors. Annu Rev Immunol. 2001;19:275–90.

17. Hernandez-Vargas P, Ortiz-Munoz G, Lopez-Franco O, Suzuki Y, Gallego-Delgado J, Sanjuan G, et al. Fcgamma receptor deficiency confers protection against atherosclerosis in apolipoprotein E knockout mice. Circ Res. 2006;99:1188–96.

18. Temma T, Saji H. Radiolabeled probes for imaging of atherosclerotic plaques. Am J Nucl Med Mol Imaging. 2012;2:432–47.

19. Nakamura I, Hasegawa K, Wada Y, Hirase T, Node K, Watanabe Y. Detection of early stage atherosclerotic plaques using PET and CT fusion imaging targeting P-selectin in low density lipoprotein receptor-deficient mice. Biochem Biophys Res Commun. 2013;433:47–51.

20. Temma T, Ogawa Y, Kuge Y, Ishino S, Takai N, Nishigori K, et al. Tissue factor detection for selectively discriminating unstable plaques in an atherosclerotic rabbit model. J Nucl Med. 2010;51:1979–86.

21. Signore A, Prasad V, Malviya G. Monoclonal antibodies for diagnosis and therapy decision making in inflammation/infection. Foreword. Q J Nucl Med Mol Imaging. 2010;54:571–3.

22. Rudd JH, Warburton EA, Fryer TD, Jones HA, Clark JC, Antoun N, et al. Imaging athero-sclerotic plaque inflammation with [18F]-fluorodeoxyglucose positron emission tomography. Circulation. 2002;105:2708–11.

23. Satomi T, Ogawa M, Mori I, Ishino S, Kubo K, Magata Y, et al. Comparison of contrast agents for atherosclerosis imaging using cultured macrophages: FDG versus ultrasmall superpara-magnetic iron oxide. J Nucl Med. 2013;54:999–1004.

Part III
Cardiology

Chapter 12
Noninvasive PET Flow Reserve Imaging to Direct Optimal Therapies for Myocardial Ischemia

Robert A. deKemp and Rob SB Beanlands

Abstract Nuclear cardiology imaging with SPECT or PET is used widely in North America for the diagnosis and management of patients with coronary artery disease. Conventional myocardial perfusion imaging (MPI) can identify areas of reversible ischemia as suitable targets for coronary artery revascularization by angioplasty or bypass surgery. However, the accuracy of this technique is limited in patients with advanced disease in multiple coronary arteries, where there is no normal reference territory against which to assess the "relative" perfusion defects. We have developed methods for the routine quantification of absolute myocardial blood flow (MBF mL/min/g) and coronary flow reserve (stress/rest MBF) using rubidium-82 dynamic PET imaging. The incremental diagnostic and prognostic value of absolute flow quantification over conventional MPI has been demonstrated in several recent studies. Clinical use of this added information for patient management to direct optimal therapy and the potential to improve cardiac outcomes remains unclear, but may be informed by recent progress and widespread clinical adoption of invasive fractional flow reserve(FFR)-directed revascularization. This paper presents recent progress in this field, toward noninvasive CFR image-guided therapy with cardiac PET and SPECT.

Keywords Noninvasive cardiac imaging • Myocardial ischemia • Myocardial blood flow • Coronary flow reserve • Positron emission tomography

12.1   Introduction

Improvements in diagnostic imaging and therapeutic methods have helped to reduce the cardiac death rate in Canada and other developed nations over the past decade [16]. However, cardiovascular disease is still the number one cause of death in most industrialized countries [3]. Noninvasive diagnostic imaging is used

R.A. deKemp (✉) • R.S. Beanlands
National Cardiac PET Centre, Division of Cardiology, University of Ottawa Heart Institute, Ottawa, ON, Canada
e-mail: radekemp@ottawaheart.ca

© The Author(s) 2016   153
Y. Kuge et al. (eds.), *Perspectives on Nuclear Medicine for Molecular Diagnosis and Integrated Therapy*, DOI 10.1007/978-4-431-55894-1_12

increasingly as a "gatekeeper" to help optimize the most effective use of higher-risk invasive (and costly) diagnostic and interventional procedures, such as coronary angiography and revascularization.

This work is motivated in part by the recent FAME trials [7, 38] showing that impaired flow reserve, when used to identify "flow-limiting" epicardial stenoses for revascularization, improved clinical outcomes (reduced cardiac death and myocardial infarction rates) and lowered the total cost of treatment. The FAME trials used *invasive angiography* measurements of fractional flow reserve (FFR), but with associated risks of embolic stroke and other complications of coronary artery catheterization that may be avoided with the use of *noninvasive imaging* methods.

Myocardial perfusion reserve (MPR) imaging using positron emission tomography (PET) may enable diagnosis of patients with microvascular disease (uVD) or nonobstructive diffuse epicardial disease, who should *not* be recommended for coronary revascularization, sparing them the unnecessary risks of invasive angiography for diagnosis alone. Some enhancements to the conventional methods of PET flow reserve imaging are proposed for accurate noninvasive imaging of *ischemia*, to improve identification of hemodynamically and physiologically significant "flow-limiting" lesions that are optimal targets for invasive revascularization. According to recent AHA/NIH publications [28], "Standard tests used to diagnose CAD are not designed to detect coronary uVD. More research is needed to find the best diagnostic tests and treatments for the disease." The flow reserve concepts used in this study are illustrated in Fig. 12.1, and the specific terms are defined in Table 12.1.

Current international practice guidelines [1, 2] recommend the use of treadmill exercise-ECG testing and stress perfusion imaging for the diagnosis of ischemia (benefit class I, evidence levels A,B) and the use of invasive flow reserve (FFR) measurements to direct invasive revascularization (benefit class I, IIa, evidence level A) for the treatment of symptoms in patients with suspected ischemic heart disease. Despite a wealth of observational data, stress MPI is still not a class 1 (A) indication to direct revascularization in patients with stable ischemic heart

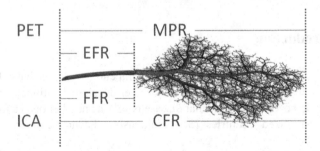

Fig. 12.1 Epicardial (EFR, FFR) ± microvascular (MPR, CFR) flow reserve measurements using PET imaging and ICA. Normal values of MPR and CFR are approximately 3–5 (average 4.0) in young healthy adults without microvascular disease. Normal epicardial vessels have FFR = 1.0, whereas "flow-limiting" stenoses with FFR < 0.75–0.80 can produce myocardial ischemia. See Table 12.1 for definitions

Table 12.1 Flow reserve terminology

Name	Definition
Coronary artery disease (CAD)	Focal or diffuse narrowing of an *epicardial* coronary artery lumen due to the formation of atherosclerotic plaque (stenosis or lesion) in the arterial wall
Microvascular disease (uVD)	Damage to the inner lining (endothelium) of the *subepicardial* small arteries or arterioles that regulate blood flow to the heart muscle
Myocardial blood flow (MBF)	*Microvascular* perfusion [mL/min/g] of blood to the heart muscle
Myocardial perfusion (flow) reserve (MPR, MFR)	**Ratio** of maximal hyperemic stress/rest perfusion (tissue flow), including the effects of *epicardial and microvascular* disease, typically measured using noninvasive PET imaging (Fig. 12.1)
Microvascular reserve (uVR)	**Ratio** of endothelium-dependent stress/rest MBF in the small resistance arteries and arterioles
Epicardial flow reserve (EFR)	**Ratio** of epicardial vessel-dependent stress/rest MBF in the large conduit arteries. The sum total of uVR + EFR is equal to MPR
Coronary flow reserve (CFR)	**Ratio** of maximal hyperemic stress/rest blood flow in the epicardial coronary arteries, reflecting the effects of *epicardial and microvascular* disease. CFR is typically measured invasively during adenosine stress using the indicator dilution technique
Fractional flow reserve (FFR)	**Fraction** of pressure maintained across an *epicardial* stenosis during hyperemic stress, measured using invasive angiography. It is analogous to the relative MPR value, in single-vessel disease without uVD

disease because there remains insufficient evidence that ischemia-directed therapy reduces the risk of death and/or myocardial infarction.

In conjunction with, or following exercise-ECG testing, stress myocardial perfusion imaging (MPI) is used widely in North America for the noninvasive diagnosis of coronary artery disease. While single-photon emission computed tomography (SPECT) is used most commonly, rubidium-82 (^{82}Rb) PET has been available in the USA since 1989 for the diagnosis of obstructive coronary artery disease (CAD). We recently completed enrolment of >15,000 patients in the Canadian multicenter trial [8] evaluating ^{82}Rb PET as an alternative radiopharmaceutical for myocardial perfusion imaging (Rb-ARMI). Initial results confirmed the high accuracy (>90 %) of low-dose ^{82}Rb PET-CT for diagnosis of obstructive coronary artery disease in patients with epicardial stenoses ≥ 50–70 % [20]. Recent meta-analyses also confirm that PET has higher accuracy for diagnosis of CAD compared to SPECT, even when using current cameras with attenuation correction and ECG-gating [24].

Stress perfusion imaging is also used for the assessment of myocardial ischemia, to identify patients that will benefit from invasive revascularization therapy procedures such as coronary angioplasty and bypass surgery [15] as shown in Fig. 12.2. The efficacy of this approach was suggested initially in the nuclear sub-study of the

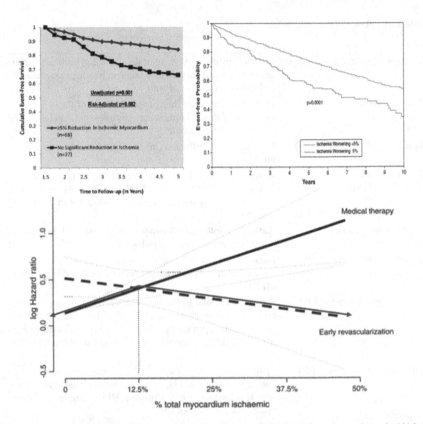

Fig. 12.2 Patients with moderate-to-severe ischemia in the COURAGE nuclear sub-study (A) had a lower rate of death or MI when there was a 5 % improvement (reduction) in ischemic burden following revascularization. In the DUKE nuclear cardiology registry (B), patients with >5 % ischemia worsening had increased risk of death or MI. Retrospective analysis of ~14,000 SPECT-MPI patients (C) indicated that the percent ischemic myocardium (>10–15 %) predicted lower risk (log hazard ratio) of death following early revascularization. In patients with less than 10–15 % ischemic myocardium, medical therapy was the most effective treatment [Reproduced from (A) [37], (B) [12], and (C) [15].]

COURAGE trial [37] and confirmed recently in patients from the DUKE registry [12], showing survival and outcome benefits from invasive revascularization using angioplasty in addition to optimal medical (drug) therapy, in patients with at least 5 % *ischemic myocardium* improvement. The ISCHEMIA trial currently in progress [23] is intended to verify prospectively, in patients with ischemia by physiological testing (for MPI: at least 10 % ischemic left ventricular (LV) myocardium), whether or not revascularization compared to medical therapy will result in improved clinical outcomes. This is a pivotal trial intended to prove conclusively the value of ischemia detection by stress perfusion imaging. However, but it is important to recognize that conventional stress MPI (using SPECT or PET) will still underestimate the extent and severity of ischemia from diffuse or multivessel disease (patients with left-main coronary artery disease are excluded) and will neither identify - nor direct treatment of - high-risk patients with disease of the coronary microvasculature.

12.2   Myocardial Blood Flow (Perfusion) Imaging

Some limitations of conventional (relative) MPI can be overcome by quantifying myocardial perfusion blood flow (MBF) in absolute units of mL/min/g. Dynamic imaging is required starting from the time of tracer injection, to capture the first-pass transit through the venous-arterial circulation as shown in Fig. 12.3. The concentration of tracer is measured over time in the arterial blood and myocardial tissues, and the rate of uptake or transfer from blood to tissue (influx rate K1 mL/min/g) is related to the absolute myocardial perfusion [21]. Flow quantification restores the true normal-to-diseased tissue contrast (Fig. 12.4), which is otherwise underestimated by measurement of the tracer retention (net uptake) alone. It also allows visualization of the stress/rest perfusion or flow reserve (MPR or MFR) as a measure of the total coronary vascular dilator capacity.

A one-tissue-compartment model is often used to describe the early kinetics (e.g., 0–5 min) of tracer exchange between the arterial blood supply and myocardial target tissues. This model has been validated for rubidium-82 (^{82}Rb) imaging in humans using nitrogen-13 (^{13}N)-ammonia PET as the reference standard [22] and

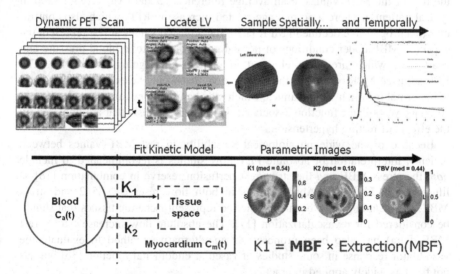

Fig. 12.3 Quantification of MBF using dynamic PET imaging. Dynamic images are acquired starting at the time of tracer injection, then activity in the LV cavity and myocardium is measured over time and fit to a one-tissue-compartment model of the tracer kinetics. The influx rate of tracer uptake or transfer from blood to tissue (K1 mL/min/g) is related to MBF, according to a tracer extraction function E(MBF)

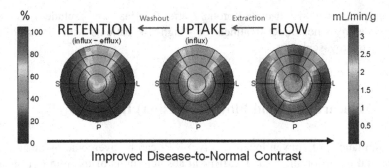

Fig. 12.4 Polar-maps of MBF (flow), [82]Rb uptake (K1 influx rate), and retention (net influx − efflux) demonstrating the effects of nonlinear tracer extraction and washout. MBF estimation restores the true disease-to-normal tissue contrast and increases the sensitivity to detect focal disease relative to areas of maximal flow

has been demonstrated to give very reproducible results using several investigational and commercial implementations as shown in Fig. 12.5a, b [9, 27, 31]. Test-retest repeatability of the method (Fig. 12.5c) is approximately 10–12 % CV (coefficient of variation) at rest and 6–7 % during pharmacologic stress [11, 30], comparable to the theoretical expected values verified recently using Monte-Carlo and analytic simulations [25].

Resting MBF is known to correlate highly with the metabolic demands of normal cardiac work [4] as shown in Fig. 12.6; therefore, it is common to adjust the rest of the MBF values to an average reference standard value (e.g., 8500 in typical patients). There a normal age-related increase in RPP, which also contributes to a progressive decline in MPR [10]. The adjusted values at rest represent the expected MBF under conditions of normal controlled systolic blood pressure and heart rate, which are often elevated in patients undergoing stress MPI. The RPP-adjusted MPR represents the flow reserve that would be expected in a patient with normal resting hemodynamics, which may be used to evaluate impairments in coronary vasodilator function associated with atherosclerosis that are unbiased by the effects of resting hypertension.

Because of the wide physiological variability in rest MBF values between patients, interpretation of absolute PET flow studies is recommended to include *both* the stress MBF *and* the stress/rest perfusion reserve in combination [18] as illustrated in Fig. 12.7. Abnormalities in both flow reserve < 1.5–2 and stress MBF < 1 mL/min/g have been suggested to represent ischemic tissues that should be considered for revascularization [17]. The absolute flow increase (stress–rest MBF delta) has also been proposed as an alternative method to evaluate the vasodilator response in some studies of vascular endothelial function [36] but has not been as widely applied in practice.

The diagnostic utility of PET MPR assessment has been confirmed in patients with multivessel disease [40]. As shown in Fig. 12.8a, there is a 50 % likelihood of three-vessel disease in patients with a global LV flow reserve that is severely

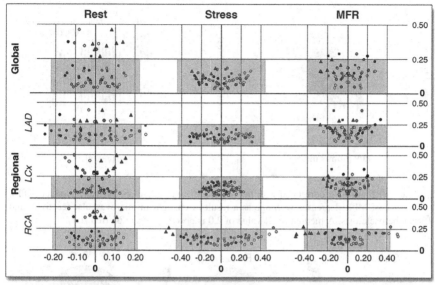

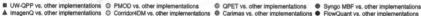

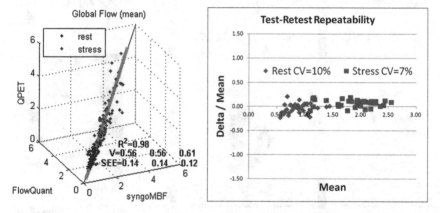

Fig. 12.5 MBF values measured using the one-tissue-compartment model are highly reproducible between several investigational (A) and commercial (B) software implementations. Rest and stress flow values are generally within 15–20 %, allowing multicenter data to be pooled or combined between vendors. Test–retest repeatability is 7–10 % at stress and rest (C), for single-session back-to-back scans

impaired (MPR = 1), whereas the balance of patients presumably have severe microvascular disease limiting their ability to increase myocardial perfusion from rest to peak stress. Measurements of absolute MPR also have prognostic value that is incremental and independent of the standard assessments of relative MPI [41], as shown in Fig. 12.8b. Patients with normal MPI (SSS < 4) but abnormal flow reserve (MFR < 2) are at increased risk of cardiac events. In the case of abnormal MPI, if

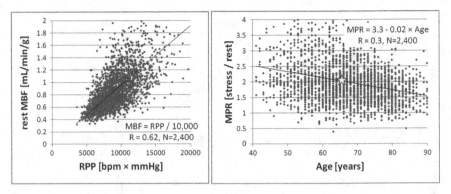

Fig. 12.6 MBF at rest is correlated with the heart rate × systolic blood pressure product (RPP). Peak stress/rest MPR decreases with age as a result of changes in microvascular reactivity and diffuse atherosclerosis. A median MPR value of 2.0 is observed at age 65 (red star)

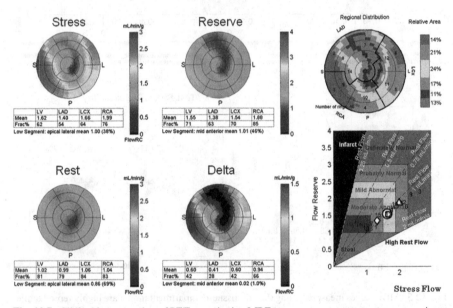

Fig. 12.7 Clinical interpretation of PET quantitative MBF measurements at rest, stress, stress/rest reserve (MPR), and stress–rest delta. The "regional distribution" map is a combination of the flow reserve and stress flow maps, according to the scheme shown on the bottom right

flow reserve is also impaired, then these patients have the highest rate of cardiac events within the following year. Similar findings have reported in a separate cohort of ischemic heart disease patients [26]; those with the lowest values of MPR had the highest cardiac event rates. Despite these observational studies, there is a lack of evidence proving that revascularization of ischemic myocardium as identified by absolute flow imaging will result in a lower risk of cardiac death or myocardial infarction.

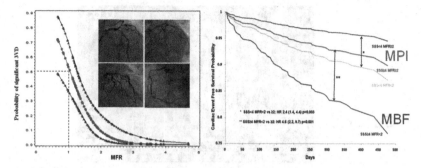

Fig. 12.8 Diagnostic utility of MPR (MFR) in multivessel disease is shown on the left [40]. Patients with global flow reserve < 1 have > 50 % probability of three-vessel disease; the remaining patients have severe microvascular disease. Patients with reductions in flow reserve (MFR < 2) have lower event-free survival, regardless of whether their relative perfusion (SSS) is normal or abnormal [41]

12.3   Fractional Flow Reserve Assessment

Invasive coronary angiography methods have been developed over the past two decades to quantify the functional or hemodynamic significance of epicardial coronary artery disease, using proximal-distal pressure measurements of the fractional flow reserve ratio (FFR) [13], as illustrated in Fig. 12.9. FFR is defined as the fractional pressure drop measured across one or more stenoses in an individual coronary artery. Interestingly, invasive measurements of FFR were originally validated against ^{15}O-water PET measurements of *relative* MPR [5]. As shown in Fig. 12.10, coronary FFR values were similar to the relative MPR on average, whereas the myocardial FFR shows a small bias of approximately +10 % vs. the PET analogous values.

Epicardial stenoses with abnormal FFR < 0.75 were initially shown to identify the presence of myocardial ischemia with high accuracy compared to a positive test on one or more of three noninvasive methods: exercise thallium planar imaging, *or* dobutamine stress echocardiography, *or* treadmill exercise ECG (Fig. 12.11) [33, 34]. This FFR threshold is therefore very sensitive for the detection of ischemia, because it correlates with ischemia on *any* of the reference standards above.

Test-retest repeatability of FFR measurements has been reported in the range of 4–7 % CV [6, 29, 32], similar to the precision of PET stress MBF (Fig. 12.12). This has led to the adoption of a 5 % "gray zone" of uncertainty in FFR measurements considered to be hemodynamically significant or flow limiting.

The pivotal FAME trial [38] showed that percutaneous coronary intervention (PCI) revascularization using coronary stenting of anatomically *and* hemodynamically significant lesions (stenosis ≥ 50 % *and* FFR ≤ 0.80) improved cardiac outcomes (Fig. 12.13) and reduced the total cost of treatment compared to the standard practice of revascularization for anatomically significant lesions only

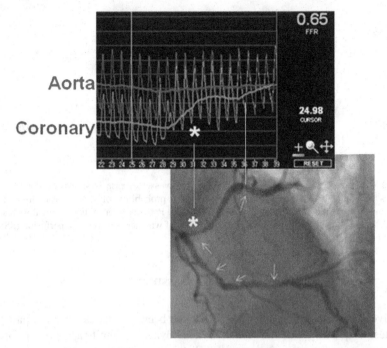

Fig. 12.9 Fractional flow reserve is measured as the ratio of intracoronary pressure distal to a stenosis and relative to the (proximal normal) aortic pressure during peak adenosine pharmacologic stress. Comparison of the FFR measurements to coronary angiography allows identification of flow-limiting stenoses that are optimal targets for revascularization

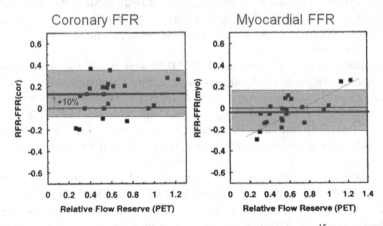

Fig. 12.10 Invasive measurements of FFR were originally validated against ^{15}O-water PET MBF studies in a group of $N = 22$ patients with single-vessel coronary artery disease. Coronary (epicardial) FFR produced values that were ~10 % higher than the relative flow reserve (relative MPR) values. The myocardial (epicardial + microvascular) FFR values corrected for atrial venous pressure were more accurate on average, but demonstrated an increasing trend versus PET. Adapted from [5]

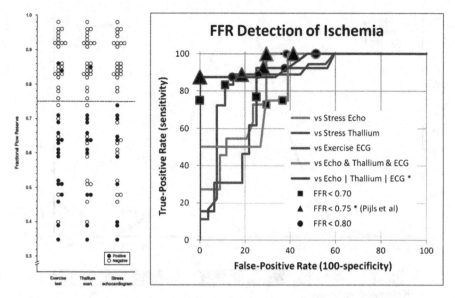

Fig. 12.11 Fractional flow reserve (FFR) compared to ischemia testing in N = 45 patients, using exercise ECG, thallium imaging, and stress echo [34]. Abnormal FFR < 0.75 was reported to have 88 % sensitivity and 100 % specificity to identify ischemia according to stress echo or exercise thallium imaging or exercise-ECG tests combined(*), but specificity decreases dramatically in the "gray zone" between the FFR cutoff values of 0.75 to 0.80 and when FFR is compared individually to the ischemia standard tests. At the FFR cutoff value < 0.80 commonly used to direct revascularization, fewer than 50 % of subjects had exercise-ECG, stress echo, and thallium tests that were all positive for ischemia

(stenosis > 50–70 %). However, there remains a significant cost (interventional pressure wires) and patient morbidity (risk of embolic strokes) associated with this invasive procedure. While FFR provides a useful physiological assessment of epicardial stenoses, it does not assess the severity of microvascular disease and actually underestimates the functional significance of epicardial lesions in the presence of microvascular disease [35]. Despite these limitations, FFR has recently been upgraded to a class I(A) indication in Europe and class IIa(A) in North America for use in directing revascularization therapy to improve clinical outcomes.

12.4   Noninvasive PET (MPR) vs. Invasive Coronary Angiography (FFR)

Reductions in the supply of blood to the myocardium are caused by two separate consequences of disease: (1) epicardial coronary stenoses and (2) microvascular dysfunction. The "flow-limiting" epicardial stenoses should be identified ideally

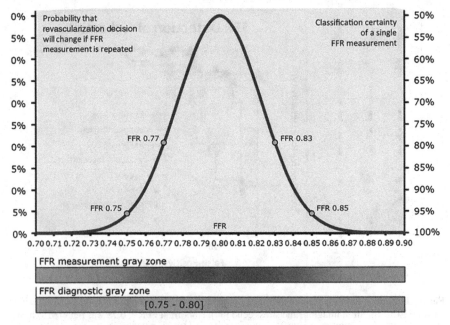

Fig. 12.12 Test-retest repeatability of back-to-back FFR measurements 10 min apart (4 % CV), reanalyzed from the DEFER study by [32]. The measurement (or classification) uncertainty is shown as the red-green colorbar, reflecting the probability that a revascularization decision would change with repeat measurement. The conventional diagnostic uncertainty or "gray zone" of 0.75–0.80 is shown as the grey-green colorbar

as targets for revascularization, whereas patients with diffuse or microvascular disease may be better treated with targeted aggressive medical therapies such as lipid-lowering statins or other novel drug treatments under development to improve endothelial function by increasing nitric-oxide bioavailability, for example.

Myocardial and fractional flow reserve measurements represent different hemodynamic effects of microvascular and epicardial disease. The interrelated physiological interpretation of PET MFR vs. invasive FFR measurements has been the subject of several recent reviews [14, 19]. The discordance between FFR and MPR is attributed to the differences in epicardial vs microvascular disease (Fig. 12.14c) and is consistent with our PET data in over 3,000 patients (Fig. 12.14a, b).

As illustrated in Fig. 12.1, noninvasive PET imaging of MPR measures the capacity to increase perfusion (and tracer delivery) in the downstream microvasculature within the myocardium, reflecting the combined "total" effects of microvascular and epicardial disease. Invasive FFR measures the pressure drop across a

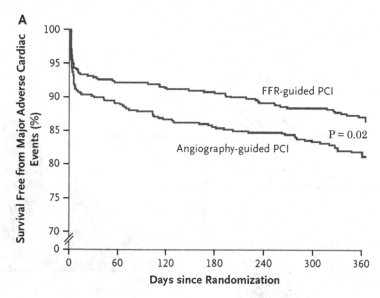

Fig. 12.13 The FAME randomized controlled trial in N = 1005 patients showed that clinical outcome was improved (87 % vs. 82 % event-free survival; p = 0.02) using FFR-guided revascularization by PCI with drug-eluting stents in patients with intermediate-grade stenosis > 50 % and FFR < 0.80. The FFR-guided approach also resulted in 30 % fewer stents placed per patient (p < 0.001) and 11 % lower overall costs including the added FFR pressure wires [38]

single epicardial stenosis during hyperemic stress, representing the peak flow compared to the (restored or expected) normal flow in the absence of stenosis. FFR determines whether a particular epicardial lesion is "flow limiting"; however, this measurement assumes that maximal peak-stress vasodilatation was achieved in the downstream microvasculature. Therefore, *in the presence of microvascular dysfunction*, FFR can be overestimated (i.e., the severity of disease underestimated) due to a submaximal stress flow response, resulting in underdiagnosis and potential undertreatment of the disease [35].

There is a wide variation in reported MFR values at a given lesion stenosis severity (Fig. 12.15a) confirming the influence of confounding variables such as peak-MFR and/or microvascular flow reserve (uVR). Measurements of *total MFR* alone cannot separate the fundamental difference in stress flow responses present in the epicardial conduit arteries vs. the microvascular resistance vessels. This effect is illustrated in Fig. 12.15b showing that a 70 % stenosis can appear to have normal *or* abnormal FFR depending on the peak hyperemic flow response (peak-MFR).

We have proposed a simple model describing MPR as the sum total of uVR and epicardial CFR as shown in Fig. 12.15c. This model is consistent with

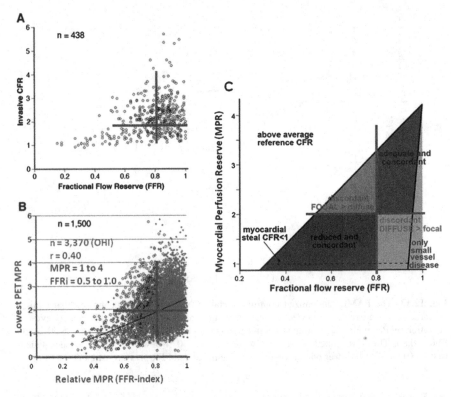

Fig. 12.14 Discordance between FFR and MPR is due to the physiological differences in focal epicardial vs. diffuse or microvascular disease. (A) Invasive [and (B) noninvasive] measures of CFR [and absolute MPR] vs. FFR [and relative MPR] measurements can be discordant in some patients, due to the different physiological consequences of focal vs. diffuse microvascular disease (C). Adapted from [19]

previous observations that MFR decreases with increasing lesion stenosis%, but at different reference levels depending on the burden of microvascular disease. uVR is presumed to be independent of epicardial stenosis severity, also consistent with previous invasive measurements of microcirculatory resistance (IMR) [39]. The model predicts that a particular threshold value (EFR = MPR − uVR) for epicardial coronary revascularization will only improve symptoms of ischemia in patients without severe microvascular disease, e.g., with uVR > 0, as shown in Fig. 12.15d. Conversely, myocardial ischemia may be overestimated in young patients without uVD, where an "apparent ischemic" stress perfusion defect in a patient with very high peak-MFR may still be above the true ischemic threshold of stress MBF.

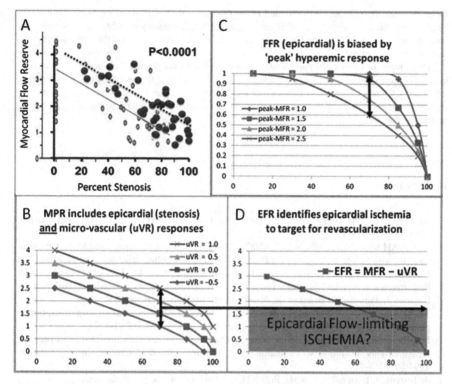

Fig. 12.15 Total myocardial perfusion (flow) reserve (MPR) is a function of epicardial stenosis severity (0–100 %) and microvascular vasodilator response (uVR) as shown in (**A, B**). In patients with severe microvascular (endothelial) dysfunction (e.g. uVR=−0.5), invasive measurement of fractional flow reserve (FFR) may appear normal in coronary lesions up to 90 % stenosis (**C**), due to the absence of hyperemic flow response (peak-MFR=1.0). Epicardial flow reserve (EFR=MPR–uVR) may be useful to identify flow-limiting lesions associated with myocardial ischemia (**D**)

12.5 Conclusion

Noninvasive nuclear imaging of myocardial blood flow (MBF) and coronary flow reserve (CFR) is now feasible as part of the clinical routine using positron emission tomography (PET) imaging. PET measurements of absolute MBF are reliable and reproducible between imaging centers and software methods, with test–retest repeatability below 10 % coefficient of variation. Ischemic thresholds have been proposed for stress MBF and coronary flow reserve in the range of 1.5 [mL/min/g] and 1.0 [stress/rest MBF], respectively. Prospective trials are needed to determine whether patient outcomes can be improved using these ischemic thresholds to direct appropriate revascularization vs. optimal medical therapies.

References

1. ACCF/AHA/SCAI Guideline for Percutaneous Coronary Intervention. J Am Coll Cardiol. 2011;58(24):e44–e122.
2. ACCF/AHA/ACP/AATS/PCNA/SCAI/STS Guideline for the Diagnosis and Management of Patients with Stable Ischemic Heart Disease. J Am Coll Cardiol. 2012;60(24):e44–e164.
3. Canadian Institutes of Health Research *Annual Report* 2010–11. Moving Forward CIHR Performance across the Spectrum: From Research Investments to Knowledge Translation.
4. Czernin J, Porenta G, Brunken R, Krivokapich J, Chen K, Bennett R, Hage A, Fung C, Tillisch J, Phelps ME. Regional blood flow, oxidative metabolism, and glucose utilization in patients with recent myocardial infarction. Circulation. 1993;88(3):884–95.
5. De Bruyne B, Baudhuin T, Melin JA, et al. Coronary flow reserve calculated from pressure measurements in humans. validation with positron emission tomography. Circulation. 1994;89:1013–22.
6. de Bruyne B, Bartunek J, Sys SU, Pijls NH, Heyndrickx GR, Wijns W. Simultaneous coronary pressure and flow velocity measurements in humans. Feasibility, reproducibility, and hemodynamic dependence of coronary flow velocity reserve, hyperemic flow versus pressure slope index, and fractional flow reserve. Circulation. 1996;94(8):1842–9.
7. De Bruyne B, Pijls NH, Kalesan B, Barbato E, Tonino PA, Piroth Z, Jagic N, Möbius-Winkler S, Rioufol G, Witt N, Kala P, MacCarthy P, Engström T, Oldroyd KG, Mavromatis K, Manoharan G, Verlee P, Frobert O, Curzen N, Johnson JB, Jüni P. Fearon WF; FAME 2 Trial Investigators. Fractional flow reserve-guided PCI versus medical therapy in stable coronary disease. N Engl J Med. 2012;367(11):991–1001.
8. deKemp RA, Wells GA, Beanlands RSB. Rubidium-82 – An Alternative Radiopharmaceutical for Myocardial Imaging (Rb-ARMI) 2009–2015. http://clinicaltrials.gov/ct2/show/NCT01128023
9. deKemp RA, DeClerck J, Klein R, Pan X-B, Nakazato R, Tonge C, Arumugam P, Berman DS, Germano G, Beanlands RS, Slomka PJ. Multi-software reproducibility study of stress and rest myocardial blood flow assessed with 3D dynamic PET-CT and a one-tissue-compartment Model of 82Rb Kinetics. J Nucl Med. 2013;54:571–577.
10. deKemp RA, Klein R, Renaud J, Garrard L, Wells GA, Beanlands R. Patient age, gender and hemodynamics are independent predictors of myocardial flow reserve as measured with dipyridamole stress PET perfusion imaging. J Nucl Med. 2014;55(S1):79.
11. Efseaff M, Klein R, Ziadi MC, Beanlands RS, deKemp RA. Short-term repeatability of resting myocardial blood flow measurements using rubidium-82 PET imaging. J Nucl Cardiol. 2012;19(5):997–1006.
12. Farzaneh-Far A, Phillips HR, Shaw LK, Starr AZ, Fiuzat M, O'Connor CM, Sastry A, Shaw LJ, Borges-Neto S. Ischemia change in stable coronary artery disease is an independent predictor of death and myocardial infarction. JACC Cardiovasc Imaging. 2012;5(7):715–24.

13. Gould KL, Kirkeeide RL, Buchi M. Coronary flow reserve as a physiologic measure of stenosis severity. J Am Coll Cardiol. 1990;15(2):459–74.
14. Gould KL. Does coronary flow trump coronary anatomy? JACC Cardiovasc Imaging. 2009;2:1009–23.
15. Hachamovitch R, Rozanski A, Shaw LJ, Stone GW, Thomson LE, Friedman JD, Hayes SW, Cohen I, Germano G, Berman DS. Impact of ischemia and scar on the therapeutic benefit derived from myocardial revascularization vs. medical therapy among patients undergoing stress-rest myocardial perfusion scintigraphy. Eur Heart J. 2011;32(8):1012–24.
16. Heart and Stroke Foundation *Annual report* on Canadians Health. A Perfect Storm of Heart Disease Looming on Our Horizon, January 25, 2010.
17. Johnson NP, Gould KL. Physiological basis for angina and ST-segment change: PET-verified thresholds of quantitative stress myocardial perfusion and coronary flow reserve. JACC Cardiovasc Imaging. 2011;4:990–8.
18. Johnson NP, Gould KL. Integrating noninvasive absolute flow, coronary flow reserve, and ischemic thresholds into a comprehensive map of physiological severity. JACC Cardiovasc Imaging. 2012;5:430–40.
19. Johnson NP, Kirkeeide RL, Gould KL. Is discordance of coronary flow reserve and fractional flow reserve due to methodology or clinically relevant coronary pathophysiology? JACC Cardiovasc Imaging. 2012;5:194–202.
20. Kaster T, Mylonas I, Renaud JM, Wells GA, Beanlands RSB, deKemp RA. Accuracy of low-dose rubidium-82 myocardial perfusion imaging for detection of coronary artery disease using 3D PET and normal database interpretation. J Nucl Cardiol. 2012.
21. Klein R, Renaud JM, Ziadi MC, Beanlands RSB, deKemp RA. Intra- and inter-operator repeatability of myocardial blood flow and myocardial flow reserve measurements using rubidium-82 pet and a highly automated analysis program. J Nucl Cardiol. 2010;17:600–16.
22. Lortie M, Beanlands RS, Yoshinaga K, Klein R, Dasilva JN, deKemp RA. Quantification of myocardial blood flow with 82Rb dynamic PET imaging. Eur J Nucl Med Mol Imaging. 2007;34:1765–74.
23. Maron D, Boden W, Ferguson B, Harrington R, Stone G, Williams D. International study of comparative health effectiveness with medical and invasive approaches (ISCHEMIA). https://clinicaltrials.gov/ct2/show/NCT01471522
24. Mc Ardle BA, Dowsley TF, deKemp RA, Wells GA, Beanlands RS. Does rubidium-82 PET have superior accuracy to SPECT perfusion imaging for the diagnosis of obstructive coronary disease? A systematic review and meta-analysis. J Am Coll Cardiol. 2012;60(18):1828–37.
25. Moody J, Murthy V, Lee B, Corbett J, Ficaro E. Variance Estimation for Myocardial Blood Flow by Dynamic PET. IEEE Trans Med Imaging. 2015 May 13. [Epub ahead of print]
26. Murthy VL, Naya M, Foster CR, Hainer J, Gaber M, Di Carli G, Blankstein R, Dorbala S, Sitek A, Pencina MJ, Di Carli MF. Improved cardiac risk assessment with noninvasive measures of coronary flow reserve. Circulation. 2011;124(20):2215–24.
27. Nesterov SV, Deshayes E, Sciagrà R, Settimo L, Declerck JM, Pan XB, Yoshinaga K, Katoh C, Slomka PJ, Germano G, Han C, Aalto V, Alessio AM, Ficaro EP, Lee BC, Nekolla SG, Gwet KL, deKemp RA, Klein R, Dickson J, Case JA, Bateman T, Prior JO, Knuuti JM. Quantification of myocardial blood flow in absolute terms using (82)Rb PET imaging: the RUBY-10 Study. JACC Cardiovasc Imaging. 2014;7(11):1119–27.
28. NIH-NHLBI website. What is Coronary Microvascular Disease? http://www.nhlbi.nih.gov/health/health-topics/topics/cmd. Accessed September 2015.
29. Ntalianis A, Sels JW, Davidavicius G, Tanaka N, Muller O, Trana C, Barbato E, Hamilos M, Mangiacapra F, Heyndrickx GR, Wijns W, Pijls NH, De Bruyne B. Fractional flow reserve for the assessment of nonculprit coronary artery stenoses in patients with acute myocardial infarction. JACC Cardiovasc Interv. 2010;3(12):1274–81.
30. Ocneanu A, Adler A, Renaud J, Beanlands R, deKemp R, Klein R. Reproducible tracer injection profile improves the test-retest repeatability of myocardial blood flow quantification with 82Rb PET. J Nucl Med. 2015;56(S3):207.

31. Pan X-B, DeClerck J. Validation *syngo* PET Myocardial Blood Flow. Siemens Healthcare: White Paper 2012.
32. Petraco R, Sen S, Nijjer S, Echavarria-Pinto M, Escaned J, Francis DP, Davies JE. Fractional flow reserve-guided revascularization: practical implications of a diagnostic gray zone and measurement variability on clinical decisions. JACC Cardiovasc Interv. 2013;6(3):222–5. doi: 10.1016/j.jcin.2012.10.014. Erratum in: JACC Cardiovasc Interv. 2013;6(4):431.
33. Pijls NH, van Son JA, Kirkeeide RL, De Bruyne B, Gould KL. Experimental basis of determining maximum coronary, myocardial, and collateral blood flow by pressure measurements for assessing functional stenosis severity before and after percutaneous transluminal coronary angioplasty. Circulation. 1993;87:1354–67.
34. Pijls NH, De Bruyne B, Peels K, Van Der Voort PH, Bonnier HJ, Bartunek J, Koolen JJ, Koolen JJ. Measurement of fractional flow reserve to assess the functional severity of coronary-artery stenoses. NEJM. 1996;334(26):1703–8.
35. Pijls NH, Tonino PA. The CRUX of maximum hyperemia: the last remaining barrier for routine use of fractional flow reserve. JACC Cardiovasc Interv. 2011;4(10):1093–5.
36. Schindler TH, Zhang X-L, Prior JO, Cadenas J, Dahlbom M, Sayre J, Schelbert HR. Assessment of intra- and inter-observer reproducibility of rest and cold-pressor-test stimulated myocardial blood flow with 13N-ammonia and PET. Eur J Nucl Med Mol Imaging. 2007;34:1178–88.
37. Shaw LJ, Berman DS, Maron DJ, et al. Optimal medical therapy with or without percutaneous coronary intervention to reduce ischemic burden: Results from the clinical outcomes utilizing revascularization and aggressive drug evaluation (COURAGE) trial nuclear sub-study. Circulation. 2008;117:1283–91.
38. Tonino PA, De Bruyne B, Pijls NH, et al. Fractional flow reserve versus angiography for guiding percutaneous coronary intervention. N Engl J Med. 2009;360:213–24.
39. Yong ASC, Ho M, Shah MG, Ng MKC, Fearon WF. Coronary microcirculatory resistance is independent of epicardial stenosis. Circ Cardiovasc Interv. 2012;5:103–8.
40. Ziadi MC, deKemp RA, Williams K, Beanlands RSB. Does quantification of myocardial flow reserve using rubidium-82 positron emission tomography facilitate detection of multi-vessel coronary artery disease? J Nucl Cardiol. 2012;19:670–80.
41. Ziadi MC, deKemp RA, Williams K, Beanlands RSB. Impaired myocardial flow reserve on rubidium-82 positron emission tomography imaging predicts adverse outcomes in patients assessed for myocardial ischemia. J Am Coll Cardiol. 2011;58:740–8.

Chapter 13
The Clinical Value of Cardiac PET in Heart Failure

Chi-Lun Ko and Yen-Wen Wu

Abstract Heart failure (HF) is a complex clinical syndrome that results from any structural or functional impairment of ventricular filling or ejection of blood [1]. Approximately 5 million patients in the USA and 15 million patients in Europe have HF. It is the leading cause of hospitalization in elderly people. Despite treatment advances, the mortality rate of HF has increased steadily. More patients are surviving myocardial infarction (MI) due to better standards of care, and consequently this may increase numbers of patients who subsequently develop HF. HF places a significant burden on patients, carers, and healthcare systems.

Limited progress has been made in identifying evidence-based, effective treatments for HF over the last decades. Potential contributors include an incomplete understanding of pathophysiology and poor matching of therapeutic mechanisms.

Positron emission tomography (PET), as a molecular imaging technique, with various tracers allows noninvasive evaluation of contractile function, myocardial perfusion, metabolism, and innervation. Molecular imaging approaches using PET could be further used to evaluate inflammation, angiogenesis, cell death, and ventricular remodeling. It could provide new insights on the chemotherapy-related cardiotoxicity and the roles of stem cell monitoring in living bodies for cell-based therapy from preclinical studies to clinical trials. In conclusion, cardiac PET is a promising tool to understand the physiologic consequences of HF, resulting in early detection of patients with HF at risk, improvement of risk stratification, and

C.-L. Ko, MD
Department of Nuclear Medicine, National Taiwan University Hospital Yun-Lin Branch, Yunlin County, Taiwan

Department of Nuclear Medicine, National Taiwan University Hospital and National Taiwan University College of Medicine, Taipei, Taiwan

Y.-W. Wu, MD, PhD (✉)
Department of Nuclear Medicine, National Taiwan University Hospital and National Taiwan University College of Medicine, Taipei, Taiwan

Cardiology Division of Cardiovascular Medical Center, Far Eastern Memorial Hospital, No.21, Sec.2, Nanya S. Rd., Banciao Dist., New Taipei City 220, Taiwan

Department of Nuclear Medicine, Far Eastern Memorial Hospital, New Taipei City, Taiwan

National Yang-Ming University School of Medicine, Taipei, Taiwan
e-mail: wuyw0502@gmail.com

© The Author(s) 2016
Y. Kuge et al. (eds.), *Perspectives on Nuclear Medicine for Molecular Diagnosis and Integrated Therapy*, DOI 10.1007/978-4-431-55894-1_13

therapeutic strategy planning and treatment response monitoring. Therefore, in order to give the readers a brief and concise overview, we will mainly review the latest advances in cardiac PET studies in heart failure.

Keywords Heart failure • Positron emission tomography • Myocardial perfusion • Myocardial metabolism • Neuroautonomic system

13.1 Perfusion

13.1.1 Coronary Artery Disease (CAD) and Microvascular Dysfunction

Patients presenting with HF are initially classified based on the etiology of their disease, i.e., ischemic or nonischemic cardiomyopathy. The diagnosis of HF is clear if prior MI is reliably documented. With the wide availability of single-photon emission computed tomography (SPECT) cameras and perfusion tracers, SPECT is currently the preferred imaging modality of cardiac radionuclide imaging with good diagnostic accuracy and prognostic significance.

PET provides better image quality because of higher spatial resolution, less scatter, and fewer attenuation artifacts and may be superior to SPECT with respect to imaging quality, interpretative confidence, and inter-reader agreement. In addition, PET allows quantitative measurement of myocardial perfusion (MP) and metabolism. Cardiac PET with perfusion tracers, such as $[^{15}O]$-water, $[^{13}N]$-ammonia, ^{82}rubidium, and $[^{18}F]$-flurpiridaz [2], allows noninvasive and absolute assessment of regional and global myocardial blood flow (MBF) in ml/min/g. In conjunction with stress, regional and global coronary flow reserve (CFR) can also be calculated, which is the ratio between MBF at peak stress and MBF at rest.

CFR measures not only vasodilator capacity but also endothelial reactivity of the coronary circulation, allowing noninvasive quantitative assessment for patients with diffuse coronary luminal narrowing or microvascular dysfunction.

Coronary microvascular dysfunction is highly prevalent among at-risk individuals and is associated with adverse outcomes regardless of sex, even in the absence of overt coronary atherosclerosis [3]. It may reflect the functional alteration of endothelium, such as hypertension, dyslipidemia, diabetes mellitus, smoking, obesity, or metabolic syndrome, or structural alteration of microangiopathy, myocardial fibrosis, or loss of capillaries. The portion of HF consists predominantly of older age and high prevalence of comorbidities. The systemic pro-inflammatory state may induce coronary endothelial inflammation, microvascular dysfunction, myocardial substrate shift, myocardial and interstitial fibrosis that contribute to high diastolic left ventricular stiffness, and HF development, even with preserved LVEF. The potential roles of myocardial perfusion abnormalities in subjects with cardiovascular risks, metabolic disease, and HF warrant further investigations.

In patients with CAD, a reduced CFR was shown to have prognostic implications, being a more sensitive predictor for cardiac death than was reduced left ventricular ejection fraction (LVEF). CFR in patients with CAD was found to be also reduced in areas supplied by non-stenotic vessels, suggesting a microvascular component. A recent study showed an association between global CFR and major adverse cardiovascular events (MACE) independently of angiographic CAD prognostic index (CADPI) [4]. This may attribute to diffuse atherosclerosis or microvascular dysfunction. In addition, global CFR also modified the effect of coronary revascularization in terms of event-free survival. These emphasize the utility of cardiac PET in patient risk stratification and the role in decision-making for coronary revascularization.

13.1.2 Transplant Vasculopathy

Cardiac allograft vasculopathy (CAV) is one of the leading causes of late mortality after heart transplantation. It is characterized by the diffuse concentric intima thickening of both epicardial and intramyocardial arteries, which is difficult to be assessed by traditional coronary angiogram. Intravascular ultrasound (IVUS) has been proposed to be the most sensitive method for diagnosis of early CAV. Due to the progressive and diffuse process involving the epicardial and microvascular coronary system, traditional stress myocardial perfusion SPECT frequently underestimates disease severity and extent in patients with CAV. With the absolute-quantitative nature, PET provides a noninvasive way to deal with this problem. A good correlation was observed between plaque burden as determined by IVUS and CFR as assessed by ^{13}N-ammonia PET in recipients with normal coronary angiography findings. Quantitative measurement of myocardial flow using dynamic ^{13}N-ammonia PET is thus clinically feasible [5]. A recent study enrolled 140 posttransplant recipients with median follow-up of 18.2 months; the relative perfusion defects, mean myocardial flow reserve, and mean stress MBF using dipyridamole rubidium-82 PET were significant predictors of adverse outcome [6].

13.2 Sympathetic Innervation

Neurohormonal activation is considered as a compensatory mechanism in HF and maintains perfusion to the heart, yet in the meanwhile is also responsible for the progression of HF. From a long-term point of view, it is associated with cardiac remodeling, progressive impairment of ventricular function, symptoms, and lethal arrhythmia. Despite their critical role in regulation of the heart, local neurohormonal statuses of patients are not routinely and closely monitored in clinical practice. Innervation imaging may provide prognostic information as well as guide selection of therapies. Both a decreased cardiac [^{123}I]-meta-iodobenzylguanidine (MIBG) activity and an increased washout rate are indicative of a poor prognosis in patients with chronic heart failure [7]. Several PET tracers, including

[^{11}C]-meta-hydroxyephedrine (HED), a norepinephrine analog, and [^{11}C]-CGP12177, a beta-adrenoceptor antagonist, not only can be used to visualize global but also regional defects in myocardial sympathetic innervation. A pilot study enrolled 10 patients with dilated cardiomyopathy who underwent PET with [^{11}C]-HED before, acutely and 3 months after cardiac resynchronization (CRT) [8]. It showed CRT improves cardiac sympathetic nerve activity in responders and seems to be more effective in those with functionally preserved neuroautonomic system.

Decreased cardiac beta-adrenoceptor density measured by [^{11}C]-CGP12177 PET was observed in a study of patients with nonischemic cardiomyopathy. In addition the receptor density was significantly correlated with systolic function [9]. Receptor density correlated with [^{123}I]-MIBG washout rate and delayed heart-to-mediastinum (H/M) ratio, but not early H/M ratio. Another study showed that reduced myocardial beta-adrenoceptor density measured by [^{11}C]-CGP12177 early after myocardial infarction is associated with the incidence of congestive heart failure on long-term follow-up [10]. Besides [^{11}C]-labeled tracers, [^{18}F]-N-[3-Bromo-4-(3-fluoro-propoxy)-benzyl]-guanidine (LMI1195), an ^{18}F-labeled analog of [^{123}I]-MIBG SPECT agent, is a new PET tracer retained in the heart through the norepinephrine transporter (NET) and allowing evaluation of the cardiac sympathetic neuronal function by PET imaging [11–13].

13.3 Noninvasive Assessment of Myocardial Metabolism

13.3.1 Myocardial Viability

Myocardial viability, the evaluation of dysfunctional but viable myocardium, can be assessed by several imaging techniques. In conjunction with dobutamine, contractile reserve can be evaluated by either echocardiography or cardiac magnetic resonance imaging (MRI). Delayed contrast-enhanced (DCE) MRI and contrast-enhanced CT can assess scar tissue. Myocardial perfusion SPECT evaluates either cell membrane or mitochondria integrity. [^{18}F]-fluorodeoxyglucose (FDG) can be used to assess glucose metabolism and to differentiate the hibernating myocardium from scar tissue. Dual-isotope simultaneous acquisition (DISA) viability testing, the combination of [^{99m}Tc]-sestamibi and [^{18}F]-FDG SPECT, provides more accurate prediction of post-revascularization functional recovery than thallium-201 [14]. PET using FDG remains the most reliable and noninvasive tool to assess myocardial viability [15] and tends to replace Tl-201 SPECT imaging in centers equipped with a PET/CT camera.

For patients with CAD-associated chronic LV dysfunction, noninvasive detection of myocardial viability is crucial for decision-making of the treatment. Myocardial viability imaging can be used to inform the often difficult clinical decision regarding revascularization in patients with CAD and left ventricular systolic dysfunction, providing data on the potential benefit to balance against the known risks [15]. FDG PET has a higher sensitivity than DCE MRI, but comparable specificity, in predicting functional recovery [16]. The post hoc subgroup analysis of the PET and Recovery Following Revascularization (PARR-2) trial suggested that FDG PET-guided management reduces the composite of cardiovascular events in patients with ischemic cardiomyopathy in a center with an experienced imaging team [17].

Despite that several studies have emphasized the utility of viability imaging in identifying patients who may benefit from revascularization, a recent meta-analysis shows confusing results [18]. Patients with viable myocardium appear to benefit from revascularization, but the same benefits were observed in patients without viable myocardium. Some suggested this might be resulted from mixed traditional (SPECT and dobutamine echocardiography) and the advanced (MRI and PET) imaging techniques, but this was still not conclusive [19, 20]. A large prospective randomized trial regarding Alternative Imaging Modalities in Ischemic Heart Failure (AIMI-HF) has conducted in 2013 [21], which will complement the results of the Surgical Treatment for Ischemic Heart Failure (STICH) viability substudy and the PET and PARR-2 trial to answer this unsolved issue.

13.3.2   Cardiac Efficiency

$[^{11}C]$-acetate, a well-known myocardial PET tracer, is directly metabolized into $[^{11}C]$-acetyl-CoA in mitochondria and enters the Krebs cycle. $[^{11}C]$-acetate PET imaging provides noninvasive and reproducible measurements of cardiac oxidative metabolism (MVO_2) [22]. Heterogeneously decreased oxidative metabolism was observed in patients with ischemic and nonischemic cardiomyopathy [23]. In chronic HF MI porcine model, myocardial perfusion and oxygen consumption in the remote non-infarcted myocardium were preserved in HF pigs as compared to controls. Global LV work and efficiency were significantly lower in HF than controls and were associated with increased wall stress [24]. It can also be used to evaluate cardiac efficiency under variable conditions, especially after treatments of heart failure. Surgical intervention with LV volume reduction and mitral regurgitation correction significantly improved cardiac efficiency in patients with end-stage heart failure, which is observed in both nonischemic and ischemic etiologies [25].

On the other hand, myocardial oxygen metabolism was increased in patients with aortic stenosis (AS), which was decreased after aortic valve replacement [26]. It is suggested that the increased myocardial oxidative metabolism in AS was largely attributable to the pressure overload of the left ventricle and normalized after unload.

In a study of diastolic heart failure patients, decreased cardiac efficiency is associated with increased LV filling pressure but does not primarily cause diastolic dysfunction or diastolic heart failure in normal hearts [27]. They suggest that improvement of cardiac efficiency may be a target for the treatment of heart failure with preserved ejection fraction (HFpEF).

13.3.3 Cardiac Resynchronization Therapy (CRT)

CRT can correct cardiac dyssynchrony and augment LV systolic function. PET is the only noninvasive imaging technique that can provide information on alternations of myocardial blood flow, glucose utilization, and oxygen consumption. $[^{11}C]$-acetate PET can also be used to evaluate the efficacy of CRT in patients with severe heart failure [8, 28–31]. CRT could improve cardiac systolic function, but global resting MBF and global MVO_2 are not always altered by CRT, even under stress condition [28]. A more homogeneous myocardial glucose uptake was observed, which implies CRT may induce a more balanced wall stress and energy requirement. Another study demonstrated that decreased oxygen consumption was observed in patients showing good response to CRT. The decrease in oxygen consumption assessed by PET in the early period after CRT is useful to predict improvement of cardiac function and major cardiac events during the first year of follow-up [31].

13.3.4 Chemotherapy-Related Heart Failure

$[^{11}C]$-acetoacetate, a ketone body tracer, is expected to have some similarities to $[^{11}C]$-acetate. In mitochondria, acetoacetate is first converted into acetoacetyl-CoA and then into acetyl-CoA. In cytoplasm, acetoacetate can also be directly incorporated into the lipogenesis pathway. Contrary to $[^{11}C]$-acetate and other MBF PET tracers, $[^{11}C]$-acetoacetate together with dynamic gated PET imaging was able to identify doxorubicin-induced heart failure at an early stage in a resting state. Thus, $[^{11}C]$-acetoacetate is promising for the assessment of cardiomyopathy [32].

13.3.5 Metabolic Therapy

Heart failure severity, substrate availability, hormonal status, and coexisting insulin resistance contribute to the metabolic change. Optimizing myocardial energy metabolism has been studied as a novel form of therapy [33]. Metabolic therapy is a promising new avenue for the treatment of heart failure. Suitable targets for therapy include substrate utilization, oxidative phosphorylation, and the availability of high-energy phosphates [34].

Insulin resistance is a recognized phenomenon leading to heart failure. The change in myocardial metabolism can be visualized using PET with metabolic tracers. A prospective study utilized $[^{15}O]$-water, $[^{11}C]$-acetate, $[^{11}C]$-glucose, and $[^{11}C]$-palmitate PET studies and found that obesity and gender independently modulate MBF and MVO_2. Moreover, gender and obesity may interact in predicting myocardial glucose uptake and insulin sensitivity [35]. FDG PET can also be used in evaluation of the effect of therapy on glucose metabolism. In a transgenic mice model, G protein-coupled receptor kinase 2 inhibition delays the reduction in glucose uptake and protects insulin signaling in the heart, preserving cardiac dimension and function [36].

13.4 Molecular Imaging Approaches of Cardiac Remodeling

13.4.1 Imaging of Matrix Metalloproteinases

The matrix metalloproteinases (MMPs) play a role in physiologic extracellular matrix (ECM) turnover and response to cardiac disease. During the progression of HF, the level of MMPs is increased. The excessive degradation of ECM may result in wall thinning, dilatation, and heart failure. Post-MI myocardial LV remodeling is also associated with changes within the myocardial extracellular matrix and often leads to heart failure. MI results in the activation of the renin-angiotensin-aldosterone system, which in turn results in the activating of MMPs within the heart. Molecular imaging of MMPs has the potential to allow early and serial evaluation of underlying alterations that accompany progression of LV remodeling [37]. The activation of MMPs in infarcted murine myocardium can be imaged by [^{111}In]- and [^{99m}Tc]-labeled single-photon ligands [38]. Several PET tracers have also been synthesized [39]. However, to date there are only limited publications, especially in the field of HF.

13.4.2 Angiogenesis

Angiogenesis occurs in response to ischemia and inflammation being part of the healing process after ischemic tissue injury. [^{18}F]-galacto-RGD allows noninvasive imaging of the expression of $\alpha_v\beta_3$ integrin that is highly expressed in the endothelium of angiogenic vessels. Noninvasive imaging using [^{18}F]-galacto-RGD PET appears promising for the monitoring of therapies aiming to stimulate angiogenesis in ischemic heart disease and preventing the development of HF [40].

13.4.3 Myocardial Inflammation

FDG PET may be useful in the study of inflammatory process since inflammatory cells accumulate glucose. However, a recent study showed some limitations to study the inflammatory process after myocardial infarction even when active uptake of FDG in normal myocardial tissue is suppressed. In the presence of large region of microvascular obstruction, FDG may not reliably and accurately represent the degree of inflammatory cell activity. Even in areas without microvascular obstruction, the degree of inflammation may be underestimated or even overestimated [41].

Besides the usefulness as a molecular target for neuroendocrine tumor imaging, some of the somatostatin receptors are also expressed by activated macrophage. A recent animal study compared [^{68}Ga]-citrate, [^{68}Ga]-DOTATATE, and [^{18}F]-FDG in a postinfarction mouse model [42]. They conclude that FDG with myocardial suppression is the most practical imaging marker of postinfarction inflammation. However, there are also some studies in human that emphasize the usefulness of the somatostatin receptor imaging in the assessment of sarcoidosis [43] and infarction [44]-related myocardial inflammation. Compared with the nonspecific FDG, this is a new potential biomarker that may be useful in evaluation of myocardial inflammation and predicting cardiac remodeling and progression toward heart failure.

13.5   Conclusions

Advances in the application of cardiac PET may play an increasingly critical role in diagnosis, prognosis, and clinical treatment of cardiovascular diseases. Molecular imaging approaches using PET could evaluate myocardial pathophysiology at different stages of HF. It further provides insights on the HF preventive strategies, tracking patients' clinical status, novel drug therapies, expanding indications for HF therapeutic devices, and gene or cell-based therapies (Fig. 13.1 and Table 13.1).

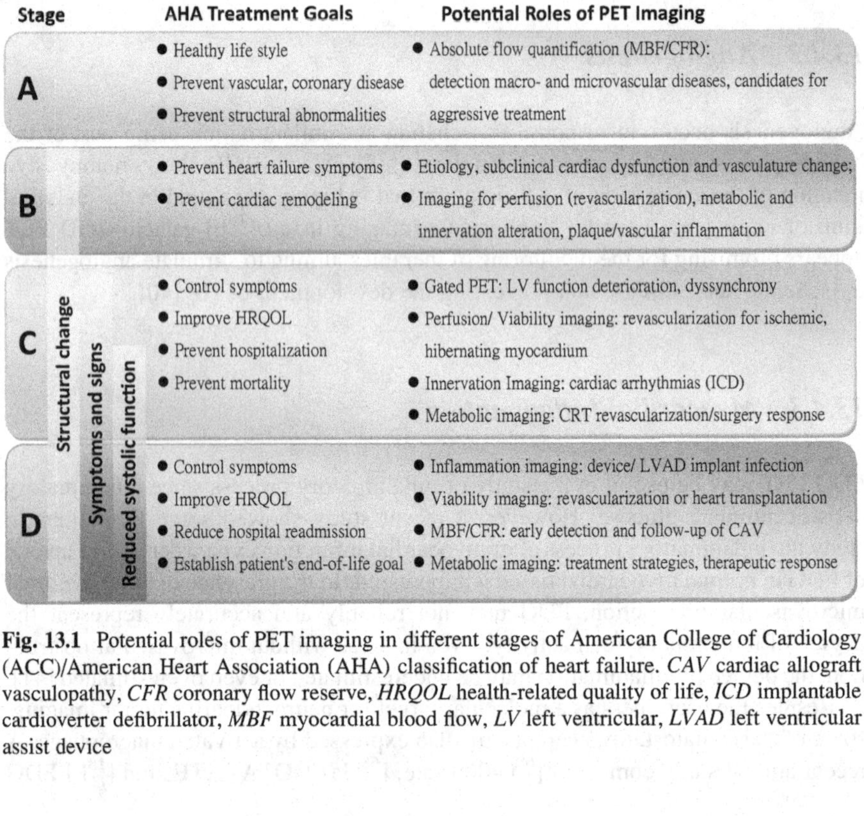

Stage	AHA Treatment Goals	Potential Roles of PET Imaging
A	• Healthy life style • Prevent vascular, coronary disease • Prevent structural abnormalities	• Absolute flow quantification (MBF/CFR): detection macro- and microvascular diseases, candidates for aggressive treatment
B	• Prevent heart failure symptoms • Prevent cardiac remodeling	• Etiology, subclinical cardiac dysfunction and vasculature change; • Imaging for perfusion (revascularization), metabolic and innervation alteration, plaque/vascular inflammation
C	• Control symptoms • Improve HRQOL • Prevent hospitalization • Prevent mortality	• Gated PET: LV function deterioration, dyssynchrony • Perfusion/ Viability imaging: revascularization for ischemic, hibernating myocardium • Innervation Imaging: cardiac arrhythmias (ICD) • Metabolic imaging: CRT revascularization/surgery response
D	• Control symptoms • Improve HRQOL • Reduce hospital readmission • Establish patient's end-of-life goal	• Inflammation imaging: device/ LVAD implant infection • Viability imaging: revascularization or heart transplantation • MBF/CFR: early detection and follow-up of CAV • Metabolic imaging: treatment strategies, therapeutic response

Left margin labels: Structural change | Symptoms and signs | Reduced systolic function

Fig. 13.1 Potential roles of PET imaging in different stages of American College of Cardiology (ACC)/American Heart Association (AHA) classification of heart failure. *CAV* cardiac allograft vasculopathy, *CFR* coronary flow reserve, *HRQOL* health-related quality of life, *ICD* implantable cardioverter defibrillator, *MBF* myocardial blood flow, *LV* left ventricular, *LVAD* left ventricular assist device

Table 13.1 Examples of PET tracers useful in heart failure patients [12, 37, 39]

Substrate	
Glucose	^{18}F-fluorodeoxyglucose
	^{11}C-glucose
Free fatty acid	^{11}C-palmitate
	^{18}F-fluoro-6-thiaheptadecanoic acid
Oxidative metabolism	^{11}C-acetate
Apoptosis	^{18}F-annexin V
Interstitial fibrosis	
Angiotensin-converting enzyme	^{18}F-captopril, ^{18}F-fluorobenzyl-lisinopril
Angiotensin II type 1 receptor	^{11}C-MK-996, ^{11}C-L-159884, ^{11}C-KR31173
Matrix metalloproteinase	^{18}F-FB-ML5
	^{11}C-labeled compounds
Sympathetic innervation	
Presynaptic	^{11}C-meta-hydroxyephedrine (HED)
	^{18}F-fluorodopamine
	^{11}C-epinephrine
	^{11}C-phenylephrine
Postsynaptic	^{11}C-CGP 12177/12388
	^{18}F-fluorocarazolol
Parasympathetic innervation	
Acetylcholine transporter	^{18}F-fluoroethoxybenzovesamicol
Nicotinic receptor	^{18}F-fluoro-A85380
Muscarinic receptor	^{11}C-methylquinuclidiny benzilate

References

1. Yancy CW, Jessup M, Bozkurt B, Butler J, Casey Jr DE, Drazner MH, et al. 2013 ACCF/AHA guideline for the management of heart failure: a report of the American College of Cardiology Foundation/American Heart Association Task Force on Practice Guidelines. J Am Coll Cardiol. 2013;62(16):e147–239. doi:10.1016/j.jacc.2013.05.019.
2. Packard RR, Huang SC, Dahlbom M, Czernin J, Maddahi J. Absolute quantitation of myocardial blood flow in human subjects with or without myocardial ischemia using dynamic

flurpiridaz F 18 PET. J Nucl Med: Off Publ Soc Nucl Med. 2014;55(9):1438–44. doi:10.2967/jnumed.114.141093.

3. Murthy VL, Naya M, Taqueti VR, Foster CR, Gaber M, Hainer J, et al. Effects of sex on coronary microvascular dysfunction and cardiac outcomes. Circulation. 2014;129 (24):2518–27. doi:10.1161/circulationaha.113.008507.

4. Taqueti VR, Hachamovitch R, Murthy VL, Naya M, Foster CR, Hainer J, et al. Global coronary flow reserve is associated with adverse cardiovascular events independently of luminal angiographic severity and modifies the effect of early revascularization. Circulation. 2015;131(1):19–27. doi:10.1161/circulationaha.114.011939.

5. Wu YW, Chen YH, Wang SS, Jui HY, Yen RF, Tzen KY, et al. PET assessment of myocardial perfusion reserve inversely correlates with intravascular ultrasound findings in angiographically normal cardiac transplant recipients. J Nucl Med: Off Publ Soc Nucl Med. 2010;51 (6):906–12. doi:10.2967/jnumed.109.073833.

6. Mc Ardle BA, Davies RA, Chen L, Small GR, Ruddy TD, Dwivedi G, et al. Prognostic value of rubidium-82 positron emission tomography in patients after heart transplant. Circ Cardiovasc Imaging. 2014;7(6):930–7. doi:10.1161/circimaging.114.002184.

7. Kuwabara Y, Tamaki N, Nakata T, Yamashina S, Yamazaki J. Determination of the survival rate in patients with congestive heart failure stratified by (1)(2)(3)I-MIBG imaging: a meta-analysis from the studies performed in Japan. Ann Nucl Med. 2011;25(2):101–7. doi:10.1007/s12149-010-0452-0.

8. Martignani C, Diemberger I, Nanni C, Biffi M, Ziacchi M, Boschi S, et al. Cardiac resynchronization therapy and cardiac sympathetic function. Eur J Clin Investig. 2015;45(8):792–9. doi:10.1111/eci.12471.

9. Tsukamoto T, Morita K, Naya M, Inubushi M, Katoh C, Nishijima K, et al. Decreased myocardial beta-adrenergic receptor density in relation to increased sympathetic tone in patients with nonischemic cardiomyopathy. J Nucl Med: Off Publ Soc Nucl Med. 2007;48 (11):1777–82. doi:10.2967/jnumed.107.043794.

10. Gaemperli O, Liga R, Spyrou N, Rosen SD, Foale R, Kooner JS, et al. Myocardial beta-adrenoceptor down-regulation early after infarction is associated with long-term incidence of congestive heart failure. Eur Heart J. 2010;31(14):1722–9. doi:10.1093/eurheartj/ehq138.

11. Yu M, Bozek J, Lamoy M, Guaraldi M, Silva P, Kagan M, et al. Evaluation of LMI1195, a novel 18F-labeled cardiac neuronal PET imaging agent, in cells and animal models. Circ Cardiovasc Imaging. 2011;4(4):435–43. doi:10.1161/circimaging.110.962126.

12. Werner RA, Rischpler C, Onthank D, Lapa C, Robinson S, Sammnick S, et al. Retention Kinetics of the 18F-labeled Sympathetic Nerve PET Tracer LMI1195: Comparison with 11C-HED and 123I-MIBG. J Nucl Med: Off Publ Soc Nucl Med. 2015. doi:10.2967/jnumed.115.158493.

13. Chen X, Werner RA, Javadi MS, Maya Y, Decker M, Lapa C, et al. Radionuclide imaging of neurohormonal system of the heart. Theranostics. 2015;5(6):545–58. doi:10.7150/thno.10900.

14. Wu YW, Huang PJ, Lee CM, Ho YL, Lin LC, Wang TD, et al. Assessment of myocardial viability using F-18 fluorodeoxyglucose/Tc-99m sestamibi dual-isotope simultaneous acquisition SPECT: comparison with Tl-201 stress-reinjection SPECT. J Nucl Cardiol. 2005;12 (4):451–9. doi:10.1016/j.nuclcard.2005.04.007.

15. Schinkel AF, Poldermans D, Elhendy A, Bax JJ. Assessment of myocardial viability in patients with heart failure. J Nucl Med: Off Publ Soc Nucl Med. 2007;48(7):1135–46. doi:10.2967/jnumed.106.038851.

16. Allman KC, Shaw LJ, Hachamovitch R, Udelson JE. Myocardial viability testing and impact of revascularization on prognosis in patients with coronary artery disease and left ventricular dysfunction: a meta-analysis. J Am Coll Cardiol. 2002;39(7):1151–8.

17. Abraham A, Nichol G, Williams KA, Guo A. deKemp RA, Garrard L et al. 18F-FDG PET imaging of myocardial viability in an experienced center with access to 18F-FDG and integration with clinical management teams: the Ottawa-FIVE substudy of the PARR 2 trial. J Nucl Med: Off Publ Soc Nucl Med. 2010;51(4):567–74. doi:10.2967/jnumed.109.065938.

18. Orlandini A, Castellana N, Pascual A, Botto F, Cecilia Bahit M, Chacon C, et al. Myocardial viability for decision-making concerning revascularization in patients with left ventricular dysfunction and coronary artery disease: a meta-analysis of non-randomized and randomized studies. Int J Cardiol. 2015;182:494–9. doi:10.1016/j.ijcard.2015.01.025.

19. Srichai MB, Jaber WA. Viability by MRI or PET would have changed the results of the STICH trial. Prog Cardiovasc Dis. 2013;55(5):487–93. doi:10.1016/j.pcad.2013.01.005.

20. Asrani NS, Chareonthaitawee P, Pellikka PA. Viability by MRI or PET would not have changed the results of the STICH trial. Prog Cardiovasc Dis. 2013;55(5):494–7. doi:10. 1016/j.pcad.2012.09.004.

21. O'Meara E, Mielniczuk LM, Wells GA. deKemp RA, Klein R, Coyle D et al. Alternative Imaging Modalities in Ischemic Heart Failure (AIMI-HF) IMAGE HF Project I-A: study protocol for a randomized controlled trial. Trials. 2013;14:218. doi:10.1186/1745-6215-14-218.

22. Nesterov SV, Turta O, Han C, Maki M, Lisinen I, Tuunanen H, et al. C-11 acetate has excellent reproducibility for quantification of myocardial oxidative metabolism. Eur Heart J Cardiovasc Imaging. 2015;16(5):500–6. doi:10.1093/ehjci/jeu289.

23. Wu YW, Naya M, Tsukamoto T, Komatsu H, Morita K, Yoshinaga K, et al. Heterogeneous reduction of myocardial oxidative metabolism in patients with ischemic and dilated cardiomyopathy using C-11 acetate PET. Circ J: Off J Jpn Circ Soc. 2008;72(5):786–92.

24. Tarkia M, Stark C, Haavisto M, Kentala R, Vahasilta T, Savunen T, et al. Cardiac remodeling in a new pig model of chronic heart failure: Assessment of left ventricular functional, metabolic, and structural changes using PET, CT, and echocardiography. J Nucl Cardiol. 2015. doi:10.1007/s12350-015-0068-9.

25. Sugiki T, Naya M, Manabe O, Wakasa S, Kubota S, Chiba S, et al. Effects of surgical ventricular reconstruction and mitral complex reconstruction on cardiac oxidative metabolism and efficiency in nonischemic and ischemic dilated cardiomyopathy. J Am Coll Cardiol Img. 2011;4(7):762–70. doi:10.1016/j.jcmg.2011.04.010.

26. Naya M, Chiba S, Iwano H, Yamada S, Katoh C, Manabe O, et al. Myocardial oxidative metabolism is increased due to hemodynamic overload in patients with aortic valve stenosis: assessment using 11C-acetate positron emission tomography. Eur J Nucl Med Mol Imaging. 2010;37(12):2242–8. doi:10.1007/s00259-010-1540-z.

27. Hasegawa S, Yamamoto K, Sakata Y, Takeda Y, Kajimoto K, Kanai Y, et al. Effects of cardiac energy efficiency in diastolic heart failure: assessment with positron emission tomography with 11C-acetate. Hypertens Res. 2008;31(6):1157–62. doi:10.1291/hypres.31.1157.

28. Henneman MM, van der Wall EE, Ypenburg C, Bleeker GB, van de Veire NR, Marsan NA, et al. Nuclear imaging in cardiac resynchronization therapy. J Nucl Med: Off Publ Soc Nucl Med. 2007;48(12):2001–10. doi:10.2967/jnumed.107.040360.

29. Ypenburg C, Bax JJ. The role of positron emission tomography in evaluation of alterations in cardiac efficiency after cardiac resynchronization therapy. J Cardiovasc Electrophysiol. 2008;19(2):133–5. doi:10.1111/j.1540-8167.2007.01032.x.

30. Kitaizumi K, Yukiiri K, Masugata H, Shinomiya K, Ohara M, Takinami H, et al. Positron emission tomographic demonstration of myocardial oxidative metabolism in a case of left ventricular restoration after cardiac resynchronization therapy. Circ J: Off J Jpn Circ Soc. 2008;72(11):1900–3.

31. Kitaizumi K, Yukiiri K, Masugata H, Takinami H, Iwado Y, Noma T, et al. Acute improvement of cardiac efficiency measured by 11C-acetate PET after cardiac resynchronization therapy and clinical outcome. Int J Cardiovasc Imaging. 2010;26(3):285–92. doi:10.1007/s10554-009-9549-8.

32. Croteau E, Tremblay S, Gascon S, Dumulon-Perreault V, Labbe SM, Rousseau JA, et al. [(11)C]-Acetoacetate PET imaging: a potential early marker for cardiac heart failure. Nucl Med Biol. 2014;41(10):863–70. doi:10.1016/j.nucmedbio.2014.08.006.

33. Tuunanen H, Ukkonen H, Knuuti J. Myocardial fatty acid metabolism and cardiac performance in heart failure. Curr Cardiol Rep. 2008;10(2):142–8.

34. Knaapen P, Knuuti J, van Rossum AC. The failing heart. N Engl J Med. 2007;356(24):2545. author reply 6.

35. Peterson LR, Soto PF, Herrero P, Mohammed BS, Avidan MS, Schechtman KB, et al. Impact of gender on the myocardial metabolic response to obesity. J Am Coll Cardiol Img. 2008;1 (4):424–33. doi:10.1016/j.jcmg.2008.05.004.

36. Ciccarelli M, Chuprun JK, Rengo G, Gao E, Wei Z, Peroutka RJ, et al. G protein-coupled receptor kinase 2 activity impairs cardiac glucose uptake and promotes insulin resistance after myocardial ischemia. Circulation. 2011;123(18):1953–62. doi:10.1161/circulationaha.110. 988642.

37. Shirani J, Dilsizian V. Molecular imaging targets of cardiac remodeling. Curr Cardiol Rep. 2009;11(2):148–54.

38. Su H, Spinale FG, Dobrucki LW, Song J, Hua J, Sweterlitsch S, et al. Noninvasive targeted imaging of matrix metalloproteinase activation in a murine model of postinfarction remodeling. Circulation. 2005;112(20):3157–67. doi:10.1161/circulationaha.105.583021.

39. Matusiak N, van Waarde A, Bischoff R, Oltenfreiter R, van de Wiele C, Dierckx RA, et al. Probes for non-invasive matrix metalloproteinase-targeted imaging with PET and SPECT. Curr Pharm Des. 2013;19(25):4647–72.

40. Higuchi T, Bengel FM, Seidl S, Watzlowik P, Kessler H, Hegenloh R, et al. Assessment of alphavbeta3 integrin expression after myocardial infarction by positron emission tomography. Cardiovasc Res. 2008;78(2):395–403. doi:10.1093/cvr/cvn033.

41. Prato FS, Butler J, Sykes J, Keenliside L, Blackwood KJ, Thompson RT, et al. Can the inflammatory response be evaluated using 18F-FDG within zones of microvascular obstruction after myocardial infarction? J Nucl Med: Off Publ Soc Nucl Med. 2015;56(2):299–304. doi:10. 2967/jnumed.114.147835.

42. Thackeray JT, Bankstahl JP, Wang Y, Korf-Klingebiel M, Walte A, Wittneben A, et al. Targeting post-infarct inflammation by PET imaging: comparison of (68)Ga-citrate and (68)Ga-DOTATATE with (18)F-FDG in a mouse model. Eur J Nucl Med Mol Imaging. 2015;42(2):317–27. doi:10.1007/s00259-014-2884-6.

43. Reiter T, Werner RA, Bauer WR, Lapa C. Detection of cardiac sarcoidosis by macrophage-directed somatostatin receptor 2-based positron emission tomography/computed tomography. Eur Heart J. 2015. doi:10.1093/eurheartj/ehv278.

44. Lapa C, Reiter T, Li X, Werner RA, Samnick S, Jahns R, et al. Imaging of myocardial inflammation with somatostatin receptor based PET/CT – A comparison to cardiac MRI. Int J Cardiol. 2015;194:44–9. doi:10.1016/j.ijcard.2015.05.073.

Chapter 14
Emerging Trends and Future Perspective of Novel Cardiac SPECT Technology

Masao Miyagawa, Yoshiko Nishiyama, Hayato Ishimura, Rami Tashiro, Kana Ide, and Teruhito Mochizuki

Abstract In response to concerns about overuse and increasing radiation exposure of myocardial perfusion imaging, nuclear medicine societies have declared statements aimed at lowering its radiation dose and costs. Simultaneously, two vendors have launched novel SPECT scanners with solid-state semiconductor detectors. Discovery NM 530c and D-SPECT utilize the same cadmium zinc telluride (CZT) detectors with a different combination of high-sensitivity multi-pinhole or parallel-hole collimator which focuses on the heart. The physical performance of those is dramatically higher than that of conventional Anger cameras; however, 2 CZT cameras are inherently different.

Although ^{99m}Tc-labeled myocardial perfusion tracers might not be ideal agents, estimation of absolute myocardial blood flow or myocardial flow reserve (MFR) using dynamic CZT SPECT is a challenging subject and attracts a great deal of interest in the field. Thus, novel software which allows automatic calculation of MFR index with dynamic CZT SPECT is currently under development and validated in our institution. This technology will hold promise if the several issues can be solved through future studies.

Keywords Cadmium zinc telluride • Cardiac SPECT • Coronary flow reserve • Effective dose • Dynamic imaging

14.1 Introduction

The overall utilization for stress myocardial perfusion imaging (MPI) reached its height in 2006 with over 10 million studies and Medicare payment over 1 billion dollars [1]. The National Council on Radiation Protection and Measurements

M. Miyagawa, MD, Ph.D. (✉) • Y. Nishiyama, MD, Ph.D. • H. Ishimura, RT •
R. Tashiro, MD, Ph.D. • K. Ide, MD, Ph.D. • T. Mochizuki, MD, Ph.D.
Department of Radiology, Ehime University Graduate School of Medicine, Shitsukawa,
Toon-city, Ehime 791-0295, Japan
e-mail: miyagawa@m.ehime-u.ac.jp

© The Author(s) 2016
Y. Kuge et al. (eds.), *Perspectives on Nuclear Medicine for Molecular Diagnosis and Integrated Therapy*, DOI 10.1007/978-4-431-55894-1_14

reported that since the early 1980s, a six-fold increase in radiation exposure to the US population from medical procedures [2] emphasizes that more than 10 % of the entire radiation burden was related to MPI [3]. In response to these concerns, professional societies have declared statements aimed at lowering its radiation dose and costs [4, 5].

Simultaneously, vendors have developed dedicated cardiac SPECT scanners with solid-state semiconductor detectors in order to do something about radiation dose and long imaging time. Two vendors have introduced novel scanners: Discovery NM 530c, (D530c); GE Healthcare and D-SPECT; and Spectrum Dynamics utilizing the same cadmium zinc telluride (CZT) detectors, with a different combination of high-sensitivity multi-pinhole or parallel-hole collimators which focuses on the myocardium [6, 7]. More than 300 of such cardiac CZT SPECT scanners are currently available in the world, and the number is increasing by more than 100 per year.

Firstly, we focus on the latest advances in MPI procedures which ought to be able to maximize the value of SPECT cameras with CZT detectors. Secondly, we try to develop a novel software for calculating the myocardial flow reserve (MFR) index using these cameras and to validate its utility for screening patients with multi-vessel coronary artery disease (CAD).

14.2   Materials and Methods

Initially, we conducted a comparative study using ^{99m}Tc line-source phantoms with and without photon scattering caused by water in the cylinder [8]. D530c had a more than two-fold spatial resolution than did the conventional Anger camera with a dual detector (Infinia; GE Healthcare). We also found that a D530c has better energy resolution compared to Infinia, which is as narrow as 5 %. Therefore, energy window width could be narrowed enough to be feasible for performing dual radioisotope simultaneous SPECT with ^{99m}Tc-tetrofosmin and ^{123}I-BMIPP [9].

MPI protocol for routine clinical practice of our institution at present is summarized in Fig. 14.1. We adopt a stress-first one-day protocol with ^{99m}Tc-perfusion tracers. CZT camera has a 5-times higher sensitivity; therefore, patients are given an injection of only 3 MBq/kg body weight (4–5 mCi) of ^{99m}Tc-perfusion tracers at peak stress. Supine and prone imaging with 5 min each is routinely performed [10]. Same-day rest imaging was performed after 9 MBq/kg of tracer injection. If we apply a strategy of stress-only protocol to our routine clinical practice, we will get further reduction in the effective radiation dose of patients and higher laboratory throughput.

Dynamic MPI starting with the bolus administration of ^{99m}Tc-perfusion tracers as described above was also performed during adenosine stress and at rest using the CZT camera. We intravenously injected saline followed by radionuclide, using an

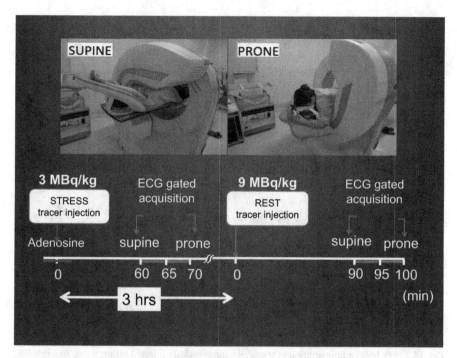

Fig. 14.1 We adopt a stress/rest one-day protocol with Tc-99m perfusion radiotracers. Supine and prone positioning are routinely performed. The total effective dose ranged 3.4–6.7 mSv. Stress-only MPI can be performed with the effective dose averaging 1 mSv

automatic injector at a constant rate of 1 milliliter per second for 30 s (Fig. 14.2). Before dynamic imaging, we carefully detected the border of the heart by chest percussion or test injection of 0.5 mCi of tracers in order to adjust the position of the heart appropriately in the quality field of view [11]. The interval between stress and rest imaging was 3 h and a 30-s pre-scan count was subtracted from the dynamic data at rest. 10-min dynamic SPECT data with list mode acquisition were reconstructed using a maximum likelihood expectation maximization (MLEM) algorithm with 40–50 iterations. We generated 200 3-D volumes integrating 3-s time frames in the course of 600 s. Routine MPI were also acquired thereafter.

The software allows the automatic edge detection of volume of interest for the blood pool in the left ventricle and the myocardium. Global time-activity curves were fitted to a one-tissue two-compartment kinetic model (2-com), a Patlak plot analysis (PPA), and a dose uptake ratio of MPI (DUR) with input function. K1 and K2 were calculated for the stress and rest images. MFR index was calculated as follows: MFR index = K1 stress/K1 at rest.

The validation study included 64 consecutive pts who underwent CZT SPECT and invasive coronary angiography within 2 weeks (35 males, 67 ± 10 years old). 15 pts had single-vessel CAD, and 22 pts had multi-vessel CAD (10 had two-vessel and 12 had three-vessel CAD) and 27 pts with no significant coronary stenosis less than 70 %.

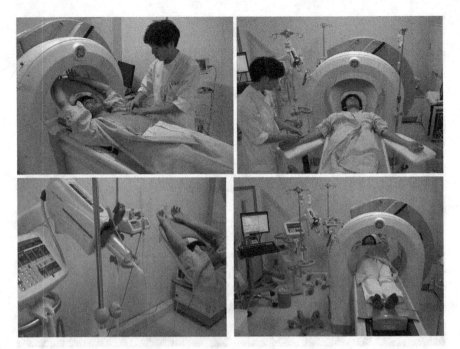

Fig. 14.2 For bolus administration of tracer, we intravenously injected saline, using an automatic injector at a constant rate of 1 milliliter per second for 30 s. We started the dynamic data acquisition just after the bolus injection

14.3 Results and Discussion

14.3.1 Reduction in Injection Dose of Radiopharmaceuticals

The introduction of CZT cameras has opened the possibility of reducing radiation dose of SPECT MPI. Oddstig et al. [12] reported that they performed a 1-day ^{99m}Tc-tetrofosmin stress-rest protocol using D530c in 150 patients who were divided into three subgroups (50 patients in each group) with 4, 3, and 2.5 MBq/kg body weight of administered activity in the stress MPI, respectively. The total effective dose (stress and rest) decreased from 9.3 mSv in the 4 MBq/kg group to 5.8 mSv in the 2.5 MBq/kg group. The image acquisition times for 2.5 MBq/kg were 8 and 5 min (stress and rest, respectively) compared to 15 min for each when using conventional SPECT. The average image quality for the stress and the rest showed no statistically significant difference among the 4, 3, and 2.5 MBq/kg groups.

Starting the MPS protocol with examination at stress and analyzing the stress images before deciding of the need for rest examination (i.e., to say "stress-only protocol") reduce the effective dose [13, 14]. The effective dose was no more than 1.4 mSv for a patient receiving 2.5 MBq/kg, who underwent the stress-only protocol. The total effective radiation dose ranged 3 to 6 mSv with the stress-rest protocol in our institution. If applied, stress-only protocol would be performed with the effective dose averaging 1 mSv. Novel CZT technology can considerably decrease the effective dose for MPI with preserved high image quality.

Moreover, the high sensitivity of D530c allows for a shorter acquisition time; actually, 5 min is sufficient for QGS in the clinical setting. Although CZT detectors are higher in cost, they have been shown to provide an eight- to ten-fold increase in sensitivity, coupled with a two-fold improvement in spatial resolution, and higher energy resolution enabling a significant reduction in imaging time and dose of isotopes and a dual radionuclide simultaneous SPECT with ^{99m}Tc and ^{123}I [6, 7].

Imbert et al. also conducted analyses of phantom and human SPECT images, comparing the D530c and D-SPECT CZT cameras with Anger cameras, and reported that the physical performance of CZT cameras is dramatically higher than that of Anger cameras; however, 2 CZT cameras are inherently different. Spatial resolution and contrast-to-noise ratio are better with the Discovery NM 530c, whereas detection sensitivity is markedly higher with the D-SPECT [15].

14.3.2   Attempts to Estimate Coronary Flow Reserve Using CZT SPECT

At present, coronary flow reserve (CFR) has been mostly replaced by FFR primarily due to its technical simplicity in the catheterization lab. In contrast, in the noninvasive field, PET-derived CFR is an emerging index used for improving both the diagnosis and risk stratification in patients with suspected CAD. And with the increased use, reliable evidences have been suggested that CFR is a powerful independent predictor of cardiac events and mortality [16–19].

In parallel to the work on these PET studies, some studies have continuously reported that using first-pass planar scintigraphy in humans [20–24] or dynamic SPECT in animals [25] provides evidences that the estimates of CFR can be also derived from conventional SPECT MPI. Although fair agreements have been noted between CFR estimated by SPECT and PET or intracoronary Doppler flow studies, they also highlighted the limitations of conventional gamma camera for the dynamic data collection during rapidly changing radiotracer concentrations [26].

The CZT cameras provide higher temporal and spatial resolution. Dynamic SPECT imaging during the first pass of a tracer was attained with the use of these cameras. From the list data, time-activity curves (TAC) would be generated for the left ventricular cavity (input function) and for myocardial tissue (output function) during stress and rest. Ben-Haim et al. [27] firstly reported the feasibility of dynamic ^{99m}Tc-MIBI SPECT and quantitation of global and regional CFRs using the D-SPECT. They calculated CFR index as the ratio of the stress and rest K1 values. Global CFR index was higher in patients with normal MPI than in patients

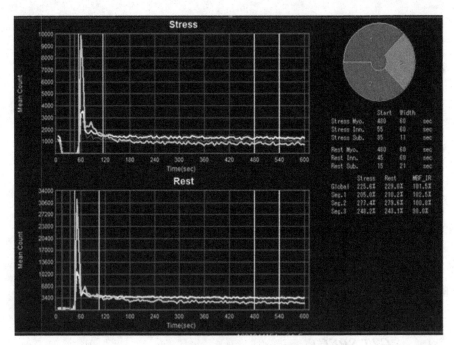

Fig. 14.3 Dynamic acquisition images were transferred to a workstation for analysis using a novel software. It allows an automatic definition of a volume of interest (VOI) for the blood pool in the left ventricle and the left ventricular myocardium. The time-activity curve (TAC) can be extracted by averaging the signal intensity in the VOI in each time frame and then expressed in counts per mm^3/s

with abnormal MPI. The CFR index was lower in territories supplied by stenotic coronary arteries than in non-stenotic arteries.

Novel software is currently under development in our institution [28]. TACs by dynamic ^{99m}Tc-tetrofosmin SPECT using the D530c during adenosine stress and rest are shown in Fig. 14.3. TAC can be extracted by averaging the signal intensity in the volume of interest (VOI) in each time frame and then expressed in counts per cubic mm^3/s. Global TAC was fitted to a 2-com model with input functions which was served by the blood pool curves. In the validation study, Global MFR index estimated by the 2-com model is significantly lower in patients with multi-vessel disease, than those without the disease. In addition, MFR index in the segments of vascular territories with significant coronary stenosis is significantly lower than those without coronary stenosis.

Most recently, Wells et al. applied the D530c to a study with a pig model for quantitation of absolute myocardial blood flow (MBF) using common perfusion tracers as ^{99m}Tc-MIBI, ^{99m}Tc-tetrofosmin, and thallium-201 [29]. Dynamic images were reconstructed with CT-based attenuation correction and energy window-based scatter correction and then processed with kinetic analysis using a 1-tissue 2-com model to obtain the uptake rate constant K1 as a function of microsphere MBF. Converting K1 back to MBF using the measured extraction fractions produced accurate values and good correlations with microsphere MBF. They have demonstrated that dynamic SPECT by the CZT camera may be feasible to estimate absolute MBF.

14.3.3 Advantages and Disadvantages of the Measurement of CFR with SPECT

At the current moment, PET plays a major role in accurate estimation of MBF or CFR. However, it has limited value for routine clinical studies because of its higher cost and more complicated procedures, including the production of short-half-lived positron tracers by in-house cyclotrons. Therefore, the advantage of SPECT-measured technique utilizing common technetium-99 m perfusion tracers is that it would increase the utility of CFR measurement in the clinical setting with a much smaller financial cost.

On the other hand, the disadvantage of quantifying CFR with SPECT may be the underestimation of the CFR value, compared to that with PET. The reasons for this underestimation could be mainly due to the limited extraction of technetium-99 m perfusion tracers at high flow rates, at which the extraction of the tracer becomes limited by membrane transport [26].

14.4 Conclusions

We need to explore patient-centered, radiation exposure-controlled, and appropriately designed protocols which do not sacrifice image quality or diagnostic accuracy of the new modality. Although ^{99m}Tc-labeled radiotracers might not be ideal flow agents, estimation of absolute MBF or CFR using dynamic CZT SPECT is challenging and of great interest. This technology will hold great promise if the several issues can be solved through future studies.

References

1. McNulty EJ, Hung Y, Almers LM, Go AS, Yeh RW. Population trends from 2000–2011 in nuclear myocardial perfusion imaging use. JAMA. 2014;311:1248–9.
2. National Council on Radiation Protection and Measurements. Report No. 160, Ionizing Radiation Exposure of the Population of the United States: National Council on Radiation Protection and Measurements; 2009.
3. Einstein AJ. Effects of radiation exposure from cardiac imaging: how good are the data? J Am Coll Cardiol. 2012;59:553–65.
4. Cerqueira MD, Allman KC, Ficaro EP, et al. Recommendations for reducing radiation exposure in myocardial perfusion imaging. J Nucl Cardiol. 2010;17:709–18.
5. DePuey EG, Mahmarian JJ, Miller TD, et al. Patient-centered imaging, ASNC Preferred Practice Statement. J Nucl Cardiol. 2012;19:185–215.
6. Bocher M, Blevis IM, Tsukerman L, Shrem Y, Kovalski G, Volokh L. A fast cardiac gamma camera with dynamic SPECT capabilities: design, system validation and future potential. Eur J Nucl Med Mol Imaging. 2010;37:1887–902.
7. Patton J, Slomka P, Germano G, Berman D. Recent technologic advances in nuclear cardiology. J Nucl Cardiol. 2007;14:501–13.
8. Takahashi Y, Miyagawa M, Nishiyama Y, Ishimura H, Mochizuki T. Performance of a semiconductor SPECT system: comparison with a conventional Anger-type SPECT instrument. Ann Nucl Med. 2013;27:11–6.
9. Takahashi Y, Miyagawa M, Nishiyama Y, Kawaguchi N, Ishimura H, Mochizuki T. Dual radioisotopes simultaneous SPECT of ^{99m}Tc-tetrofosmin and ^{123}I-BMIPP using a semiconductor detector. Asia Oceania J Nucl Med Biol. 2014;3:43–9.
10. Nishiyama Y, Miyagawa M, Kawaguchi N, et al. Combined supine and prone myocardial perfusion single-photon emission computed tomography with a cadmium zinc telluride camera for detection of coronary artery disease. Circ J. 2014;78:1169–75.
11. Hindorf C, Oddstig J, Hedeer F, Hansson MJ, Jögi J, Engblom H. Importance of correct patient positioning in myocardial perfusion SPECT when using a CZT camera. J Nucl Cardiol. 2014;21:695–702.
12. Oddstig J, Hedeer F, Jogi J, Carlsson M, Hindorf C, Engblom H. Reduced administered activity, reduced acquisition time, and preserved image quality for the new CZT camera. J Nucl Cardiol. 2013;20:38–44.
13. Duvall WL, Wijetunga MN, Klein TM, et al. Stress-only Tc-99m myocardial perfusion imaging in an Emergency Department Chest Pain Unit. J Emerg Med. 2011;42:642–50.
14. Einstein AJ, Johnson LL, DeLuca AJ, et al. Radiation dose and prognosis of ultra-low-dose stress-first myocardial perfusion SPECT in patients with chest pain using a high-efficiency camera. J Nucl Med. 2015;56:545–51.
15. Imbert L, Poussier S, Franken PR, et al. Compared performance of high-sensitivity cameras dedicated to myocardial perfusion SPECT: a comprehensive analysis of phantom and human images. J Nucl Med. 2012;53:1897–903.
16. Yoshinaga K, Chow BJ, Williams K, et al. What is the prognostic value of myocardial perfusion imaging using rubidium-82 positron emission tomography? J Am Coll Cardiol. 2006;48:1029–39.
17. Herzog BA, Husmann L, Valenta I, et al. Long-term prognostic value of ^{13}N ammonia myocardial perfusion positron emission tomography added value of coronary flow reserve. J Am Coll Cardiol. 2009;54:150–6.
18. Murthy VL, Naya M, Foster CR, et al. Improved cardiac risk assessment with noninvasive measures of coronary flow reserve. Circulation. 2011;124:2215–24.
19. Naya M, Murthy VL, Taqueti VR, et al. Preserved coronary flow reserve effectively excludes high-risk coronary artery disease on angiography. J Nucl Med. 2014;55:248–55.

20. Taki J, Fujino S, Nakajima K, et al. Tc-99m retention characteristics during pharmacological hyperemia in human myocardium: comparison with coronary flow reserve measured by Doppler flowire. J Nucl Med. 2001;42:1457–63.
21. Sugihara H, Yonekura Y, Kataoka K, Fukai D, Kitamura N, Taniguchi Y. Estimation of coronary flow reserve with the use of dynamic planar and SPECT images of Tc-99m tetrofosmin. J Nucl Cardiol. 2001;8:575–9.
22. Ito Y, Katoh C, Noriyasu K, et al. Estimation of myocardial blood flow and myocardial flow reserve by 99mTc-sestamibi imaging: comparison with the results of O-15 H_2O PET. Eur J Nucl Med Mol Imaging. 2003;30:281–7.
23. Storto G, Cirillo P, Vicario ML, et al. Estimation of coronary flow reserve by Tc-99m sestamibi imaging in patients with coronary artery disease: comparison with the results of intracoronary Doppler technique. J Nucl Cardiol. 2004;11:682–8.
24. Daniele S, Nappi C, Acampa W, et al. Incremental prognostic value of coronary flow reserve assessed with single-photon emission computed tomography. J Nucl Cardiol. 2011;18:612–9.
25. Iida H, Eberl S, Kim KM, et al. Absolute quantitation of myocardial blood flow with ^{201}Tl and dynamic SPECT in canine: optimization and validation of kinetic modeling. Eur J Nucl Med Mol Imaging. 2008;35:896–905.
26. Petretta M, Soricelli A, Storto G, Cuocolo A. Assessment of coronary flow reserve using single photon emission computed tomography with technetium 99m-labeled tracers. J Nucl Cardiol. 2008;15:456–65.
27. Ben-Haim S, Murthy VL, Breault C, et al. Quantification of myocardial perfusion reserve using dynamic SPECT imaging in humans: a feasibility study. J Nucl Med. 2013;54:873–9.
28. Miyagawa M, Nishiyama Y, Kawaguchi N, et al. Estimation of myocardial flow reserve using a cadmium-zinc telluride (CZT) SPECT in patients with multi-vessel coronary artery disease. J Nucl Med 2013:54;Supplement 157P.
29. Wells RG, Timmins R, Klein R, et al. Dynamic SPECT measurement of absolute myocardial blood flow in a porcine model. J Nucl Med. 2014;55:1685–91.

Chapter 15
Right Ventricular Metabolism and Its Efficiency

Clinical Aspects and Future Directions

Keiichiro Yoshinaga, Hiroshi Ohira, Ichizo Tsujino, Osamu Manabe, Takahiro Sato, Chietsugu Katoh, Katsuhiko Kasai, Yuuki Tomiyama, Masaharu Nishimura, and Nagara Tamaki

Abstract *Background*: Elevated pulmonary arterial pressure may increase right ventricular (RV) oxidative metabolism in patients with pulmonary hypertension (PH) and heart failure (HF). [11]C- acetate positron emission tomography (PET) can be used to measure RV oxidative metabolism noninvasively. The combination of RV oxidative metabolism and cardiac work, as estimated by cardiac magnetic resonance imaging (CMR), indicates RV efficiency and can provide new insights. However, the clinical importance of these markers has not been fully studied. The purpose of this study was to investigate the possible impacts of these markers in patients with PH through ^{11}C-acetate PET.

Methods: Ventricular function was assessed using magnetic resonance imaging (MRI). Dynamic ^{11}C-acetate PET was used to simultaneously measure RV and

K. Yoshinaga, MD, Ph.D., FACC (✉)
Department of Nuclear Medicine, Hokkaido University Graduate School of Medicine, Kita15 Nishi7, Kita-Ku, Sapporo 060-8638, Hokkaido, Japan

Molecular Imaging Research Center, National Institute of Radiological Sciences, 4-9-1 Anagawa, Inage-Ku, Chiba 263-8555, Japan
e-mail: kyoshi@nirs.go.jp

H. Ohira, MD, Ph.D. • I. Tsujino, MD, Ph.D. • T. Sato, MD, Ph.D. • M. Nishimura, MD, Ph.D.
First Department of Medicine, Hokkaido University Graduate School of Medicine, Sapporo, Japan

O. Manabe, MD, Ph.D. • Y. Tomiyama, MSc
Department of Nuclear Medicine, Hokkaido University Graduate School of Medicine, Sapporo, Japan

C. Katoh, MD, Ph.D. • K. Kasai, MSc
Hokkaido University Graduate School of Health Sciences, Sapporo, Japan

N. Tamaki, MD, Ph.D.
Department of Nuclear Medicine, Hokkaido University Graduate School of Medicine, Sapporo, Japan

Department of Nuclear Medicine, Graduate School of Medicine, Hokkaido University, Sapporo, Japan

Y. Kuge et al. (eds.), *Perspectives on Nuclear Medicine for Molecular Diagnosis and Integrated Therapy*, DOI 10.1007/978-4-431-55894-1_15

left ventricular (LV) oxidative metabolism (k_{mono}). The RV myocardial work per oxygen consumption index was calculated as follows: [RV stroke volume index (SVI)/RV k_{mono}]. PH patients who had additional or increased doses of PH-specific vasodilator(s), based on the joint guidelines of the European Society of Cardiology (ESC) and European Respiratory Society (ERS) for the diagnosis and management of PH, were compared with five PH patients who had no treatment modification (control group).

Results: PH patients showed higher RV k_{mono} than did controls ($P < 0.05$). RV oxidative metabolism was correlated with the mean pulmonary arterial pressure (mPAP) ($r = 0.44$, $P = 0.021$), pulmonary vascular resistance (PVR) ($R = 0.56$, $P = 0.002$), and brain natriuretic peptide (BNP) ($R = 0.42$, $P = 0.029$). Members of the PH therapy group had reduced RV oxidative metabolism ($P = 0.002$) and improved RV work/oxygen consumption index ($P < 0.001$).

Conclusions: RV oxidative metabolism increased as the correlation between mPAP and PVR increased. PH-specific treatments reduced RV oxidative metabolism. Therefore, RV metabolism and its efficiency can provide new pathophysiological insights and will be a new therapeutic marker in patients with PH.

Keywords Metabolism • Pulmonary hypertension • Right ventricle • Tomography

15.1 Introduction

The right ventricle (RV) is the anterior cardiac chamber located just behind the sternum. The RV receives systemic venous return and pumps it into the pulmonary arteries [1]. Under normal conditions, the RV requires little energy to pump venous blood to the pulmonary arteries since pulmonary circulation has a much lower vascular resistance than does systemic circulation [2]. The RV therefore usually has low oxygen consumption.

Until recently, most cardiology research was concerned with left ventricle (LV) physiologies and pathologies. In fact, in the early twentieth century, some groups hypothesized that human circulation could be maintained without RV function [3]. However, cardiovascular surgeons recognized the importance of RV function, and RV dysfunction appeared to be associated with major cardiovascular events in heart failure (HF) [4]. In addition, development of state-of-the-art cardiovascular imaging modalities such as echocardiography, cardiac magnetic resonance (CMR) imaging, and positron emission tomography (PET) have made it possible to noninvasively evaluate the functional and physiological characteristics of RV myocardium [5, 6]. Based on this background, research on the RV has progressed intensively in recent years.

One of the major causes of RV dysfunction is pulmonary hypertension (PH). PH is categorized into five groups as follows: Group 1, pulmonary artery hypertension (PAH); Group 2, PH with LV disease; Group 3, PH associated with lung disease and/or hypoxia; Group 4, PH due to chronic thrombosis and/or embolism; and Group 5, miscellaneous [7]. Elevated pulmonary arterial pressure (PAP) and pulmonary vascular resistance (PVR) may induce RV dysfunction in patients with PH

[7]. However, the RV has a high capacity to adapt to pressure or volume overload before failing in its function [8]. Before myocardial fibrosis and RV heart failure develop, moderate to severe PH often leads to initial RV adaptation [9]. Given the increased arterial pressure in pulmonary circulation, the RV may require a significant power output in response to increased afterload, and this may increase the demand for oxygen in the RV [10]. In this circumstance, the RV may require improved mechanical efficiency in order to increase the power output. A study by Wong et al. showed that idiopathic PH with RV dysfunction was associated with increased RV myocardial oxygen consumption (MVO_2) and reduced RV efficiency [11], a situation possibly mirroring the case of LV energetics in heart failure [12–14]. However, the study by Wong et al. lacked control subjects [11]. Yoshinaga et al. evaluated the RV oxidative metabolism in patients with PH and showed that patients with PH had increased oxidative metabolism in comparison with that of normal individuals [15]. Increasing RV oxidative metabolism was associated with several prognostic markers such as mean PAP (mPAP), PVR, and brain natriuretic peptide (BNP). These findings suggest that elevated RV oxidative metabolism may be a prognostic marker.

[11]C-acetate PET is a noninvasive technique for measuring regional and global myocardial oxidative metabolism [13, 16–19], which is correlated with tricarboxylic acid cycle flux and MVO_2 [16]. RV myocardial oxidative metabolism can also be measured noninvasively using ^{11}C-acetate PET [15, 17, 20–22]. HF therapies such as beta-blockers that reduce MVO_2 are considered to improve the survival of patients with HF [23]. LV cardiac efficiency can be estimated noninvasively [12] by combining the mechanical work with the oxidative metabolism as measured by ^{11}C-acetate PET. This form of LV efficiency measurement has been applied to evaluate several new HF treatments including beta-blockers, cardiac resynchronized therapy, surgical reconstruction therapy, and obstructive sleep apnea (OSA) syndrome treatments [13, 14, 24–26].

PH-specific vasodilators such as endothelin receptor antagonists, phosphodiesterase-5 inhibitors, and prostacyclin decrease pulmonary arterial pressure [7, 27]. These new vasodilators indeed improve survival in PH patients. Oikawa et al. reported that reducing mPAP through the use of epoprostenol was associated with reduced RV glucose metabolism observed by ^{18}F-fluorodeoxyglucose (FDG) PET [28]. However, it is not clear whether such a treatment favorably affects RV myocardial oxidative metabolism.

The purpose of this study was to investigate the possible impacts of the intensified PH-specific vasodilator therapy on myocardial energetics using ^{11}C-acetate PET.

15.2   Materials and Methods

15.2.1   Study Subjects

Study subjects were recruited from the first department of medicine at the Hokkaido University Hospital. The patient inclusion criteria were as follows: (1) a resting mPAP ≥ 25 mmHg and a pulmonary capillary wedge pressure (PCWP) $\leq$

15 mmHg [7], (2) symptoms of PH in accordance with World Health Organization (WHO) functional class II or III, (3) PH subtypes chronic thromboembolic pulmonary hypertension (CTEPH) or PAH [29], and (4) stable condition (unchanged for > 4 weeks).

Exclusion criteria were secondary PH due to LV disease, unstable condition of patients, and permanent pacemaker implantation.

The study was approved by the Hokkaido University Graduate School of Medicine Human Research Ethics Board. Written informed consent was obtained from all patients.

15.2.2 Experimental Protocol

14 PH patients underwent right heart catheterization. Precapillary PH was diagnosed based on a mPAP $\geq$ 25 mmHg at rest and a PCWP $\leq$ 15 mmHg [7]. Among the 14 PH patients, nine patients started or added the PH-specific vasodilators based on the combined guidelines of the European Society of Cardiology (ESC) and the European Respiratory Society (ERS), and these nine patients were categorized as the intensified treatment group [30]. The remaining five patients did not change their treatments and served as a control group.

Within 7 days of right heart catheterization, all patients underwent blood sampling, CMR, and ^{11}C-acetate PET at rest on the same day [15]. CMR and ^{11}C-acetate PET were repeated after 10.7 ± 6.5 months for the intensified treatment group (Fig. 15.1). Patients with PH but without OSA served as the control group

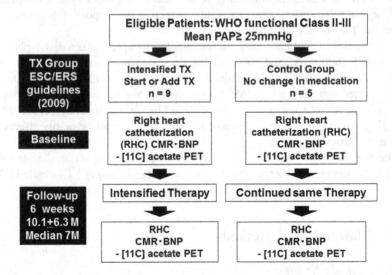

Fig. 15.1 Study design of the current study. *BNP* brain natriuretic peptide, *CMR* cardiac magnetic resonance, *RHC* right heart catheterization, *TX* treatment

and underwent CMR and ^{11}C-acetate PET at rest at baseline and after 10.6 ± 6.3 months $(P = NS)$.

WHO functional class evaluation and blood tests including BNP were measured at baseline and follow-up.

15.2.3 Right Heart Catheterization

A complete hemodynamic evaluation was performed in all PH patients using the standard technique for right heart catheterization. The hemodynamic measurements included mean right atrial pressure, mPAP, and mean PCWP. Cardiac output was determined through thermodilution. PVR was calculated as (mPAP – mean PCWP) divided by cardiac output.

15.2.4 Measurements of BNP

Blood samples were obtained for fasting conditions the morning before the PET studies. BNP data were obtained for all patients. Plasma BNP was measured using immunoradiometric assay [31].

15.2.5 Cardiac Magnetic Resonance Imaging

CMR imaging studies were performed using a 1.5-T Achieva magnetic resonance imaging system (Philips Medical Systems, Best, the Netherlands) equipped with master gradients (maximum gradient amplitude 33 mT/m and maximum slew rate 100 mT/m/msec). CMR data acquisition was performed on patients in the supine position with breath-holding in expiration. We used a five-element cardiac phased-array coil and a vector cardiographic method for electrocardiogram (ECG)-gating images. We performed localizing scans with breath-hold cine imaging and axial orientation. Coronal images were used for cardiac anatomy evaluation. CMR images spanned from bronchial bifurcation to diaphragm level thus allowing for whole-heart analysis. We obtained 12 short-axis cine slices during a steady-state free precession pulse sequence. The precession pulse sequence was as follows: repetition time $= 2.8$ msec, echo time $= 1.4$ msec, flip angle $= 60$, acquisition matrix $= 192 \times 256$, field of view $= 380$ mm, slice thickness $= 10$ mm, inter-slice gap $= 0$ mm, and phases/cardiac cycle $= 20$ [32].

15.2.6 CMR Data Analysis

CMR images were analyzed using commercially available software (Extended MR Work Space: version 2.6.3, Philips Medical Systems, Amsterdam, the Netherlands). RV and LV volumes were measured using cine long-axis images. RV and LV endocardial borders were semiautomatically traced. We then calculated the RV ejection fraction (EF), LVEF, and RV volumes using this information [15]. RVEF was measured in transverse (axial) orientation. LVEF was measured in short-axial orientation [33]. All CMR images were analyzed by clinicians blinded to the clinical and imaging data.

15.2.7 Positron Emission Tomography

All patients were instructed to fast overnight. PH patients who had vasodilator treatments took their morning medications before the PET and CMR studies. Patients were positioned with the heart centered in the field of view in a whole-body PET scanner (ECAT HR+, Siemens/CTI Knoxville, TN) [34]. Dynamic PET acquisition was initiated (10×10 s (s); 2×30s; 5×100 s; 3×180 s; 2×300 s) [14] followed by intravenous administration of 20 mCi (mCi) [740 megabecquerel (MBq)] ^{11}C-acetate.

15.2.8 ^{11}C-Acetate PET Data Analysis

The reconstructed dynamic PET images were analyzed by applying a region of interest over the whole LV and free wall of the RV myocardium in 3–5 mid-ventricular transaxial planes [15, 20, 26]. A mono-exponential function was fit to the myocardial time-activity data. The clearance rate constant (k_{mono}) was determined as described previously [13, 14, 34]. The mono-exponential fit began at the point when the blood pool was stable (usually 2–4 min after injection) (Fig. 15.2).

All data were analyzed by clinicians blinded to the clinical and imaging data.

15.2.9 RV Work Per MVO₂ Index Calculation

The ^{11}C-acetate clearance data were combined with the stroke work data to derive myocardial efficiency using the LV work metabolic index (WMI) using the following equation [13, 14, 26].

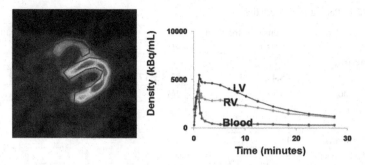

Fig. 15.2 Example of left and right myocardial time-activity data from a ^{11}C-acetate PET acquisition. A mono-exponential function fit to the myocardial clearance yields a clearance rate constant; k_{mono} represents the rate of oxidative metabolism and reflects MVO$_2$. Blue line represents left ventricular (LV) myocardium time-activity curve. Orange line represents right ventricular (RV) myocardium time-activity curve. Red line indicates blood time-activity curve

WMI $=$ SVI $\times$ SBP $\times$ HR/k_{mono}; where SVI is the stroke volume index determined by CMR, SBP is systolic blood pressure, HR is heart rate, and k_{mono} is the mono-exponential rate constant for ^{11}C-acetate clearance from the myocardium.

As a modified LV work metabolic index equation, the RV work per MVO$_2$ index was calculated as the ratio of RV SVI measured by CMR divided by RV MVO$_2$. The equation was as follows [35]:

$$RV \text{ work per MVO}_2 \text{ index} = RV \text{ SVI} / RV \text{ } k_{mono} \times RV \text{ mass} \times 20$$

15.2.10   Statistical Analysis

Continuous variables (using a logarithmic transformation on skewed distributions as appropriate) are presented as mean and standard deviations. Categorical variables are presented as frequencies with percentages. Differences in results for the PH group and the control group were examined for statistical significance with a two-sample t-test for continuous variables. A P value of less than 0.05 was considered indicative of a statistically significant difference. Statistical calculations were carried out using SAS software version 9.2 (SAS Institute, Inc., Cary, NC).

15.3   Results

15.3.1   Patient Characteristics

A total of 14 WHO functional class II or III PH patients were prospectively enrolled in the study between December 2009 and July 2011, and all PH patients completed the study protocol.

Table 15.1 Patient characteristics

	Intensified treatment ($n=9$)	Control ($n=5$)	P value intensified treatment vs. control
Characteristics			
Age (y)	48.4 ± 12.9	52.8 ± 17.5	NS
Male/female	3/6	2/3	NS
Medications			
Vasodilators			
No vasodilators	1	5	
Hemodynamics	8	0	
Right heart catheterization			
Systolic PAP (mmHg)	60.9 ± 19.5	53.2 ± 8.8	0.14
Diastolic PAP (mmHg)	24.8 ± 6.4	19.4 ± 8.0	0.54
Mean PAP (mmHg)	37.8 ± 9.2	32.6 ± 7.4	0.7
PVR (dynes $+s^{-1}+cm^{-5}$)	564.4 ± 246.93	514.6 ± 149.4	0.35

Values are mean $\pm$ SD when appropriate
PAP pulmonary arterial pressure, *PVR* pulmonary vascular resistance

The baseline characteristics of the participants are shown in Table 15.1. There was no significant difference in mean age between members of the intensified PH treatment patient group and those of the control group.

15.3.2 Right Heart Catheterization

The baseline right heart catheterization data is shown in Table 15.1. There was no significant difference in the systolic PAP, diastolic PAP, mPAP, and PVR of the intensified PH treatment group and those of the control group.

15.3.3 LV and RV Systolic Function

The RVEF and LVEF were similar in both the intensified PH treatment group and the control group (Table 15.2).

Table 15.2 LV and RV functional measurements

	Intensified treatment ($n = 9$)	Control ($n = 5$)	P value intensified treatment vs. control
LVEF (%)	57.5 ± 10.5	61.0 ± 7.3	0.50
RVEF (%)	32.1 ± 13.0	34.7 ± 9.7	0.59
LV k_{mono} (min^{-1})	0.052 ± 0.008	0.058 ± 0.006	0.72
RV k_{mono} (min^{-1})	0.043 ± 0.008	0.044 ± 0.01	0.18
SVI/RV k_{mono} (mL/min^{-1}·m^2)	730.8 ± 253.6	829.1 ± 362.9	0.31

Values are mean $\pm$ SD when appropriate
LV left ventricular, *LVEF* left ventricular ejection fraction, *RV* right ventricular, *RVEF* right ventricular ejection fraction, *RVSV* right ventricular stroke volume

15.3.4 LV and RV Oxidative Metabolism

There was no statistically significant difference between the LV oxidative metabolism, k_{mono}, of the intensified PH treatment group and that of the controls ($P = 0.72$). There was also no statistically significant difference between the RV oxidative metabolism, k_{mono}, of the intensified PH treatment group and that of the controls ($P = 0.18$) (Table 15.2). In addition, the RV SVI per RV k_{mono} was similar in both the intensified PH treatment group and the control group ($P = 0.31$).

15.3.5 Longer-Term Effects of Intensified PH-Specific Therapy on RV Metabolism and Work per Oxygen Consumption

The intensified PH therapy group tended to have reduced PVR compared with that of the control group (-20.6 ± 41.7 vs. -3.4 ± 33.2 %, $P = 0.29$). Intensified PH therapy tended to reduce BNP (377.2 ± 694.5 to 70.8 ± 132.6 mol/mL, $P = 0.18$).

Intensified PH therapy significantly reduced RV oxidative metabolism (0.044 ± 0.008 to 0.039 ± 0.007/min, $P = 0.002$) while increasing SVI (31.4 ± 10.1 to 39.3 ± 9.6 mL/m^2, $P = 0.017$) (Fig. 15.3). As a result, the intensified PH-specific therapy significantly improved the RV work/oxygen consumption index (730.8 ± 253.6 to 1038.5 ± 262.7 mL/min + m^2, $P < 0.001$) (Fig. 15.4). There was no significant change in LV k_{mono} in this group (0.052 ± 0.008 to 0.050 ± 0.006/min, $P = 0.35$). The control group showed no changes in these parameters (RV k_{mono}: 0.041 ± 0.006 to 0.049 ± 0.01/min, $P = 0.15$, RV work/oxygen consumption index: 829.1 ± 362.9 to 721.5 ± 241.2 mL/min + m^2, $P = 0.69$).

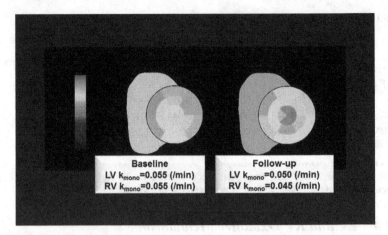

Fig. 15.3 Representative case of PAH patient who had intensified PH-specific vasodilator therapy. LV k_{mono} did not change after the intensified PH-specific vasodilator treatment. In contrast, RV k_{mono} was markedly reduced after the intensified PH-specific vasodilator therapy

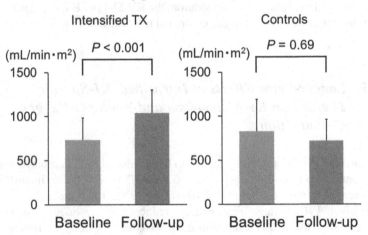

Fig. 15.4 Effects of intensified PH-specific vasodilator therapy on RV work per oxygen consumption index. Patients who had intensified PH-specific vasodilator therapy had a significantly improved RV work per oxygen consumption index. In contrast, there was no significant difference in RV work per oxygen consumption index in control group. *PH* pulmonary hypertension, *RV* right ventricle, *TX* therapy

15.4 Discussion

Intensified PH-specific vasodilator therapy tended to reduce PVR and BNP. The intensive PH-specific therapy led to reduction in right ventricular oxidative metabolism and a significant improvement in right ventricular work per oxygen consumption index in patients with pulmonary hypertension.

15.4.1 Increased RV Oxidative Metabolism in Patients with PH

The major determinants of myocardial metabolism are heart rate, contractility, and wall stress [36, 37]. Oxygen demand in the RV may also increase with elevated PAP [10].

In LV, heart failure is considered to be an energy-depleted state. Improved survival through the use of beta-blockers and vasodilator therapy is in part associated with the energy-sparing effects of these medications [38].

RV MVO_2 was originally measured through right coronary venous blood sampling [10]. As noninvasive approaches, ^{11}C-acetate and ^{15}O-labeled tracers PET have also been applied for RV oxidative measurements in HF and PH [15, 17, 22, 26, 39, 40]. The current data revealed increased RV oxidative metabolism in patients with PH and reduced RV contraction. The current data agreed with findings of our previous study and the study by Wong et al. [15, 39].

15.4.2 Study Population and Effects of PH-Specific Vasodilator Therapy

In the current study, eight PH patients did not have PH-specific vasodilator therapy. One patient had a PH-specific vasodilator, but the PH control did not reach the standard control level. Therefore, these nine patients either started or added the PH-specific vasodilator. The remaining five patients already received PH-specific vasodilator treatments and they were stable. These five patients did not meet the criteria to add further vasodilators to control their PH based on ESC and ERS guidelines [30].

The intensified PH therapy group tended to have reduced mPAP. Although the mPAP did not reach statistically significant levels, this finding may be due to the small sample size, but it may still indicate that intensified PH-specific therapy had beneficial effects. In fact, BNP also tended to be reduced after the therapy, a finding that may indicate a secondary reduction in wall stress due to reduced mPAP. It may therefore be appropriate to evaluate the therapeutic effects on RV energetics in this study population.

15.4.3 Effects of PH-Specific Vasodilator Therapy on RV Oxidative Metabolism and Work per MVO₂ Index

In the previous study, we evaluated RV power and RV efficiency using the following equation: RV efficiency $= HR \times mPAP \times SV \times 1.33 \times 10^{-4}/RV$ $k_{mono} \times RV$ mass $\times 20$ [35]. Using this equation, WHO functional classification II and III PH patients actually had increased RV power and RV efficiency compared to patients in the control group [15]. The increasing power and RV efficiency may be adaptive processes associated with increasing mPAP. In the LV, the LV efficiency is estimated using the WMI. The WMI was calculated as follows: WMI $= SVI \times SBP \times HR/k_{mono}$ [13]. LVHF treatments usually do not significantly change the HR and SBP [14]. In contrast, PH-specific vasodilators significantly reduce the mPAP [27]. Therefore, if the equation proposed by Sun et al. is simply applied to RV efficiency measurements [35], RV efficiency may be reduced after PH-specific vasodilator therapy since the reduction of mPAP would play a significant role over the increasing SVI. The afterload of pulmonary circulation is usually lower than that of systemic circulation [1, 41]. Therefore, the RV may have volume efficiency rather than pressure efficiency as would apply in the case of the LV. Therefore, we applied SVI per MVO₂ index instead of Sun's equation in the current study.

The SVI per MVO₂ index shows that the intensified PH-specific vasodilator therapy significantly improved this parameter in comparison with that of controls. The trend of mPAP reduction may contribute to these improvements. Therefore, improving volume efficiency in the RV may be one of the therapeutic effects of PH-specific vasodilators, and doing so may contribute to the improvement of outcomes in patients with PH. This hypothesis should be tested in a larger study population in the future.

15.4.4 Limitations

The thickness of the RV free wall is usually 4–5 mm, which is thinner than the LV free wall. However, the current study population had thicker RV walls. When radiotracer uptake is measured, the partial volume effect may significantly attenuate the data. However, we analyzed the oxidative metabolism using mono-exponential fitting. This approach measures clearance of the radiotracer from the myocardium. Thus, the partial volume effect should be minimal.

15.5 Conclusion

Intensified PH-specific vasodilator therapy led to a reduction in right ventricular oxidative metabolism and a significant improvement in right ventricular work per oxygen consumption index in patients with pulmonary hypertension. These effects may contribute to the benefits of intensified PH-specific vasodilator therapy.

Conflicts of Interest None

Acknowledgments The authors thank Keiichi Magota, PhD; Ken-ichi Nishijima, PhD; Daisuke Abo, MSc; and Eriko Suzuki for their support for this study. This manuscript has been reviewed by a North American English-language professional editor, Ms. Holly Beanlands. The authors also thank Ms. Holly Beanlands for critical reading of the manuscript.

This study was supported in part by grants from the Japanese Ministry of Education, Culture, Sports, Science and Technology (Category B, No. 23390294), Hokkaido Heart Association (H-20) (Sapporo, Japan), Adult Vascular Disease Research Foundation (#H22-23) (Kyoto, Japan), North-Tech Research Foundation (#H23-S2-17, Sapporo, Japan), and grants from the Innovation Program of the Japan Science and Technology Agency. Dr. Yoshinaga is supported by the Imura Clinical Research Award (Adult Vascular Disease Research Foundation).

References

1. Haddad F, Hunt SA, Rosenthal DN, Murphy DJ. Right ventricular function in cardiovascular disease, part I: Anatomy, physiology, aging, and functional assessment of the right ventricle. Circulation. 2008;117:1436–48. doi:10.1161/CIRCULATIONAHA.107.653576.
2. Dell'Italia LJ. The right ventricle: anatomy, physiology, and clinical importance. Curr Probl Cardiol. 1991;16:653–720.
3. Lee FA. Hemodynamics of the right ventricle in normal and disease states. Cardiol Clin. 1992; 10:59–67.
4. Meyer P, Filippatos GS, Ahmed MI, Iskandrian AE, Bittner V, Perry GJ, et al. Effects of right ventricular ejection fraction on outcomes in chronic systolic heart failure. Circulation. 2010;121:252–8. doi:10.1161/CIRCULATIONAHA.109.887570.
5. Champion HC, Michelakis ED, Hassoun PM. Comprehensive invasive and noninvasive approach to the right ventricle-pulmonary circulation unit: state of the art and clinical and research implications. Circulation. 2009;120:992–1007. doi:10.1161/CIRCULATIONAHA. 106.674028.
6. Valsangiacomo Buechel ER, Mertens LL. Imaging the right heart: the use of integrated multi-modality imaging. Eur Heart J. 2012;33:949–60. doi:10.1093/eurheartj/ehr490.

7. Chin KM, Rubin LJ. Pulmonary arterial hypertension. J Am Coll Cardiol. 2008;51:1527–38.
8. Haddad F, Doyle R, Murphy DJ, Hunt SA. Right ventricular function in cardiovascular disease, part II: pathophysiology, clinical importance, and management of right ventricular failure. Circulation. 2008;117:1717–31. doi:10.1161/CIRCULATIONAHA.107.653584.
9. Chin KM, Kim NH, Rubin LJ. The right ventricle in pulmonary hypertension. Coron Artery Dis. 2005;16:13–8.
10. Zong P, Tune JD, Downey HF. Mechanisms of oxygen demand/supply balance in the right ventricle. Exp Biol Med (Maywood). 2005;230:507–19.
11. Wong YY, Ruiter G, Lubberink M, Raijmakers PG, Knaapen P, Marcus JT, et al. Right ventricular failure in idiopathic pulmonary arterial hypertension is associated with inefficient myocardial oxygen utilization. Circ Heart Fail. 2011;4:700–6. doi:10.1161/CIRCHEART FAILURE.111.962381.
12. Ukkonen H, Beanlands R. Oxidative metabolism and cardiac efficiency. In: Wahl R, editor. Principles and practice of PET and PET/CT. 2nd ed. Philadelphia: Lippincott Williams & Wilkins; 2009. p. 589–606.
13. Beanlands RS. Nahmias C, Gordon E, Coates G, deKemp R, Firnau G, et al. The effects of beta(1)-blockade on oxidative metabolism and the metabolic cost of ventricular work in patients with left ventricular dysfunction: A double-blind, placebo-controlled, positron-emission tomography study. Circulation. 2000;102:2070–5.
14. Yoshinaga K, Burwash IG, Leech JA, Haddad H, Johnson CB. deKemp RA, et al. The effects of continuous positive airway pressure on myocardial energetics in patients with heart failure and obstructive sleep apnea. J Am Coll Cardiol. 2007;49:450–8.
15. Yoshinaga K, Ohira H, Tsujino I, Oyama-Manabe N, Mielniczuk L, Beanlands RS, et al. Attenuated right ventricular energetics evaluated using (1)(1)C-acetate PET in patients with pulmonary hypertension. Eur J Nucl Med Mol Imaging. 2014;41:1240–50. doi:10.1007/s00259-014-2736-4.
16. Armbrecht JJ, Buxton DB, Brunken RC, Phelps ME, Schelbert HR. Regional myocardial oxygen consumption determined noninvasively in humans with [1-11C]acetate and dynamic positron tomography. Circulation. 1989;80:863–72.
17. Stolen KQ, Kemppainen J, Ukkonen H, Kalliokoski KK, Luotolahti M, Lehikoinen P, et al. Exercise training improves biventricular oxidative metabolism and left ventricular efficiency in patients with dilated cardiomyopathy. J Am Coll Cardiol. 2003;41:460–7.
18. Yoshinaga K, Chow BJ, Dekemp RA, Thorn S, Ruddy TD, Davies RA, et al. Application of cardiac molecular imaging using positron emission tomography in evaluation of drug and therapeutics for cardiovascular disorders. Curr Pharm Des. 2005;11:903–32.
19. Yoshinaga K, Tamaki N. Imaging myocardial metabolism. Curr Opin Biotechnol. 2007;18: 52–9. doi:10.1016/j.copbio.2006.11.003.
20. Ukkonen H, Saraste M, Akkila J, Knuuti J, Karanko M, Iida H, et al. Myocardial efficiency during levosimendan infusion in congestive heart failure. Clin Pharmacol Ther. 2000;68: 522–31.
21. Wong YY, Raijmakers P, van Campen J, van der Laarse WJ, Knaapen P, Lubberink M, et al. 11C-Acetate clearance as an index of oxygen consumption of the right myocardium in idiopathic pulmonary arterial hypertension: a validation study using 15O-labeled tracers and PET. J Nucl Med. 2013;54:1258–62. doi:10.2967/jnumed.112.115915.
22. Ohira H, Beanlands RS, Davies RA, Mielniczuk L. The role of nuclear imaging in pulmonary hypertension. J Nucl Cardiol. 2015;22:141–57. doi:10.1007/s12350-014-9960-y.
23. Packer M, Bristow MR, Cohn JN, Colucci WS, Fowler MB, Gilbert EM, et al. The effect of carvedilol on morbidity and mortality in patients with chronic heart failure. U.S. Carvedilol Heart Failure Study Group. N Engl J Med. 1996;334:1349–55. doi:10.1056/NEJM199605233342101.
24. Chiba S, Naya M, Iwano H, Yoshinaga K, Katoh C, Manabe O, et al. Interrelation between myocardial oxidative metabolism and diastolic function in patients undergoing surgical ventricular reconstruction. Eur J Nucl Med Mol Imaging. 2013;40:349–55. doi:10.1007/s00259-012-2297-3.

25. Hall AB, Ziadi MC, Leech JA, Chen SY, Burwash IG, Renaud J, et al. Effects of short-term continuous positive airway pressure on myocardial sympathetic nerve function and energetics in patients with heart failure and obstructive sleep apnea: a randomized study. Circulation. 2014;130:892–901. doi:10.1161/CIRCULATIONAHA.113.005893.
26. Ukkonen H, Beanlands RS, Burwash IG, de Kemp RA, Nahmias C, Fallen E, et al. Effect of cardiac resynchronization on myocardial efficiency and regional oxidative metabolism. Circulation. 2003;107:28–31.
27. Galie N, Corris PA, Frost A, Girgis RE, Granton J, Jing ZC, et al. Updated treatment algorithm of pulmonary arterial hypertension. J Am Coll Cardiol. 2013;62:D60–72. doi:10.1016/j.jacc. 2013.10.031.
28. Oikawa M, Kagaya Y, Otani H, Sakuma M, Demachi J, Suzuki J, et al. Increased [18F] fluorodeoxyglucose accumulation in right ventricular free wall in patients with pulmonary hypertension and the effect of epoprostenol. J Am Coll Cardiol. 2005;45:1849–55.
29. Simonneau G, Robbins IM, Beghetti M, Channick RN, Delcroix M, Denton CP, et al. Updated clinical classification of pulmonary hypertension. J Am Coll Cardiol. 2009;54:S43–54. doi:10. 1016/j.jacc.2009.04.012.
30. Task Force for D, Treatment of Pulmonary Hypertension of European Society of C, European Respiratory S, International Society of H, Lung T, Galie N, et al. Guidelines for the diagnosis and treatment of pulmonary hypertension. Eur Respir J. 2009;34:1219–63. doi:10.1183/09031936.00139009.
31. Nagaya N, Nishikimi T, Uematsu M, Satoh T, Kyotani S, Sakamaki F, et al. Plasma brain natriuretic peptide as a prognostic indicator in patients with primary pulmonary hypertension. Circulation. 2000;102:865–70.
32. Alfakih K, Plein S, Bloomer T, Jones T, Ridgway J, Sivananthan M. Comparison of right ventricular volume measurements between axial and short axis orientation using steady-state free precession magnetic resonance imaging. J Magn Reson Imaging. 2003;18: 25–32. doi:10.1002/jmri.10329.
33. Oyama-Manabe N, Sato T, Tsujino I, Kudo K, Manabe O, Kato F, et al. The strain-encoded (SENC) MR imaging for detection of global right ventricular dysfunction in pulmonary hypertension. Int J Cardiovasc Imaging. 2013;29:371–8. doi:10.1007/s10554-012-0105-6.
34. Yoshinaga K, Katoh C, Beanlands RS, Noriyasu K, Komuro K, Yamada S, et al. Reduced oxidative metabolic response in dysfunctional myocardium with preserved glucose metabolism but with impaired contractile reserve. J Nucl Med. 2004;45:1885–91.
35. Sun KT, Yeatman LA, Buxton DB, Chen K, Johnson JA, Huang SC, et al. Simultaneous measurement of myocardial oxygen consumption and blood flow using [1-carbon-11]acetate. J Nucl Med. 1998;39:272–80.
36. Braunwald E. Control of myocardial oxygen consumption: physiologic and clinical considerations. Am J Cardiol. 1971;27:416–32.
37. Laine H, Katoh C, Luotolahti M, Yki-Jarvinen H, Kantola I, Jula A, et al. Myocardial oxygen consumption is unchanged but efficiency is reduced in patients with essential hypertension and left ventricular hypertrophy. Circulation. 1999;100:2425–30.
38. Katz AM. Potential deleterious effects of inotropic agents in the therapy of chronic heart failure. Circulation. 1986;73:III184–90.
39. Wong YY, Westerhof N, Ruiter G, Lubberink M, Raijmakers P, Knaapen P, et al. Systolic pulmonary artery pressure and heart rate are main determinants of oxygen consumption in the right ventricular myocardium of patients with idiopathic pulmonary arterial hypertension. Eur J Heart Fail. 2011;13:1290–5. doi:10.1093/eurjhf/hfr140.
40. Knaapen P, Germans T, Knuuti J, Paulus WJ, Dijkmans PA, Allaart CP, et al. Myocardial energetics and efficiency: current status of the noninvasive approach. Circulation. 2007;115: 918–27. doi:10.1161/CIRCULATIONAHA.106.660639.
41. Sheehan F, Redington A. The right ventricle: anatomy, physiology and clinical imaging. Heart. 2008;94:1510–5. doi:10.1136/hrt.2007.132779.

Chapter 16
Usefulness of ^{18}F-FDG PET in Diagnosing Cardiac Sarcoidosis

Osamu Manabe, Keiichiro Yoshinaga, Hiroshi Ohira,
and Noriko Oyama-Manabe

Abstract Sarcoidosis is a multisystem granulomatous disorder of unknown etiology. The number of patients with cardiac involvement is considered to be limited, but cardiac sarcoidosis is a very serious and unpredictable aspect of sarcoidosis resulting in conduction-system abnormalities and heart failure. The severity of cardiac involvement depends on the extent and location of the granulomatous lesions.

When establishing a diagnosis, ^{18}F-fluorodeoxyglucose (^{18}F-FDG) positron emission tomography (PET) is a useful tool to detect active inflammatory lesions associated with sarcoidosis. The heart uses different energy sources including free fatty acids (FFA), glucose, and others. The ^{18}F-FDG is an analog of glucose, and for the precise evaluation of the extent and severity of cardiac involvement, recent studies have focused on reducing physiological myocardial ^{18}F-FDG uptake. Long fasting and dietary modification, such as observing a low-carbohydrate or high-fat diet, are the recommended regimens for preparations to make a precise evaluation. The FFA level before the PET scan could be a predictor of the success to the suppression of the physiological ^{18}F-FDG accumulation.

With ^{18}F-FDG PET therapy monitoring or risk stratification based on quantitative ^{18}F-FDG accumulation becomes possible. The quantification of the volume and intensity of ^{18}F-FDG uptake could assist in predicting the clinical outcomes and in evaluating the efficiency of steroid treatments.

O. Manabe (✉)
Department of Nuclear Medicine, Hokkaido University Graduate School of Medicine, Sapporo, Japan
e-mail: osamumanabe817@med.hokudai.ac.jp

K. Yoshinaga
Department of Nuclear Medicine, Hokkaido University Graduate School of Medicine, Kita15 Nishi7, Kita-Ku, Sapporo 060-8638, Hokkaido, Japan

Molecular Imaging Research Center, National Institute of Radiological Sciences, 4-9-1 Anagawa, Inage-Ku, Chiba 263-8555, Japan

H. Ohira
First Department of Medicine, Hokkaido University Hospital, Sapporo, Japan

N. Oyama-Manabe
Diagnostic and Interventional Radiology, Hokkaido University Hospital, Sapporo, Japan

© The Author(s) 2016   209
Y. Kuge et al. (eds.), *Perspectives on Nuclear Medicine for Molecular Diagnosis and Integrated Therapy*, DOI 10.1007/978-4-431-55894-1_16

This report provides a summary of the usefulness of ^{18}F-FDG PET in its current status as a diagnostic modality for cardiac sarcoidosis.

Keywords Cardiac   sarcoidosis   •   Positron   emission   tomography   •
Fluorodeoxyglucose

16.1 Background

Sarcoidosis is a multisystem granulomatous disorder of unknown etiology. It is characterized by noncaseating, epithelioid granulomas. Typically, young or middle-aged adults are affected. In Japan, the annual incidence ranges from 1 to 2 cases per 100,000 of the population. The bilateral hilar and mediastinal lymph nodes, lungs, skin, musculoskeletal system, and eyes are well known to be involved in lesions. Essentially all organs, including the heart, may potentially be involved [1, 2].

Sarcoidosis patient treatment generally follows a favorable clinical course. However, about 30 % of patients suffer chronically or experience recurrence. Granulomas forming in an organ can affect how the organ functions and be a cause of signs and symptoms. Especially, prognosis is related to the presence of cardiac lesions [3].

The frequency of cardiac involvement varies and is significantly influenced by ancetstry. In Japan over 25 % of cases with sarcoidosis experience symptomatic cardiac involvement, whereas in the USA and Europe, only about 5 % of cases present cardiac involvement. Autopsy studies in the USA have shown the frequency of cardiac involvement to be about 20 %, whereas autopsy studies in Japan have shown a frequency above 50 % [4–6].

16.2 Diagnostic Criteria for Cardiac Sarcoidosis

Histologic analysis of operative or endomyocardial biopsy specimens could be the irrefutably best standard in diagnosing cardiac sarcoidosis. However, it is not feasible to perform endomyocardial biopsies on all suspected regions, and myocardial biopsies tend to have lower sensitivity in the diagnosis of cardiac sarcoidosis. Therefore, the Japanese Ministry of Health and Welfare (JMHW) guidelines for diagnostic imaging have been used as the diagnostic standard since early times [7]. The JMHW criteria include both the histologic and the clinical diagnosis groups. For the clinical diagnosis group, the positive findings of electrocardiography, echocardiography, and ^{67}Ga scintigraphy are the major criteria; minor criteria include findings of electrocardiography, echocardiography, perfusion images, and cardiac magnetic resonance images. Among the criteria, ^{18}F-fluorodeoxyglucose (^{18}F-FDG) positron emission tomography (PET) is not included in the 2006 criteria; it is only noted as a comment that abnormal ^{18}F-FDG accumulation in the heart is a diagnostically useful finding. However, the usefulness of ^{18}F-FDG PET has been increasingly recognized; the Japanese health insurance system

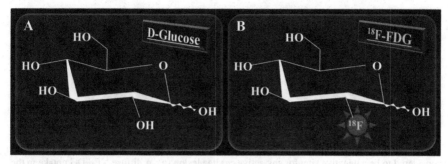

Fig. 16.1 Chemical structural formula of D-glucose and ^{18}F-FDG.
The chemical structural formulas of the glucose and ^{18}F-fluorodeoxyglucose (^{18}F-FDG) are shown in panels A and B, respectively. ^{18}F-FDG is a glucose analog widely used in PET studies of glucose metabolism. ^{18}F-FDG is taken up by plasma-membrane transporters and phosphorylated by the intracellular enzymes in the same manner as glucose. The metabolism of ^{18}F-FDG stops after 6-phosphorylation which is different from glucose and provides an advantage in metabolism studies

approved it for detection of inflammation sites in cardiac sarcoidosis on April 2012. Recently, the Heart Rhythm Society of the USA also proposed the diagnosis and management of cardiac sarcoidosis with ^{18}F-FDG PET and MRI recommended for the evaluation of cardiac sarcoidosis, if there is a cardiac history and abnormality in the electrocardiogram or echocardiography in sarcoidosis patients [8].

16.3 Cardiac Metabolism

For the cardiac metabolism, under long fasting conditions, glucose production and glucose oxidation would decrease. As a result, free fatty acid (FFA) is mobilized from adipose tissue, and the increase in available FFA becomes an alternative source of energy in the myocardium. The ^{18}F-FDG is a glucose analog used clinically in PET to indicate glucose utilization (Fig. 16.1), and physiological myocardial uptake has been reported. The levels of the cardiac uptake vary regardless of blood glucose levels [9].

16.4 ^{18}F-FDG Uptake Patterns in Evaluations of Cardiac Sarcoidosis

To evaluate cardiac sarcoidosis, uptake patterns of ^{18}F-FDG were divided into four kinds as suggested in Fig. 16.2 [7]. Without myocardial ^{18}F-FDG uptake is considered to be negative in active cardiac lesions. A distinct diffuse ^{18}F-FDG uptake in the entire left ventricular wall without localized high ^{18}F-FDG uptake generally is

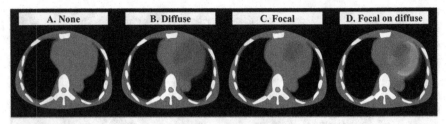

Fig. 16.2 ¹⁸F-FDG uptake patterns to evaluate cardiac sarcoidosis.
Uptake patterns were divided into four groups. No ^{18}F-fluorodeoxyglucose (^{18}F-FDG) uptake is considered to be a negative sign for any active cardiac lesion (**a**). A diffuse ^{18}F-FDG uptake in the entire left ventricular wall without any localized high ^{18}F-FDG uptake is generally thought to be a physiological uptake (**b**). With slight accumulation in (**b**), it was not possible to determine if this was caused by cardiac sarcoidosis. Focal uptake (**c**) and focal on diffuse uptakes (**d**) of ^{18}F-FDG in the left ventricular wall are considered to be positive signs for cardiac sarcoidosis

thought to represent a physiological uptake, not indicating an abnormality. Focal and focal on diffuse ^{18}F-FDG uptakes in the left ventricular wall are considered to be positive indicators of cardiac sarcoidosis.

16.5   Preparation for the ^{18}F-FDG PET to Evaluate Cardiac Lesions

The physiological myocardial ^{18}F-FDG uptake may mislead when attempting to establish cardiac sarcoidosis. Proper preparation such as extended fasting with a low-carbohydrate diet before the scan is needed to suppress the physiological cardiac uptake [10]. We have confirmed the usefulness of the effect of 18 h of fasting with a low-carbohydrate diet compared to a minimum 6-h fasting preparation [9]. Patients with at least 6 h of fasting showed a higher diffuse left ventricular (LV) ^{18}F-FDG uptake than patients with longer fasting and low-carbohydrate diets. Patients who fasted for longer and observed a low-carbohydrate diet showed higher FFA levels than a shorter fasting group. In the shorter fasting group, patients with diffuse LV ^{18}F-FDG uptake showed significantly lower FFA levels than patients without a diffuse LV uptake. This shows that the FFA level is an important marker to suppress physiological ^{18}F-FDG uptake. The protocol to obtain better ^{18}F-FDG PET images in cardiac sarcoidosis patients is shown in Fig. 16.3.

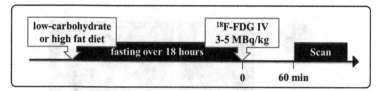

Fig. 16.3 The protocol for the ^{18}F-FDG PET scanning for cardiac sarcoidosis.
Patients were instructed to observe a low-carbohydrate or high-fat diet on the day prior to the scanning, with additional fasting for more than 18 h. The PET images were acquired 60 min after injection of the ^{18}F-FDG

16.6   Location of the ^{18}F-FDG Uptake

Cardiac sarcoidosis provoked the conduction disturbance such as atrioventricular block. There is a relationship between electrocardiogram abnormalities and myocardial ^{18}F-FDG uptake. In particular, the focal ^{18}F-FDG uptake in the interventricular septum in cardiac sarcoidosis is associated with atrioventricular blockage. Therefore, to identify the location of the ^{18}F-FDG uptake is an important issue of potentially great benefit in treatment planning [11].

The ^{18}F-FDG uptake due to inflammation in the LV wall is sometimes difficult to distinguish from the physiological uptake. On the other hand, the physiological uptake in the right ventricle (RV) is less common and less intense. Therefore, although less frequent of the sarcoidosis involvement, the ^{18}F-FDG uptake in the RV due to cardiac sarcoidosis may be useful in diagnosing in sarcoidosis [12].

16.7   Relationship Between ^{18}F-FDG Accumulation and Activity of Sarcoidosis

The significant ^{18}F-FDG accumulation in cardiac sarcoidosis is caused by active inflammatory changes involving activated inflammatory cells like neutrophils, macrophages, and lymphocytes [13], and the ^{18}F-FDG uptake may reflect an active inflammation condition. This makes ^{18}F-FDG PET useful both for the detection of cardiac sarcoidosis as well as for monitoring the treatment response and early recurrence [14].

The maximum standardized uptake value (SUVmax) has been used for semi-quantitative measurements to assess the intensity of ^{18}F-FDG uptake. Recently, the availability of volume-based analysis, such as metabolic volume and total lesion glycolysis, has been widely used to evaluate the extent and activity of the ^{18}F-FDG uptake in malignant tumors [15]. Ahmadian et al. applied volume-based analysis to cardiac sarcoidosis and reported that the metabolic activity estimated by ^{18}F-FDG PET was a reliable independent predictor of cardiac events in cardiac sarcoidosis patients [16]. A volume-based quantification of ^{18}F-FDG uptake could be of value

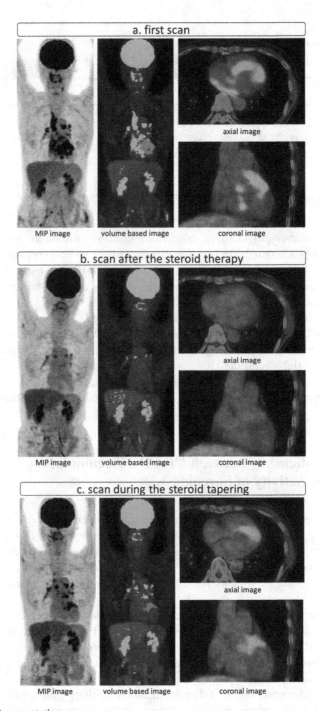

Fig. 16.4 Representative case.
This is a case of a cardiac sarcoidosis patient with uveitis and respiratory discomfort. She had a
right bundle branch block and right axis deviation on the electrocardiograph and thinning of the

in a number of fields of cardiac and inflammation diseases like it is for malignant tumors (Fig. 16.4).

16.8 Conclusions

Observations from ^{18}F-FDG PET images are a useful diagnostic tool to detect active inflammatory lesions associated with cardiac sarcoidosis. For a precise evaluation of the extent and severity of cardiac involvement, long fasting and dietary modifications, such as observing a low-carbohydrate or a high-fat diet, are recommended approaches to reduce physiological myocardial ^{18}F-FDG uptake. The FFA level before the PET data acquisition could be a predictor for success in the suppression of physiological ^{18}F-FDG accumulation. Such ^{18}F-FDG PET images also enable therapy monitoring or risk stratification based on the quantitative accumulation determination. The quantification of the volume and intensity of ^{18}F-FDG uptake may also help predict the clinical outcomes and evaluate the efficiency of steroid treatment.

Conflicts of Interest None

Acknowledgments This study was supported in part by grants from the Innovation Program of the Japan Science and Technology Agency and a Hokkaido Heart Association Grant for Research.

←_____

Fig. 16.4 (continued) septal wall with severe hypokinesis on the echocardiograph. There was a clearly abnormal ^{18}F-FDG uptake in the LV wall as well as in the lymph nodes which indicated active inflammatory changes associated with sarcoidosis (**a**). The estimated maximum standardized uptake value (SUVmax) was 10.6, and the volume of the uptake was 76.1 ml (the threshold was obtained from the liver uptake) at the cardiac lesion. The ^{18}F-FDG PET [revealed the dramatic] showed a nearly total disappearance of the abnormal cardiac uptake after 4 weeks of therapy with prednisolone (**b**). However, the ^{18}F-FDG PET during the tapering of the prednisolone showed renewed ^{18}F-FDG uptake. Here, the estimated maximum standardized uptake value (SUVmax) was 6.2, and the volume of the uptake was 7.83 ml (the threshold was obtained from the liver uptake). This case indicates that ^{18}F-FDG was useful to evaluate the sarcoidosis activity and indicated the improvement during the therapy as well as the recurrence of the active sarcoidosis

References

1. Hunninghake GW, Costabel U, Ando M, et al. ATS/ERS/WASOG statement on sarcoidosis. American Thoracic Society/European Respiratory Society/World Association of Sarcoidosis and other Granulomatous Disorders. Sarcoidosis Vasc Diffuse Lung Dis. 1999;16:149–73.
2. Iannuzzi MC, Rybicki BA, Teirstein AS. Sarcoidosis. N Engl J Med. 2007;357:2153–65.
3. Sekhri V, Sanal S, Delorenzo LJ, Aronow WS, Maguire GP. Cardiac sarcoidosis: a comprehensive review. Arch Med Sci. 2011;7:546–54.
4. Baughman RP, Teirstein AS, Judson MA, et al. Clinical characteristics of patients in a case control study of sarcoidosis. Am J Respir Crit Care Med. 2001;164:1885–9.
5. Silverman KJ, Hutchins GM, Bulkley BH. Cardiac sarcoid: a clinicopathologic study of 84 unselected patients with systemic sarcoidosis. Circulation. 1978;58:1204–11.
6. Iwai K, Sekiguti M, Hosoda Y, et al. Racial difference in cardiac sarcoidosis incidence observed at autopsy. Sarcoidosis. 1994;11:26–31.
7. Ishida Y, Yoshinaga K, Miyagawa M, et al. Recommendations for (18)F-fluorodeoxyglucose positron emission tomography imaging for cardiac sarcoidosis: Japanese Society of Nuclear Cardiology recommendations. Ann Nucl Med. 2014;28:393–403.
8. Birnie DH, Sauer WH, Bogun F, et al. HRS expert consensus statement on the diagnosis and management of arrhythmias associated with cardiac sarcoidosis. Heart Rhythm. 2014;11:1305–23.
9. Manabe O, Yoshinaga K, Ohira H, et al. The effects of 18-h fasting with low-carbohydrate diet preparation on suppressed physiological myocardial (18)F-fluorodeoxyglucose (FDG) uptake and possible minimal effects of unfractionated heparin use in patients with suspected cardiac involvement sarcoidosis. J Nucl Cardiol. 2015. Aug. [Epub ahead of print]
10. Ohira H, Tsujino I, Yoshinaga K. (1)(8)F-Fluoro-2-deoxyglucose positron emission tomography in cardiac sarcoidosis. Eur J Nucl Med Mol Imaging. 2011;38:1773–83.
11. Manabe O, Ohira H, Yoshinaga K, et al. Elevated (18)F-fluorodeoxyglucose uptake in the interventricular septum is associated with atrioventricular block in patients with suspected cardiac involvement sarcoidosis. Eur J Nucl Med Mol Imaging. 2013;40:1558–66.
12. Manabe O, Yoshinaga K, Ohira H, et al. Right ventricular (18)F-FDG uptake is an important indicator for cardiac involvement in patients with suspected cardiac sarcoidosis. Ann Nucl Med. 2014;28:656–63.
13. Koiwa H, Tsujino I, Ohira H, Yoshinaga K, Otsuka N, Nishimura M. Images in cardiovascular medicine: Imaging of cardiac sarcoid lesions using fasting cardiac 18F-fluorodeoxyglucose positron emission tomography: an autopsy case. Circulation. 2010;122:535–6.
14. Manabe O, Oyama-Manabe N, Ohira H, Tsutsui H, Tamaki N. Multimodality evaluation of cardiac sarcoidosis. J Nucl Cardiol. 2012;19:621–4.
15. Hirata K, Kobayashi K, Wong KP, et al. A semi-automated technique determining the liver standardized uptake value reference for tumor delineation in FDG PET-CT. PLoS One. 2014;9, e105682.
16. Ahmadian A, Brogan A, Berman J, et al. Quantitative interpretation of FDG PET/CT with myocardial perfusion imaging increases diagnostic information in the evaluation of cardiac sarcoidosis. J Nucl Cardiol. 2014;21:925–39.

Part IV
Neurology

Chapter 17
PET Quantification in Molecular Brain Imaging Taking into Account the Contribution of the Radiometabolite Entering the Brain

Masanori Ichise, Yasuyuki Kimura, Hitoshi Shimada, Makoto Higuchi, and Tetsuya Suhara

Abstract A good understanding of the in vivo pharmacokinetics of radioligands is important for accurate PET quantification in molecular brain imaging. For many reversibly binding radioligands for which there exists a brain region devoid of molecular target binding sites called "reference tissue," data analysis methods that do not require blood data including the standardized uptake value ratio of target-to-reference tissue at a "fixed time point" (SUVR) and reference tissue model to estimate binding potential (BP_{ND}) are commonly used, the latter being directly proportional to the binding site density (B_{avail}). Theoretically, BP_{ND} is the tissue ratio minus 1 at equilibrium. It is generally believed that radioligands should not ideally produce radiometabolites that can enter the brain because they might complicate accurate quantification of specific binding of the parent radioligand. However, the tissue ratio that contains the contribution of radiometabolite can also be theoretically a valid parameter that reflects the target binding site density. This article describes the validation of the tissue ratio concept using, as an example of our recent PET data analysis approach for a novel radioligand, ^{11}C-PBB3, to quantify pathological tau accumulations in the brain of Alzheimer's disease patients in which the SUVR and reference tissue model methods using the cerebellar cortex as the reference tissue were validated by the dual-input graphical analysis model that uses the plasma parent and radiometabolite activity as input functions in order to take into account the contribution of the radiometabolite entering the brain.

Keywords PET quantification • SUVR • Binding potential • Radiometabolites • Tau • ^{11}C-PBB3 • Alzheimer's disease

M. Ichise, MD, Ph.D. (✉) • Y. Kimura, MD, Ph.D. • H. Shimada, MD, Ph.D. • M. Higuchi, MD, Ph.D. • T. Suhara, MD, Ph.D.
Molecular Imaging Center, National Institute of Radiological Sciences, 4-9-1 Anagawa, Inage-ku, Chiba, Chiba 263-8555, Japan
e-mail: ichisem@nirs.go.jp

© The Author(s) 2016   219
Y. Kuge et al. (eds.), *Perspectives on Nuclear Medicine for Molecular Diagnosis and Integrated Therapy*, DOI 10.1007/978-4-431-55894-1_17

17.1 Introduction

Molecular brain imaging with positron emission tomography (PET) using radiolabeled ligands (radioligands) that target neuroreceptors/transporters and neuropathological biomarker proteins such as amyloid β (Aβ) proteins and pathological tau proteins has many exciting clinical and research applications. The major advantage of PET imaging is that PET using suitable radioligands allows for the accurate quantification of the target binding site density. For accurate PET quantification, however, a good understanding of the in vivo pharmacokinetics of radioligands is important.

For many reversibly binding radioligands for which there exists a brain region devoid of molecular target binding sites called "reference tissue," data analysis methods that do not require blood data including the standardized uptake value ratio (SUVR) method and reference tissue models to estimate binding potential (BP_{ND}) are commonly used to quantify specific molecular target binding sites. The validity of these simple methods can be evaluated by detailed pharmacokinetic modeling of dynamically acquired PET data and radiometabolite corrected arterial plasma parent radioligand activity as an input function. In this respect, it is generally believed that radioligands should not ideally produce metabolites that can enter the brain because they might complicate accurate quantification of specific binding of the parent radioligand.

The purpose of this article is to show that PET quantification using the SUVR and reference tissue model methods can also be valid even when the metabolite contributes to the measured brain radioactivity. In the theory section, the concept of PET measured "brain tissue ratios" in the context of radiometabolites entering the brain will be explored first, and then our recent PET data analysis approach for a novel radioligand, ^{11}C-PBB3 (2-((1E,3E)-4-(6-(^{11}C-methylamino)pyridin-3-yl) buta-1,3-dienyl) benzo[d]thiazol-6-ol) [1], to quantify pathological tau accumulations in the brain of Alzheimer's disease (AD) [2] will be highlighted as an example in which the SUVR and reference tissue model methods were validated by the dual-input graphical analysis model [3] that takes into account the contribution of the radiometabolite entering the brain.

17.2 Materials and Methods

17.2.1 Theory

PET data in molecular brain imaging are commonly analyzed by applying kinetic compartment models, which assume a compartmental system and derive the target binding parameters that reflect the densities of target binding sites in brain regions of interest (ROIs) [4]. Brain regions containing target binding sites (target tissue) have at least three compartments (or two-tissue (2T) compartments) (Fig. 17.1a

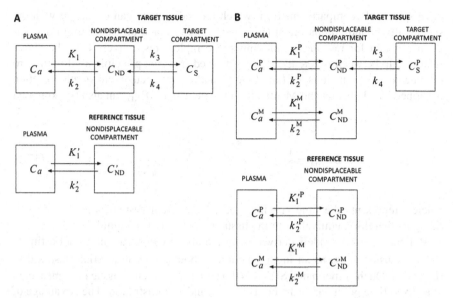

Fig. 17.1 Compartment configurations used to model in vivo radioligand kinetics when the parent only enters the brain (**a**) and both the parent and metabolite enter the brain (**b**). Terms are defined in the text

top). The first compartment is the arterial plasma (C_a), from which the unmetabolized parent radioligand passes into the second compartment or the first tissue compartment known as the nondisplaceable compartment (C_{ND}). The third compartment or the second tissue compartment (C_S) is the specific target binding sites. Reference tissue regions do not have the specific binding compartment (C_S) (Fig. 17.1a bottom). In Fig. 17.1a, K_1 (mL·mL^{-1}·min^{-1}) is the delivery rate constant; k_2 (min^{-1}), k_3 (min^{-1}), and k_4 (min^{-1}) are the first-order kinetic rate constants. Throughout the text, the prime sign is used to indicate the reference tissue. $C_B(t) = C_{ND}(t) + C_S(t)$ and $C'_B(t) = C'_{ND}(t)$ represent the target and reference tissue time activity, respectively, and $C_a(t)$ is the plasma parent radioligand activity at time t after the bolus radioligand administration.

Using $C_a(t)$ as an input function, compartment model approaches allow for the estimation of the distribution volume, V, which is the brain-to-plasma radioactivity ratio, $C_B(t)/C_a(t)$, at equilibrium in which there is no net transfer of radioligand activity between all compartments. Of note is that this equilibrium condition cannot be achieved in the PET experimental paradigm with a bolus radioligand administration. However, the compartment model analysis allows for the estimation of parameters defined at equilibrium. By assuming that the nondisplaceable distribution volume in the target tissue (V_{ND}) is the same as in the reference tissue (V'_{ND}), the target binding parameter, binding potential (BP_{ND}), is calculated as $V - V'/V' = V_S/V_{ND}$, which is directly proportional to the binding site density B_{avail}, i.e., $BP_{ND} = f_{ND}(B_{avail}/K_D)$, where f_{ND} and K_D represent the fraction of nondisplaceable compartment from which the radioligand can exchange with the specifically bound compartment (free tissue fraction) and the equilibrium dissociation constant for radioligand-binding site complex, respectively [5]. The above relationship between BP_{ND} and B_{avail} is derived from the principle used in in vitro binding assays, which is in turn based on the bimolecular enzymatic reaction described by Michaelis and Menten [6]. Of note is that BP_{ND} can also be expressed as

$$BP_{ND} = \frac{V - V'}{V'} = \frac{\frac{C_B(t)}{C_a(t)} - \frac{C'_B(t)}{C_a(t)}}{\frac{C'_B(t)}{C_a(t)}} = \frac{C_B(t)}{C'_B(t)} - 1 \qquad (17.1)$$

where t represents the time at which the compartment system is in equilibrium. BP_{ND} is, therefore, equivalent to the tissue ratio minus 1 at equilibrium.

Reference tissue models derived from the above compartment model estimate BP_{ND} by using $C'_B(t)$ as an input function without requiring arterial plasma data ($C_a(t)$) [4]. On the other hand, SUVR is the target-to-reference tissue ratio measured at a "fixed time point" after the bolus radioligand administration. The advantage of SUVR is that it can be calculated from static PET imaging data without the requirement of arterial data. SUVR $= C_B(t)/C'_B(t)$ is, therefore, closely related to BP_{ND} (Eq. 17.1), the differences between the two being that BP_{ND} is independent of radioligand delivery (blood flow) or its systemic clearance because it is defined at equilibrium,

On the other hand, in the situation where the metabolite enters the brain, the compartment system is more complex as shown in Fig. 17.1b in which superscripts P and M refer to "parent" and "metabolite," respectively, and the metabolite is assumed not to bind specifically to targets (see the discussion about the situation where the metabolite also binds specifically) [3]. Here, let's consider the tissue ratio minus 1 at equilibrium assuming that V_{ND} is the same in the reference and target tissues, which is given by

$$\begin{aligned} BP_{ND}^* &= \frac{C_B(t)}{C'_B(t)} - 1 = \frac{C_B^P(t) + C_B^M(t)}{C'^P_B(t) + C'^M_B(t)} - 1 = \frac{V^P + \delta V^M}{V'^P + \delta V'^M} - 1 \\ &= \frac{V_S}{V_{ND}^P + \delta V_{ND}^M} \end{aligned} \qquad (17.2)$$

where δ is the metabolite-to-parent activity ratio in plasma at equilibrium $\left(\delta = C_a^M(t)/C_a^P(t)\right)$ and it is a constant value. This tissue ratio minus 1 at equilibrium has an additional term, δV_{ND}^M, the contribution of the metabolite nondisplaceable distribution volume in the denominator of Eq. 17.2, and it is here denoted by BP_{ND}^* to distinguish it from BP_{ND}, which is the tissue ratio minus 1 at equilibrium when only the parent enters the brain. To estimate this tissue ratio minus 1 by the reference tissue model, in fact, no knowledge of the metabolite status is needed because it uses $C_B(t)$ as an input function. The same argument applies to the SUVR. Importantly, BP^*_{ND} like BP_{ND} is directly proportional to the target binding site density, B_{avail}, as shown below.

$$BP^*_{ND} = \frac{V_S}{V^P_{ND} + \delta V^M_{ND}} = \frac{f^P_P}{\frac{f^P_P}{f^P_{ND}} + \delta \frac{f^M_P}{f^M_{ND}}} \times \frac{B_{avail}}{K_D} \tag{17.3}$$

where f^P_P or f^M_P the free fraction of parent (P) or metabolite (M) in plasma is a constant and so are f^P_{ND}, f^M_{ND}, and δ in the same individual. Note that $V_S = f^P_P B_{avail} / K_D$ and V_{ND} can be expressed as f_P/f_{ND} because the free radioligand or metabolite activity in the plasma and the tissue compartments are the same at equilibrium $(f_P C_a(t) = f_{ND} C_{ND}(t))$ [4, 5]. The validation of the reference tissue model BP^*_{ND} can be accomplished by the dual-input graphical analysis model derived from the model illustrated by Fig. 17.1b that takes into account the contribution of radiometabolites entering the brain using the combined plasma radioactivity $(C^P_a(t) + C^M_a(t))$ as an input function [3]. The operational equation is given by

$$\frac{\int_0^t C_B(t)dt}{C_B(t)} = \alpha(t) \frac{\int_0^t \left(C^P_a(t) + C^M_a(t)\right) dt}{C_B(t)} + \beta(t) \tag{17.4}$$

Eq. 17.4 becomes linear when the system reaches transient equilibrium between the brain and plasma compartments at time t^* and both the slope α and intercept β can be considered constant beyond t^*. The tissue ratio minus 1 at equilibrium is calculated as

$$BP^*_{ND} = \frac{V_S}{V^P_{ND} + \delta V^M_{ND}} = \frac{\alpha_{target\ tissue}}{\alpha_{reference\ tissue}} - 1.$$

The tissue ratio minus 1 at equilibrium can also be estimated by the traditional compartment model (Fig. 17.1a) using the parent-only input function $(C^P_a(t))$ if data fitting can be adequately accomplished. However, it may not match the tissue ratio minus 1 estimated by the reference tissue model or the dual-input model if a significant amount of the metabolite is entering the brain because the tissue radioactivity includes the metabolite contribution, which is not accounted for by the traditional compartment model (Fig. 17.1a).

17.2.2   Radioligand

[11]C-PBB3 is a novel radioligand developed at the National Institute of Radiological Sciences, Chiba, Japan, for PET imaging of pathological tau aggregates in the brain [1]. Neurofibrillary tau tangles are one of the two pathological hallmarks of AD, the

other being the senile plaques containing Aβ deposition [7]. ^{11}C-PBB3 binds reversibly to neurofibrillary tau tangles of a wide range of isoform compositions with high affinity ($K_D = 2.5$ nM) and selectivity [1]. ^{11}C-PBB3 upon intravenous administration is rapidly converted in plasma to one major radiometabolite identical chemically in both humans and mice, a significant amount of which enters the mouse brain (30% of radioactivity in brain 5 min after injection) [8]. ^{11}C-PBB3 SUVR in AD patients has previously been shown to reflect the known pathological tau distribution at various stages of AD [9].

17.2.3 PET Data

The reader is referred to our recent ^{11}C-PBB3 PET data analysis study [2] regarding the detail of PET data acquisition and full data analysis. Here, the description is limited to information relevant to illustrating the concept of tissue ratio estimation considering the contribution of radiometabolite to the brain activity.

[11]C-PBB3 PET data consisted of 70 min dynamic scans after a bolus injection of approximately 400 MBq of ^{11}C-PBB3 in 7 AD patients (76 ± 7 y) and 7 elderly healthy control subjects (70 ± 6 y). Input functions ($C_a^P(t)$ and $C_a^M(t)$) were obtained from multiple arterial samples by determining plasma fractions of the parent and its radiometabolites with high-performance liquid chromatography.

To improve the statistical quality of PET ROI data, we generated cerebral cortical ROIs pooling all voxels of high (>0.3, high), medium (0.15–0.3, middle), low (0–0.15, low), and non-binding (<0) BP_{ND}^* values on preliminarily generated parametric images by the original multilinear reference tissue model (MRTM$_O$)[10] using the cerebellar cortex as the reference tissue because tau accumulation is known to be histopathologically absent in the cerebellar cortex of either normal or AD brains [11].

17.2.4 Data Analysis

The tissue ratio minus 1 was estimated in four ways using cerebral cortical ROI data with the cerebellar cortex as the reference tissue:

1) BP_{ND}^* estimation by the dual-input graphical analysis using $\left(C_a^P(t) + C_a^M(t)\right)$ as an input function (Eq. 17.4)
2) BP_{ND} estimation by 2T compartment kinetic analysis using $C_a^P(t)$ as an input function (Fig. 17.1a)
3) BP_{ND}^* estimation by the reference tissue model MRTM$_O$ using $C_B'(t)$ as an input function
4) SUVR minus 1 at a fixed time point (50 min–70 min)

The tissue ratio minus 1 values obtained by the above 4 methods were then compared to validate the use of SUVR and the reference tissue model BP^*_{ND}. Additionally, parametric images of MRTM$_O$ and (SUVR-1) were generated and compared.

17.3 Results

The brain ^{11}C-PBB3 time activity curves (TACs) quickly peaked within a few minutes of intravenous injection of ^{11}C-PBB3 with gradual decreases thereafter with a significantly slower washout for high binding cerebral cortex in ADs than in HCs (Fig. 17.2a). Plasma parent TACs peaked very quickly and decreased also quickly thereafter (Fig. 17.2b). One major radiometabolite of ^{11}C-PBB3 appeared very quickly in the plasma and slowly decreased thereafter (Fig 17.2b). Both plasma parent and metabolite TACs in ADs and HCs were very similar (Fig. 17.2b)

Graphical plots (Eq. 17.4) with a combined $C^P_a(t) + C^M_a(t)$ plasma input became linear beyond t* = 11 min when both α and β could be considered constant. BP^*_{ND} estimations were very stable for all regions. On the other hand, the 2T kinetic analysis to estimate BP_{ND} was unstable in some regions with a large parameter estimation variability in the rest of the regions. The 2TC BP_{ND} values were numerically quite different from the corresponding BP^*_{ND} values with a very poor correlation between the two-tissue ratio minus 1 estimations ($BP_{ND} = 1.06 \pm 0.66$ vs. $BP^*_{ND} = 0.36 \pm 0.07$ with $r^2 = 0.04$ in the high binding region, for example.

The reference tissue model MRTM$_O$ robustly estimated BP^*_{ND} for the ROI data and enabled stable voxel-wise parametric imaging of BP^*_{ND}. The BP^*_{ND} estimated by the ROI-based MRTM$_O$ analysis closely matched the corresponding BP^*_{ND}

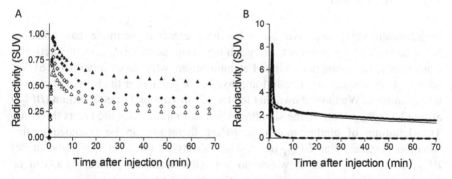

Fig. 17.2 Time activity curves (TACs) in the brain (**a**) and arterial plasma (**b**) after the injection of ^{11}C-PBB3 in AD patients and healthy controls (HCs). (**a**) TACs are shown for the high tau binding (▲) cerebral cortical region and cerebellar cortex (♦) in ADs, and the cerebral cortical region (△) and the cerebellar cortex (◇) in HCs. (B) Plasma TACs are shown for the total radioactivity (thick (ADs) and thin (HCs) solid lines), metabolite (thick (ADs) and thin (HCs) dotted lines), and parent (thick (ADs) and thin (HCs) dashed lines). Data represent mean of all 7 ADs or 7 HCs

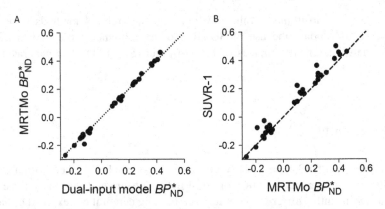

Fig. 17.3 (a) Correlation of ROI BP_{ND}^* estimated by dual-input graphical model and reference tissue model MRTM$_O$. (b) Correlation of ROI BP_{ND}^* estimated by MRTM$_O$ and SUVR minus 1 (50 min–70 min)

estimated by the dual-input graphical analysis with a perfect correlation between the two ($r^2 = 1.00$) (Fig. 17.3a). On the other hand, SUVR minus 1 values (calculated from the averaged 50 min to 70 min data) overestimated MRTM$_O$ BP_{ND}^* values by up to 38%. However, there was an excellent correlation between the two ($r^2 = 0.97$) (Fig. 17.3b). Both the MRTM$_O$ BP_{ND}^* parametric images and SUVR minus 1 images showed a clear delineation of tau pathology in the cerebral cortices including the hippocampal formation in AD (Fig. 17.4a, c) compared with HC (Fig. 17.4b, d).

17.4 Discussion

In the present article, we have shown that the reference tissue model-based binding potential (BP_{ND}) that reflects the target binding site density (B_{avail}) is theoretically equivalent to the tissue ratio minus 1 at equilibrium, whereas closely related SUVR minus 1 is the tissue ratio minus 1 at a fixed time point after the bolus radioligand administration. We have shown that the tissue ratio minus 1 at equilibrium (BP_{ND}^*) also reflects B_{avail} even in the situation where the radiometabolite enters the brain. The definition of binding potential, BP_{ND}, therefore can be extended to this situation (expressed as BP_{ND}^* here). The validity of the reference tissue model BP_{ND}^* and SUVR, both of which do not require arterial plasma data, can be evaluated by the dual-input $\left(C_a^P(t) + C_a^M(t)\right)$ model but not by the conventional single input ($C_a^P(t)$) model because the tissue ratio minus 1 at equilibrium includes the radiometabolite contribution to the tissue activity, which is not accounted for by the parent-only model. Of note is that the reference tissue BP_{ND}^* or SUVR estimation

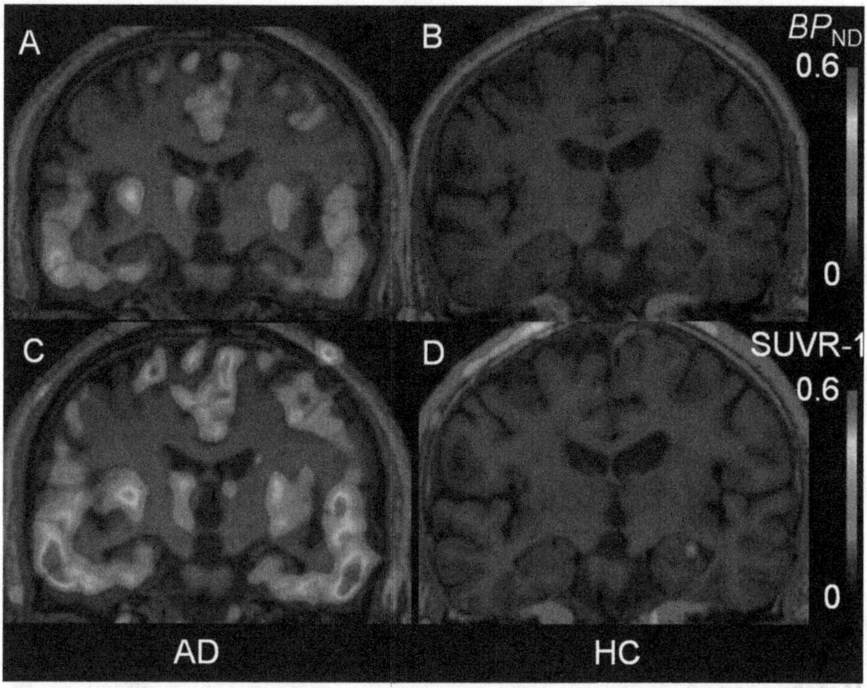

Fig. 17.4 Coronal parametric images of AD and HC. The MRTM$_O$ BP^*_{ND} images in ADs (**a**) and HCs (**b**). SUVR-1 images (50 min–70 min) in ADs (**c**) and HCs (**d**)

does not require any assumption of metabolite, because the estimation is performed without blood data.

Although we assumed here that the radiometabolite does not bind to the target site, it can be shown that BP_{ND} is also directly proportional to B_{avail} when the metabolite binds specifically (17.2). BP^*_{ND} has additional term, δV^M_{ND}, in the denominator (Eq. 17.2), which may increase the intersubject variability of BP^*_{ND} compared with BP_{ND}. In our ^{11}C-PBB3 analyses, there was no difference in the mean $\left(V^P_{ND} + \delta V^M_{ND}\right)$ values between ADs and HCs [2].

SUVR minus 1 at 50 min–70 min overestimated BP^*_{ND}. However, there was an excellent correlation between the two. SUVR is potentially affected by blood flow and systemic radioligand clearance, while BP^*_{ND} is independent of these factors because BP^*_{ND} represents the tissue ratio minus 1 at equilibrium. Therefore, a larger variability of cerebral blood flow in AD patents than in normal elderly subjects may result in a larger intersubject SUVR variability compared with BP^*_{ND}, although a longer dynamic imaging needed for BP^*_{ND} estimation might be less well tolerated for elderly patients than a shorter static imaging for SUVR measurements. The advantage of the reference tissue model-based estimation of the tissue ratio over the SUVR measurement has recently been shown for a long-term longitudinal Aβ PET imaging study [12].

17.5 Conclusions

The reference tissue-based binding potential (BP_{ND}) that reflects the target binding site density (B_{avail}) is equivalent to the tissue ratio minus 1 at equilibrium. The tissue ratio minus 1 at equilibrium (BP^*_{ND}) also reflects B_{avail} even in the situation where the radiometabolite enters the brain. The validity of the reference tissue model BP^*_{ND} and SUVR can be evaluated by the dual-input model not by the conventional single input model because the tissue ratio minus 1 at equilibrium includes the radiometabolite contribution to the tissue activity, which is not accounted for by the parent-only model.

References

1. Maruyama M, Shimada H, Suhara T, et al. Imaging of tau pathology in a tauopathy mouse model and in Alzheimer's patients compared to normal controls. Neuron. 2013;79:1094–108.
2. Kimura Y, Ichise M, Ito H, et al. PET quantification of tau pathology in human brain with ^{11}C-PBB3. J Nucl Med. 2015;56:1359–65.
3. Ichise M, Fujita M, Seibyl JP, et al. Graphical analysis and simplified quantification of striatal and extrastriatal dopamine D2 receptor binding with ^{123}I]epidepride SPECT. J Nucl Med. 1999;40:1902–12.
4. Ichise M. Neuroreceptor imaging and kinetic modeling. In: Van Heertum RL, Tikofsky R, Ichise M, editors. Cerebral SPECT and PET imaging. 4th ed. Philadelphia: Lippincott Wiliams and Wilkinson; 2009. p. 40–53. chapter 4.
5. Innis RB, Cunningham VJ, Delforge J, et al. Consensus nomenclature for in vivo imaging of reversibly binding radioligands. J Cerebr Blood F Met. 2007;27:1533–9.
6. Michaelis L, Menten ML. Die Kinetik der Invertinwirkung. Biochem Z. 1913;49:1333.
7. Braak H, Braak E. Neuropathological staging of Alzheimer-related changes. Acta Neuropathol. 1991;82:239–59.
8. Hashimoto H, Kawamura K, Igarashi N, et al. Radiosynthesis, photoisomerization, biodistribution, and metabolite analysis of ^{11}C-PBB3 as a clinically useful PET probe for imaging of tau pathology. J Nucl Med. 2014;55:1532–8.
9. Shimada H, Higuchi M, Shinotoh H, et al. In vivo visualization of tau pathology in Alzheimer's disease patients by [11C]PBB3-PET. Alzheimer's Dement. 2013;9:P845. Abstract.
10. Ichise M, Ballinger JR, Golan H, et al. Noninvasive quantification of dopamine D2 receptors in humans with iodine-123-IBF SPECT. J Nucl Med. 1996;37:513–20.
11. Herrmann M, Golombowski S, Kräuchi K, et al. ELISA-quantitation of phosphorylated tau protein in the Alzheimer's disease brain. Eur Neurol. 1999;42:205–10.
12. van Berckel BNM, Ossenkoppele R, Tolboom N, et al. Longitudinal amyloid imaging using ^{11}C-PiB: methodologic considerations. J Nucl Med. 2013;54:1570–6.

Chapter 18
Hypoxia Imaging with ^{18}F-FMISO PET for Brain Tumors

Kenji Hirata, Kentaro Kobayashi, and Nagara Tamaki

Abstract Tumor hypoxia is an important object for imaging because hypoxia is associated with tumor aggressiveness and resistance to radiation therapy. Here, ^{18}F-fluoromisonidazole (FMISO) has been used for many years as the most commonly employed hypoxia imaging tracer. Unlike F-18 fluorodeoxyglucose (FDG), FMISO does not accumulate in normal brain tissue making it able to provide images of hypoxic brain tumors with high contrast. Clinical evidence has suggested that FMISO PET can predict patient prognosis and treatment response. Among gliomas of various grades (WHO 2007), it has been known that grade IV glioblastoma resides under severe hypoxia and is a cause of development of necrosis in the tumor. For this study we tested whether FMISO can distinguish the oxygen condition of glioblastomas and lower-grade gliomas. Twenty-three glioma patients underwent FMISO PET for the study. All the glioblastoma patients ($N = 14$) showed high FMISO uptakes in the tumor, whereas none of the other patients (i.e., gliomas of grade III or lower, $N = 9$) did, demonstrated by both qualitative and quantitative assessments. The data suggest that FMISO PET may be a useful tool to distinguish glioblastomas from lower-grade gliomas. Our results, however, were slightly different from previous investigations reporting that some lower-grade gliomas (e.g., grade III) showed positive FMISO uptake. Many of these acquired the FMISO PET images 2 h after the FMISO injection, while for the study here we waited 4 h to be able to collect hypoxia-specific signals rather than perfusion signals as FMISO clearance from plasma is slow due to its lipophilic nature. No optimum uptake time for FMISO has been established, and we directly compared the 2-h vs. the 4-h images with the same patients ($N = 17$). At 2 h, the gray matter had significantly higher standardized uptake value (SUV) than the white matter, possibly due to different degrees of perfusion but not due to hypoxia. At 4 h, there were no differences between gray and white matter without any significant increase in the noise level measured by the coefficient of variation between the 2-h and the 4-h images. At 2 h, 6/8 (75 %) of glioblastoma patients

---

K. Hirata (✉) • K. Kobayashi
Department of Nuclear Medicine, Hokkaido University, Sapporo, Japan
e-mail: khirata@med.hokudai.ac.jp

N. Tamaki
Department of Nuclear Medicine, Graduate School of Medicine, Hokkaido University, Sapporo, Japan

© The Author(s) 2016   229
Y. Kuge et al. (eds.), *Perspectives on Nuclear Medicine for Molecular Diagnosis and Integrated Therapy*, DOI 10.1007/978-4-431-55894-1_18

showed higher uptakes in the tumor than in the surrounding brain tissue, whereas at 4 h this was the case for 8/8 (100 %). In addition, at 2 h, 3/4 (75 %) of patients with lower-grade gliomas showed moderate uptakes, while at 4 h none did (0/4 or 0 %). These data indicate that 4-h images are better than 2-h images for the purpose of glioma grading. In conclusion, we evaluated the diagnostic performance of FMISO PET for gliomas and suggest that FMISO PET may be able to assist in the diagnosis of glioblastomas when PET images are acquired at 4 h post injection.

Keywords Hypoxia • 18 F-Fluoromisonidazole • Glioma • Glioblastoma

18.1   Introduction

This review article summarizes our recent studies with ^{18}F-fluoromisonidazole (FMISO) positron emission tomography (PET) applied to brain tumors [1, 2]. A variety of tumors which can be divided into two categories develop in the brain: primary brain tumors that originate from the brain tissue and metastatic brain tumors that originate from malignant tumors in other organs. Gliomas account for 60 % of primary brain tumors. Gliomas comprise a range of tumors, from benign to malignant, that are derived from glial cells such as astrocytes, oligodendrocytes, and ependymal cells. Among gliomas, the glioblastoma is the most aggressive astrocytic tumor. Glioblastomas are categorized as grade IV in the WHO classification [3]. The standard treatment for glioblastomas is surgery followed by radiotherapy and chemotherapy [4]. With state-of-the-art multidisciplinary therapy, the 1-year survival rate of glioblastoma patients is reported to be 56 %, which is significantly poorer than with grade III (78 %) or less malignant gliomas [5]. A pathological diagnosis of surgical specimens by biopsy or resection is necessary to establish the diagnosis for glioblastomas [6], but brain surgery involving eloquent regions can exacerbate the prognosis by causing neurological morbidity and should be avoided if possible [7]. Patients with impaired performance status or elderly patients especially would benefit from nonsurgical methods of establishing the diagnosis, substituting surgical tissue sampling.

The basic in vivo imaging modality for brain tumors is magnetic resonance (MR) imaging. Intratumoral characteristics and tumor expansion states are shown accurately with MR imaging. The use of PET with ^{18}F-fluorodeoxyglucose (FDG) is a well-established method for many different types of tumors in the body, including lung cancer, head and neck cancers, and others. FDG PET also plays important roles in the diagnosis of glioblastomas. The diagnosis of a glioblastoma is generally suggested if there is a ringlike enhancement by gadolinium on MR images or an intense uptake of FDG [6, 8–15]. However, there are cases of false-negative MRI findings as some glioblastoma lack the ringlike enhancement [6]. In discriminating glioblastoma from grade III tumors, FDG PET is also not always adequate as a large number of patients of grade III gliomas show high FDG uptakes [13, 14]. This makes a biopsy necessary in many cases, and a noninvasive in vivo imaging tool would be of benefit to omit invasive biopsy procedures in clinical settings [11].

The WHO 2007 criteria determine the glioma grade based on microscopic characteristics present in the malignancy. Grade II tumors show cell atypia and grade III tumors tissue anaplasia and cell mitosis in addition to cell atypia. Grade IV glioblastomas have pathological features that are not found in grade III or lower-grade gliomas, particularly microvascular proliferation and necrosis [3]. Basically, necrosis is considered to be closely related to hypoxia as low oxygen concentrations do not allow the energy metabolism to proceed as in unaffected tissue. In fact, glioblastomas are known to be in a state of severe hypoxia possibly due to vascular abnormalities and high oxygen demand, whereas the hypoxia of grade III or lower-grade gliomas is less severe [16–19]. We hypothesized that imaging the hypoxia of glioblastomas could be useful to distinguish glioblastomas from lower-grade gliomas.

Measuring hypoxia in living tissue uses needle electrodes; however, this technique presents significant shortcomings. First, it is invasive to insert a needle into deep layers of tissue in humans. Second, it requires considerable skill and the reproducibility is not high. Third, needles may alter the tissue structure and so influence the local oxygen partial pressure, and for these reasons needle electrodes are not used in clinical practice. An alternative is presented by ^{18}F-fluoromiso-nidazole (FMISO) PET which is a widely used method for in vivo hypoxia imaging [20–23]. Valk et al. first introduced the use of FMISO for glioma imaging in 1992 [24], and the usefulness of FMISO for glioma imaging has been extensively investigated [25–32]. The FMISO is also known to accumulate in severe hypoxic structures but not in mildly hypoxic structures, suggesting that FMISO would be able to discriminate severe from mild hypoxia. This made us hypothesize that much FMISO may accumulate in glioblastomas and only little in lower-grade gliomas. If such a difference could be substantiated, hypoxia imaging using FMISO would provide an avenue to discriminate glioblastomas from lower-grade gliomas. The first paper of our project was to test the hypothesis [1]. We evaluated the diagnostic usefulness of FMISO PET in terms of glioma grading in comparison with diagnosis with FDG PET in patients suspected of having glioblastomas on MR images.

With FMISO there is a trade-off problem regarding uptake time (the interval between the FMISO injection and the PET emission scanning). A longer uptake time is theoretically desirable to image hypoxia with good lesion-to-background signal ratios, but the longer time leads to lower signal-to-noise ratios due to radiological decay of the F-18. Early reports by Grunbaum et al. [33] and Thorwarth et al. [34] addressing this issue suggested a 4-h acquisition as suitable. Despite this, most research adopted 2-h protocols [24, 25, 27–32], possibly because a shorter protocol would be more generally acceptable in clinical settings. Based on this, the second part of our project was to directly compare 2-h and 4-h images from the same patients [2].

18.2 Materials and Methods

The first of the studies reported here was conducted for the purpose of testing the ability to discriminate between glioblastomas and lower-grade gliomas with FMISO PET. Twenty-seven patients with possible high-grade gliomas were considered for the study [1]. The patients included showed cerebral parenchymal tumors surrounded by edematous tissue on MR images but no known malignancy in other organs. We excluded patients where previous tumorectomy, chemotherapy, or radiotherapy for lesions had been performed. The only exception was a patient with a recurrent tumor 6 years after tumorectomy combined with chemoradiotherapy for a low-grade glioma. Among the 27 patients, two were excluded because they had contraindications of surgical operations. The remaining 25 patients underwent either a tumoral resection ($n = 16$) or biopsy ($n = 9$) at most 2 weeks after the PET scanning. The surgical specimen was investigated by two experienced neuropathologists to determine the pathological diagnosis based on the 2007 WHO classification. Among the 25 patients, two were diagnosed as having metastatic adenocarcinoma and multiple sclerosis, respectively, and these two patients were excluded from the analysis. Finally 23 patients (M/F = 10:13, age 57 ± 15 years old) all with the pathological diagnosis of gliomas were included in the study.

With these 23 patients, we acquired FMISO and FDG PET images following the same protocol for all the patients. The interval between FMISO and FDG was at most 1 week. The FMISO synthesis protocol was previously described in detail elsewhere [35, 36]. On the day of FMISO, the patient was not asked to fast before the PET, and 400 MBq of FMISO was intravenously injected. Then, 4 h later, the emission scanning was initiated to acquire static PET images of the entire brain. FDG PET was performed on another day; here the dosage of FDG was also 400 MBq. The uptake time for FDG was 1 h, and the scanning range for the FDG PET was the same for the FMISO PET with a high-resolution PET scanner (ECAT HR+ scanner; Asahi-Siemens Medical Technologies Ltd., Tokyo, Japan) operated in a three-dimensional mode for 22 patients. For one patient the FMISO images were acquired using an integrated PET-CT scanner (Biograph 64 PET-CT scanner; Asahi-Siemens Medical Technologies Ltd., Tokyo, Japan). The duration of the emission scanning using the ECAT HR+ scanner was 10 min. The duration of the transmission scanning using the ECAT HR+ scanner with a ^{68}Ge/^{68}Ga retractable line source was 3 min. This acquisition protocol was the same for both FDG and FMISO. With the Biograph 64 PET-CT scanner, the duration of the emission scanning was also 10 min. The transmission scanning was performed using an X-ray CT, and the attenuation correction used the CT images. The attenuation-corrected radioactivity images from both scanners were reconstructed using a filtered back projection with a 4 mm full width at half maximum Hann filter.

For our second study, to compare the 2-h vs. 4-h images of FMISO PET, we investigated 17 different patients with brain tumors (M/F = 7:10, age 62 ± 14 years old, range 33–85 years old). The study populations for first and second studies were different, and none of the patients included in the first study were included in the second study. The PET images for each patient in the second study were acquired twice, 2 and 4 h following the injection. The injected dosage of FMISO was 399 ± 25 MBq. The first scanning took place 115.9 ± 14.6 min after the injection and the second 227.4 ± 15.1 min after injection. The scanner was a Gemini GXL 16 PET-CT (Philips). The duration of the emission scanning was 20 min. Transmission scanning was performed using the X-ray CT which was used for attenuation correction. Attenuation-corrected radioactivity images were reconstructed using ordered subset expectation maximization.

For the first study, the images were analyzed both qualitatively and quantitatively. An experienced nuclear physician who was blinded from the pathological diagnosis visually evaluated all the images in the qualitative assessment for the first study. In the qualitative assessment of the FMISO PET images, the FMISO uptake was visually categorized into three groups. Where the highest uptake in the tumor was weaker than that in the surrounding brain tissue, the patient was considered as showing *low FMISO uptake*. Where the highest uptake in the tumor was equal to that in the surrounding brain tissue, the patient was considered as showing *intermediate FMISO uptake*. Where the highest uptake in the tumor was stronger than that in the surrounding brain tissue, the patient was considered as showing *high FMISO uptake*. This grouping rule was however not efficient as no patients were assigned to show *low FMISO uptake*. As a result the *low FMISO uptake* and the *intermediate FMISO uptake* patients were combined in one group of *FMISO-negative* patients. The remaining patients, those assigned to the *high FMISO uptake* group, were designated as *FMISO-positive* patients. This binary division was presented in a previous paper [27]. Similarly, in the qualitative assessment of the FDG PET images, we evaluated the FDG accumulation in the tumor using the grouping detailed elsewhere [14]. First, the FDG uptake was visually categorized into three groups: low, intermediate, and high. Where the highest uptake in the tumor was weaker than or equal to that in the contralateral white matter, the patient was considered as showing *low FDG uptake*. Where the highest uptake in the tumor was stronger than that in the contralateral white matter but weaker than that in the contralateral gray matter, the patient was considered as showing *intermediate FDG uptake*. Where the highest uptake in the tumor was equal to or stronger than that in the contralateral gray matter, the patient was considered as showing *high FDG uptake*. Like the FMISO categorization, the *low FDG uptake* and *intermediate FDG uptake* patients were combined and termed *FDG-negative* patients, and those of *high FDG uptake* were termed FDG-positive patients.

For the second study, the grouping of the FMISO uptake in the tumor was performed slightly differently, here it was visually assessed. The degree of uptake was assigned as either high, medium, or low. Low uptake here means the uptake compared to the surrounding brain tissue.

Such qualitative assessments may be subjective and a quantitative assessment was also made. For the first study, the PET images were coregistered with individual MR images (FLAIR) using a mutual information technique implemented in the NEUROSTAT software package [37, 38]. Then, polygonal regions of interest

(ROI) were manually drawn to enclose the entire tumor on every slice that also included peritumoral edematous regions. The single voxel having the highest radioactivity concentration in the tumor was determined in the PET images using in-house software. The highest radioactivity concentration was used to calculate a maximum standardized uptake value (SUV_{max}). A SUV_{peak} value has recently come into use to overcome the shortcomings of SUV_{max}. However, the concept of SUV_{peak} is not unique as different researchers use different definitions. Here, we use the term SUV_{10mm} to explicitly show the meaning: a 10-mm-diameter circular ROI with the center at the maximum voxel was created. The averaged value for the circular ROI was assigned as SUV_{10mm}, and the SUV was calculated as (tissue radioactivity [Bq/ml])*(body weight [g])/(injected radioactivity [Bq]). Next, further ROIs were created on the following reference regions: the cerebellar cortex, the contralateral frontoparietal cortex on the level of the centrum semiovale, and the contralateral frontoparietal white matter on the level of the centrum semiovale. The lesion-to-cerebellum ratio of the FMISO was determined as the ratio of the SUV_{10mm} to the cerebellar averaged SUV. The lesion-to-gray matter and lesion-to-white matter ratios of the FDG were the ratios of SUV_{10mm} to gray matter and white matter SUV, respectively [13]. The ROI placement process was performed by an experienced nuclear physician, and where the tumor occupied bilateral lobes, the hemisphere with the larger part of the tumor was considered as the tumor side. We further measured the hypoxic tissue volume showing significant FMISO uptake in the tumor with the cerebellum used as the reference tissue for this purpose. The voxels having higher SUV than 1.3 times that of the cerebellar SUV were extracted in the tumoral polygonal ROI described above. No threshold for FMISO uptake volumes has been established, and the 1.3 value was empirically adopted from image segmentation in ^{11}C-methionine brain PET [31, 39, 40]. The FMISO uptake volumes were expressed as a percentage of the extracted voxels in the whole tumoral ROI.

For the second study, the 2-h and 4-h images were coregistered to CT. To obtain reference values from normal tissue, circular 10-mm-diameter ROIs were defined on gray matter, white matter, and the cerebellar cortex. The SUV_{mean}, standard deviation (SD), and coefficient of variation (CV) were measured within these ROIs. To express tumor uptake values, the SUV_{max} and lesion-to-cerebellum ratios were calculated in the same way as in the first study.

In the following, all parametric data are expressed as means ± SD. The patients with grade III or with less malignant gliomas were grouped together as non-glioblastoma patients to simplify the analysis. The relationship between the histo-pathological diagnosis and the visual assessment results was examined using Fisher's exact test. The differences in age, tumor size, SUVs, lesion-to-normal tissue ratios, and uptake volume for glioblastoma vs. non-glioblastoma patients were examined using the Mann-Whitney U-test. The 2-h vs. 4-h values were compared using paired t-tests; P-values smaller than 0.05 were considered statistically significant. The statistical analysis and figure drawing used R 2.14.0 and R 3.1.3 for Windows.

18.3 Results

In the first study, 14 patients were diagnosed with glioblastomas and categorized as grade IV in the WHO classification. Among the remaining nine patients, one had anaplastic astrocytoma (grade III), one had anaplastic oligodendroglioma (grade III), three had anaplastic oligoastrocytomas (grade III), one had diffuse astrocytoma (grade II), one had oligodendroglioma (grade II), and two had oligoastrocytomas (grade II). Necrosis was identified in all the glioblastoma patients, while none of the non-glioblastoma patients showed necrosis within the tumor. The age of the glioblastoma patients was 65.5 ± 9.9 years, and the age of non-glioblastoma patients was 43.7 ± 12.2 years; the age difference was statistically significant ($p < 0.01$). The tumor sizes were measured on FLAIR MR images and were not significantly different for glioblastomas vs. non-glioblastomas (64.4 ± 17.5 mm vs. 77.6 ± 22.5 mm in diameter) ($p =$ NS). Gadolinium enhancement was observed in 3/9 non-glioblastoma patients and in14/14 glioblastoma patients. By visual assessment, all of the glioblastoma patients (14/14) were classified as FMISO positive and all of the non-glioblastoma patients as FMISO negative. There was a significant association by Fisher's exact test between the histology (glioblastoma or non-glioblastoma) and FMISO uptake (FMISO positive or FMISO negative) ($p < 0.001$). This visual assessment of the FMISO PET images correctly discriminated glioblastoma patients from non-glioblastoma patients with sensitivity, specificity, and accuracy of 100 %, 100 %, and 100 %, respectively. For the FDG PET results, after excluding a diabetic patient with hyperglycemia at the time of the FDG PET, all glioblastoma patients (13/13) were FDG positive and 3/9 non-glioblastoma patients were FDG positive. This relationship reached statistical difference ($p < 0.01$), but the diagnostic performance of the FDG PET was poorer than the FMISO PET, with sensitivity, specificity, and accuracy being 100 %, 66 %, and 86 %, respectively. Figures 18.1, 18.2, 18.3, 18.4, and 18.5 show representative cases.

In the quantitative assessment of the first study, the SUV_{max} of the FMISO was 3.09 ± 0.62 (range, 2.22–4.31) in glioblastoma patients, significantly higher than in non-glioblastoma patients (1.73 ± 0.36; range, 1.36–2.39) ($p < 0.001$). As detailed above, we introduced the SUV_{10mm} term to be able to minimize noise effects. The SUV_{10mm} of FMISO was similar to the SUV_{max} of FMISO, with the values being 3.00 ± 0.61 (range, 2.15–4.18), significantly higher than in non-glioblastoma patients (1.64 ± 0.38; range, 1.29–2.35) ($p < 0.001$). The lesion-to-cerebellum ratio of the FMISO (the SUV_{10mm}/cerebellar SUV) was higher in the glioblastoma patients (2.74 ± 0.60; range, 1.71–3.81) than in the non-glioblastoma patients (1.22 ± 0.06; range, 1.09–1.29) ($p < 0.001$). The quantitative results of the FDG PET were slightly different from those of the FMISO PET. Here the diabetic patient was also excluded from the analyses of SUV and the lesion-to-normal tissue ratio of the FDG PET. The SUV_{max} of the FDG was not significantly different for the glioblastoma and non-glioblastoma patients (7.55 ± 3.72; range, 4.34–16.38, vs. 8.21 ± 6.04; range, 4.75–23.49) ($p = 0.95$). Similarly, the SUV_{10mm} of the

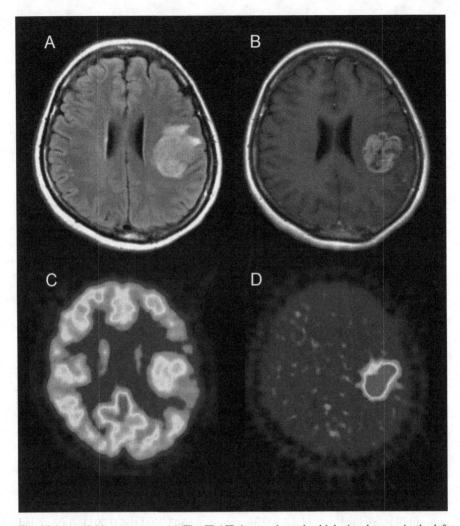

Fig. 18.1 A glioblastoma case. (**a**) The FLAIR image showed a high-signal tumor in the left hemisphere. (**b**) The tumor was enhanced by gadolinium contrast material. (**c**) The FDG uptake in the tumor was comparable to that of contralateral cerebral cortex. (**d**) The FMISO uptake was higher in the tumor than in the surrounding brain tissue

FDG was not significantly different for the glioblastoma and non-glioblastoma patients (7.41 ± 3.63; range, 4.26–15.90, vs. 8.03 ± 5.96; range, 4.64–23.12) ($p = 0.95$). The lesion-to-gray matter ratio of the FDG (the SUV_{10mm}/SUV in the contralateral gray matter) was higher in the glioblastoma patients (1.46 ± 0.75; range, 0.91–3.79) than in the non-glioblastoma patients (1.07 ± 0.62; range, 0.66–2.95, $p < 0.05$). The lesion-to-white matter ratio of the FDG (the SUV_{10mm}/ SUV in the contralateral white matter) was not significantly different for the glioblastoma (2.81 ± 1.23; range, 1.87–6.44) and non-glioblastoma (2.66 ± 1.60;

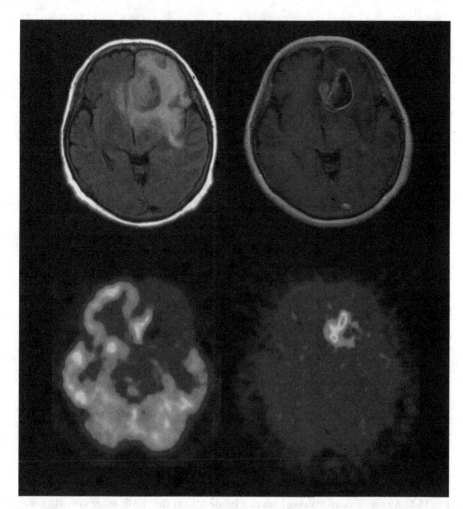

Fig. 18.2 A glioblastoma case. (**a**) The FLAIR image showed a tumor in the left frontal lobe. (**b**) The tumor showed a ringlike enhancement by gadolinium contrast material. (**c**) The FDG uptake was observed in a part of the gadolinium-enhanced area. The FDG uptake was comparable to the right cerebral cortex. (**d**) The FMISO PET showed a similar distribution of FMISO as FDG but with stronger tumor-to-background contrast than FDG

range, 1.71–6.51) ($p = 0.16$) patients. Finally, the uptake volume of FMISO was larger in the glioblastoma than in non-glioblastoma patients (27.18 ± 10.46 %; range, 14.02–46.67 %, vs. 6.07 ± 2.50 %; range, 2.12–9.22 %), ($p < 0.001$).

In the second study, the 2-h images and the 4-h images of FMISO PET were directly compared for the same subjects. Figure 18.6 shows representative images that do not show tumors. Visually, the SUV in the brain was higher at 2 h than at 4 h. More specifically, the gray matter SUV was higher at 2 h than at 4 h, whereas the white matter SUV was comparable in the images at 2 h and 4 h. Profile curves

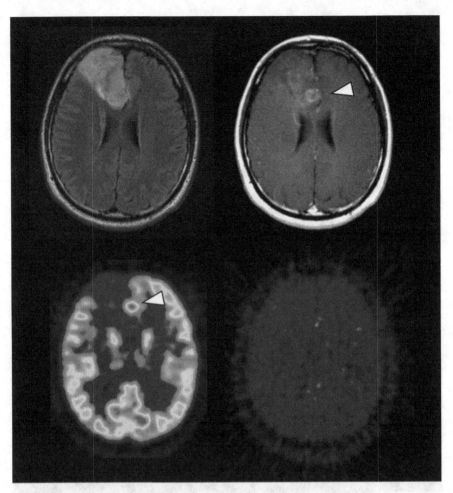

Fig. 18.3 An anaplastic oligoastrocytoma case (grade III). (**a**) The FLAIR image showed a tumor in the right frontal lobe. (**b**) A small part of the tumor is enhanced after treatment with gadolinium contrast material (arrowhead). (**c**) The FDG uptake was observed in the enhanced part (arrowhead). The FDG uptake was higher than that in the left cerebral cortex. (**d**) No FMISO accumulated in the tumor

demonstrate these differences in Figure 18.6. At 2 h, the gray matter was distinguishable from the white matter, as the gray matter showed higher SUV than the white matter while at 4 h; the curve was almost flat. Figure 18.7 shows scatter plots of gray and white matter SUV at 2 h vs. 4 h. In all cases the gray matter SUV decreased with time and all the points plot under the line of identity. White matter SUV was not significantly different at 2 and 4 h. Figure 18.8 shows the CV of gray and white matter, compared at 2 h and 4 h. The gray matter CV increased slightly from 2 to 4 h ($P = 0.0008$), while the white matter CV was not significantly different at 2 and 4 h.

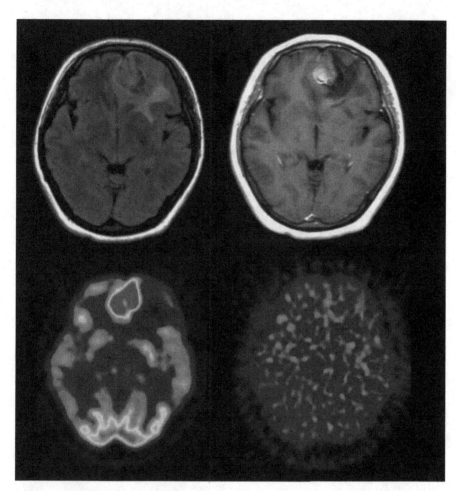

Fig. 18.4 An anaplastic oligodendroglioma case (grade III). (**a**) The FLAIR image showed a tumor in the left frontal lobe. (**b**) A part of the tumor enhanced by gadolinium contrast material. (**c**) The FDG uptake was observed even outside the enhancing area. The FDG uptake was much higher than that in the right cerebral cortex. (**d**) No FMISO uptake was observed in the tumor

In the visual assessment of the tumors, we first looked into grade IV tumors because based on the first study we believed that the grade IV tumors would have a hypoxic volume and thus should show FMISO uptake. At 2 h, six out of eight grade IV patients showed high FMISO uptakes, and the remaining two patients showed medium uptakes. At 4 h, however, eight out of eight (100 %) patients showed high FMISO uptakes. Then, we looked into grade II and III tumors that we thought would not have developed severe hypoxia and thus would not show FMISO uptake. At 2 h, three out of four patients showed medium uptakes and the fourth patient showed a low uptake. This was changed at 4 h where four out of four (100 %) patients showed low uptakes. The results of the visual assessment can be

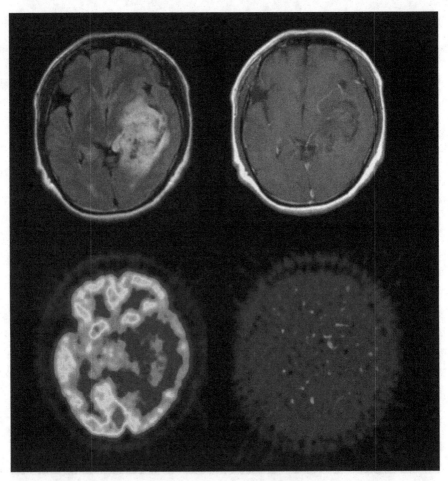

Fig. 18.5 An oligodendroglioma case (grade II). (**a**) The FLAIR image showed a tumor in the left temporal lobe. (**b**) The tumor slightly enhanced by gadolinium contrast material. (**c**) The FDG uptake was weaker than in the right cerebral cortex. (**d**) No FMISO uptake was observed in the tumor

summarized as those 4-h images provide more definitive information for discriminating grade IV tumors from lower-grade tumors. The quantitative analysis further supported this; in all the cases, the SUV_{max} and tumor-to-normal ratio increased from 2 h to 4 h (Fig. 18.9). Here, lower-grade gliomas (grades II and III) showed decreases in SUV_{max} and in the tumor-to-normal ratio from 2 h to 4 h (Fig. 18.10).

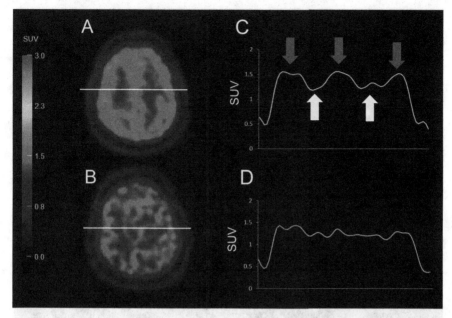

Fig. 18.6 A brain slice FMISO PET image (**a**) 2 h after administration of FMISO and (**b**) after 4 h. No tumor existed on these slices. (**c**) 2-h SUV profile corresponding to the horizontal line in (**a**). The red arrows indicate gray matter, and the white arrows indicate white matter. (**d**) 4-h profile corresponding to the horizontal line (**b**)

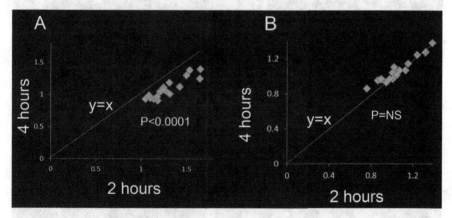

Fig. 18.7 SUV of (**a**) gray and (**b**) white matter at 2 h vs. 4 h

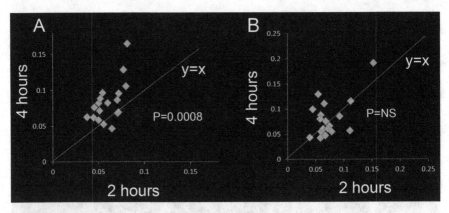

Fig. 18.8 Plot of variation (CV) of (**a**) gray and (**b**) white matter at 2 h vs. 4 h

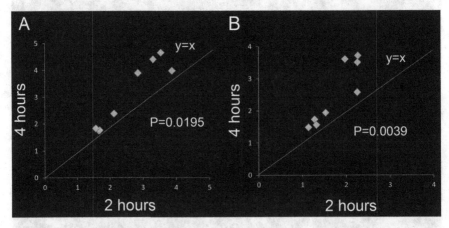

Fig. 18.9 All glioblastoma cases showed increases in both the (**a**) SUV_{max} and (**b**) tumor-to-normal ratio from 2 h to 4 h

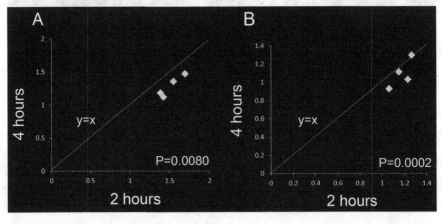

Fig. 18.10 All grade II to III cases showed decrease in (**a**) SUV_{max}, and 3/4 cases showed decrease in (**b**) tumor-to-normal ratio from 2 h to 4 h

18.4 Discussion

We have detailed two studies in this article. The results of the first indicated that much FMISO accumulated in all the glioblastomas here but not in the lower-grade gliomas. Different from this, FDG accumulated in both glioblastomas (100 %) and in some lower-grade gliomas (33 %). This suggests that FMISO PET is superior to FDG PET in a differential diagnosis. Visual analysis was confirmed by analyses of the SUV, lesion-to-normal tissue ratio, and FMISO uptake volume. The results of the second study indicated that FMISO PET 4 h after administration is superior to the images after 2 h in differentiating glioblastomas from non-glioblastomas.

In the 2007 WHO definition, grade IV gliomas show microvascular proliferation and necrosis as well as anaplasia and mitotic activity [3]; necrotic tissue is not observed in grade III or lower-grade gliomas. In brain tumor specimens, necrotic change is an important histopathological landmark that distinguishes glioblastomas from lower-grade gliomas. In previous reports, the necrosis in glioblastoma is considered to be associated with tissue hypoxia [16, 17]. The FMISO PET identification of hypoxia proceeds through several steps. Injected FMISO is first transported by the blood flow and taken up by viable cells. Then, FMISO is oxidized by intracellular oxygen if there is a sufficient amount of oxygen available in a cell, and the oxidized FMISO is excreted from the cell. The FMISO is not oxidized when there is insufficient oxygen available (hypoxic conditions) and the FMISO is here retained in the cell [41]. Considering these mechanisms, we may expect that FMISO accumulates in perinecrotic hypoxic tissue but not in the central necrotic region. We observed that only little FMISO accumulates in non-glioblastoma patients. Some studies used needle electrodes to measure oxygen partial pressures in human gliomas [18, 19, 42] and have suggested that both glioblastomas and grade II and III gliomas are present under hypoxic conditions. Lower-grade gliomas do not develop necrosis and may be expected to suffer from only a milder degree of hypoxia than that of glioblastomas [18, 19]. FMISO accumulation requires severe hypoxic conditions (pO2 < 10 mmHg) [43, 44], and the results here are consistent with this.

Cher et al. investigated FMISO uptake in various tumors and the correlation with histological findings [27]. They reported that all grade IV tumors showed high FMISO uptakes (they were FMISO positive as we define it here) and that all grade I and II tumors showed FMISO uptakes comparable to the surrounding tissue (they were FMISO negative as we define it). However, there was a slightly elevated FMISO uptake in one of three grade III patients and low uptakes in the remaining two grade III patients [27]. Our results in the first study are consistent with this previous data, except for the grade III patients, as all of our grade III gliomas were FMISO negative. Cher et al. used 2 h as the waiting time before conducting the FMISO PET scanning, while the study here used 4 h. Many FMISO PET protocols have used 2 h as the uptake time [24, 25, 27–32], while Thorwarth et al. questioned the adequacy of 2 h for imaging of FMISO [34]. There, the kinetic analysis of dynamic datasets of FMISO PET suggested that the hot spots at 2 h did not reflect actual hypoxia but rather showed a high initial influx of the FMISO due to increased blood flow to the tumor. In our first study, no grade III patients showed high FMISO uptakes, and we speculated that this was possibly because the relatively long uptake time allowed the tracer to be excreted from the tissue without severe hypoxia. To further elucidate this, we conducted the second study, to directly compare images at 2 and 4 h after FMISO injection in the same patients. At 4 h, the background gray matter SUV was lower, and the presence of the tumor uptake was fully substantiated: all the glioblastomas were FMISO positive, and all the non-glioblastomas were FMISO negative. These results are consistent with the Thorwarth observations [34].

Recent advances in molecular targeting therapies and image guided therapies are remarkable, and it may be expected that in the near future the therapy of first choice for glioblastomas will be chemo- or radiotherapy rather than surgery. In such cases, new techniques like FMISO PET may help avoid a biopsy followed by a pathological investigation. Aged patients or patients with impaired performance status would particularly benefit from such techniques.

The FDG PET reflects the histological aggressiveness of gliomas, and glioblastomas commonly show the highest FDG uptake among gliomas [12–14]. In the first study here, a high FDG uptake was unexceptionally observed in glioblastoma patients. At the same time, however, three of nine non-glioblastoma patients also showed high FDG uptakes. These findings are consistent with the previous data [13, 14], and the results indicate that FDG PET is useful for histological grading but inconclusive when a differential diagnosis of glioblastomas from lower-grade gliomas is at issue. This leads us to suggest that FMISO PET may play a more important role when a tumor shows a high FDG uptake (equal to or greater than the uptake in the surrounding gray matter). Another important PET tracer for brain tumor imaging is ^{11}C-methionine (MET). For MET the uptake intensity corresponding to each tumor grade can be summarized as in Fig. 18.11. It is well

Fig. 18.11 A scheme of the suggested roles of ^{11}C-methionine (MET), ^{18}F-FDG, and ^{18}F-FMISO PET in differential diagnosis of gliomas

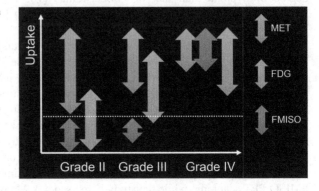

known that even grade II tumors may show high MET uptakes, especially in the case of tumors with oligodendroglial components [45, 46], and that MET is good at showing the tumor boundary. The FDG uptake increases with the tumor grade [47], and the results here suggest that FMISO uptake is absent in grades II and III, but strong in grade IV. Altogether these tracers will provide significant information to assist in distinguishing tumor type and stage.

In the first study, the FMISO PET images were evaluated in different manners by visual assessment, SUV, lesion-to-normal tissue ratio, and uptake volume. The results of these analyses were consistent in showing the relationship between FMISO uptake and glioma grade. In clinical settings the findings suggest that a visual assessment is sufficient for a diagnosis, as the numerical values provide information consistent with the visual assessment. The numerical values may however be useful for purposes like assessing the prognosis and treatment response. Both the SUV_{max} and SUV_{10mm} with FMISO were higher in glioblastoma patients than in non-glioblastoma patients; the range of the values for the groups overlaps, possibly explained by inter-subject variability in the SUV. The lesion-to-cerebellum ratio clearly distinguished glioblastoma patients from non-glioblastoma patients. The usefulness of the lesion-to-cerebellum ratio has also been demonstrated by Bruehlmeier et al. [26], by showing that lesion-to-cerebellum ratios were comparable with the distribution of FMISO volumes. It may be argued that cerebral glioma patients often show asymmetric blood flows in the cerebellum (the so-called crossed cerebellar diaschisis) and that the cerebellar value may not be uniquely useful as a reference. In the study here, FMISO accumulation of the left and right cerebellar cortex did not show significant asymmetry (data not shown); however, this may be assumed not to be a problem in using the lesion-to-cerebellum ratio.

To further confirm the findings, the uptake volume of FMISO in the tumor was measured and compared for glioblastoma and non-glioblastoma patients. This comparison showed that glioblastomas exhibited significantly larger uptake volumes of FMISO than non-glioblastomas. In general, the hypoxic volume is distinguished with tissue-to-blood ratios ≥ 1.2 in images acquired 2 h after FMISO injection with venous blood samples [28–31]. In brain tumor segmentation for MET PET, a tumor-to-normal ratio ≥ 1.3 is frequently used [31, 39, 40, 48]. The study here did not collect blood samples at the scanning but showed intratumoral volumes in excess of a 1.3-fold cerebellum mean, which we consider an adequate substitute. The method here did not directly quantify the hypoxic volume, and this is one of the limitations of the study. As another limitation, the number of patients included in this study is small, and further study with more patients is necessary to substantiate the findings. In particular, such studies need to focus on small glioblastoma lesions and aggressive grade III tumors, because these could be a source of false-negative or positive results. Third, we did not investigate specific immunohistochemical features of hypoxia, like the hypoxia-inducible factor-1α (HIF-1α). Investigating HIF-1α further reveals the oxygen condition in the tumor. Finally, in clinical settings, metastatic brain tumors and malignant lymphomas also require a diagnosis that will distinguish them from glioblastomas. Further, additional and different types of brain tumors will need to be investigated.

We also wish to briefly discuss PET tracers other than FMISO [23]. The slow clearance of FMISO from tissue is a shortcoming in clinical settings. If the uptake time could be shortened to maybe 1 h, this would improve the feasibility of hypoxia imaging. Currently, FMISO is the tracer where most evidence has been accumulated, but promising data have been published for other tracers as well. A review article by Kurihara et al. on preclinical and clinical applications of hypoxia PET tracers including FMISO also mentions ^{18}F-fluoroerythronitroimidazole (FETNIM), ^{18}F-fluoroazomycin-arabinofuranoside (FAZA), and [62]Cu or ^{64}Cu-diacetyl-bis(N^4-methylthiosemicarbazone) (Cu-ATSM) [49]. Among these, FETNIM has not been used with brain tumors, while FAZA is less lipophilic than FMISO, suggesting that background activity in the plasma could be excreted more quickly than FMISO. This point is important for shortening the uptake time. However, in an animal study, Sorger et al. have showed that faster clearance of FAZA resulted in lower FAZA uptake in the tumor than with FMISO [50]. It is not easy to solve this dilemma between uptake time and contrast. Postema et al. conducted a study of FAZA PET in 50 patients with a number of different malignant tumors, including seven glioblastoma patients [51]. Here images were acquired 2–3 h after injection, and the image quality was reported as good, but not superior to FMISO. With Cu-ATSM there is the advantage that the radionuclide [62]Cu can be provided by a [62]Zn/[62]Cu generator, which at present does not require an on-site cyclotron to image hypoxia. O'Donoghue et al. conducted an animal study using a R3327-AT tumor model and found a correlation between the 19-h images of Cu-ATSM and FMISO images at 2–4 h as well as oxygen probe measurements [52]. However, 1-h images of Cu-ATSM did not correlate with the FMISO images. A more recent study by Dence et al. compared Cu-ATSM with FMISO, FDG, and 18 F-fluorothymidine (FLT) using a 9 L gliosarcoma model. Here, autoradiography showed a strong correlation between the Cu-ATSM and FMISO distributions [53]. Tateishi et al. acquired Cu-ATSM PET for glioma patients and demonstrated a correlation between Cu-ATSM uptake and glioma grades [54]. Despite evidence, it is still not substantiated whether Cu-ATSM represents hypoxia. Further, ^{18}F-EF5, 2-(2-nitro-1[H]-imidazol-1-yl)-N-(2,2,3,3,3-pentafluoropropyl)-acetamide, was first tested in an animal study by Ziemer [55]. Evens et al. found that EF5 uptake correlated with a poor prognosis in glioma patients [18]. They also reported correlations of EF5 uptake with microscopic findings of vasculature [56] and radiation responses [57].

18.5 Conclusions

This article summarizes our recent findings in two studies related to FMISO PET for brain tumors. The first study demonstrated that much FMISO accumulated in glioblastomas but not in lower-grade gliomas. The second study demonstrated that FMISO PET images acquired 4 h after administration were better at showing hypoxic tumors than the images acquired 2 h after injection. Combining these results, the 4-h FMISO PET may be useful in preoperatively discriminating glioblastomas from lower-grade gliomas.

References

1. Hirata K, Terasaka S, Shiga T, et al. (18)F-Fluoromisonidazole positron emission tomography may differentiate glioblastoma multiforme from less malignant gliomas. Eur J Nucl Med Mol Imaging. 2012;39:760–70.
2. Kobayashi K, Hirata K, Yamaguchi S, et al. FMISO PET at 4 hours showed a better lesion-to-background ratio uptake than 2 hours in brain tumors. J Nucl Med. 2015;56:S373.
3. Louis DN, Ohgaki H, Wiestler OD, et al. The 2007 WHO classification of tumours of the central nervous system. Acta Neuropathol. 2007;114:97–109.
4. Gorlia T, van den Bent MJ, Hegi ME, et al. Nomograms for predicting survival of patients with newly diagnosed glioblastoma: prognostic factor analysis of EORTC and NCIC trial 26981-22981/CE.3. Lancet Oncol. 2008;9:29–38.
5. Cho KH, Kim JY, Lee SH, et al. Simultaneous integrated boost intensity-modulated radiotherapy in patients with high-grade gliomas. Int J Radiat Oncol Biol Phys. 2010;78:390–7.
6. Behin A, Hoang-Xuan K, Carpentier AF, Delattre JY. Primary brain tumours in adults. Lancet. 2003;361:323–31.
7. Spetzler RF, Martin NA. A proposed grading system for arteriovenous malformations. J Neurosurg. 1986;65:476–83.
8. Brasch R, Pham C, Shames D, et al. Assessing tumor angiogenesis using macromolecular MR imaging contrast media. J Magn Reson Imaging. 1997;7:68–74.
9. Law M, Oh S, Babb JS, et al. Low-grade gliomas: dynamic susceptibility-weighted contrast-enhanced perfusion MR imaging--prediction of patient clinical response. Radiology. 2006;238:658–67.
10. Cao Y, Nagesh V, Hamstra D, et al. The extent and severity of vascular leakage as evidence of tumor aggressiveness in high-grade gliomas. Cancer Res. 2006;66:8912–7.
11. Emblem KE, Nedregaard B, Nome T, et al. Glioma grading by using histogram analysis of blood volume heterogeneity from MR-derived cerebral blood volume maps. Radiology. 2008;247:808–17.
12. Di Chiro G, DeLaPaz RL, Brooks RA, et al. Glucose utilization of cerebral gliomas measured by [18F] fluorodeoxyglucose and positron emission tomography. Neurology. 1982;32:1323–9.
13. Kaschten B, Stevenaert A, Sadzot B, et al. Preoperative evaluation of 54 gliomas by PET with fluorine-18-fluorodeoxyglucose and/or carbon-11-methionine. J Nucl Med. 1998;39:778–85.
14. Padma MV, Said S, Jacobs M, et al. Prediction of pathology and survival by FDG PET in gliomas. J Neurooncol. 2003;64:227–37.
15. Borbely K, Nyary I, Toth M, Ericson K, Gulyas B. Optimization of semi-quantification in metabolic PET studies with 18F-fluorodeoxyglucose and 11C-methionine in the determination of malignancy of gliomas. J Neurol Sci. 2006;246:85–94.

16. Oliver L, Olivier C, Marhuenda FB, Campone M, Vallette FM. Hypoxia and the malignant glioma microenvironment: regulation and implications for therapy. Curr Mol Pharmacol. 2009;2:263–84.

17. Flynn JR, Wang L, Gillespie DL, et al. Hypoxia-regulated protein expression, patient characteristics, and preoperative imaging as predictors of survival in adults with glioblastoma multiforme. Cancer. 2008;113:1032–42.

18. Evans SM, Judy KD, Dunphy I, et al. Hypoxia is important in the biology and aggression of human glial brain tumors. Clin Cancer Res. 2004;10:8177–84.

19. Lally BE, Rockwell S, Fischer DB, Collingridge DR, Piepmeier JM, Knisely JP. The interactions of polarographic measurements of oxygen tension and histological grade in human glioma. Cancer J. 2006;12:461–6.

20. Rasey JS, Grunbaum Z, Magee S, et al. Characterization of radiolabeled fluoromisonidazole as a probe for hypoxic cells. Radiat Res. 1987;111:292–304.

21. Martin GV, Caldwell JH, Rasey JS, Grunbaum Z, Cerqueira M, Krohn KA. Enhanced binding of the hypoxic cell marker [3H]fluoromisonidazole in ischemic myocardium. J Nucl Med. 1989;30:194–201.

22. Rasey JS, Koh WJ, Grierson JR, Grunbaum Z, Krohn KA. Radiolabelled fluoromisonidazole as an imaging agent for tumor hypoxia. Int J Radiat Oncol Biol Phys. 1989;17:985–91.

23. Kobayashi H, Hirata K, Yamaguchi S, Terasaka S, Shiga T, Houkin K. Usefulness of FMISO-PET for glioma analysis. Neurol Med Chir (Tokyo). 2013;53:773–8.

24. Valk PE, Mathis CA, Prados MD, Gilbert JC, Budinger TF. Hypoxia in human gliomas: demonstration by PET with fluorine-18-fluoromisonidazole. J Nucl Med. 1992;33:2133–7.

25. Rajendran JG, Mankoff DA, O'Sullivan F, et al. Hypoxia and glucose metabolism in malignant tumors: evaluation by [18F]fluoromisonidazole and [18F]fluorodeoxyglucose positron emission tomography imaging. Clin Cancer Res. 2004;10:2245–52.

26. Bruehlmeier M, Roelcke U, Schubiger PA, Ametamey SM. Assessment of hypoxia and perfusion in human brain tumors using PET with 18F-fluoromisonidazole and 15O-H2O. J Nucl Med. 2004;45:1851–9.

27. Cher LM, Murone C, Lawrentschuk N, et al. Correlation of hypoxic cell fraction and angiogenesis with glucose metabolic rate in gliomas using 18F-fluoromisonidazole, 18F-FDG PET, and immunohistochemical studies. J Nucl Med. 2006;47:410–8.

28. Spence AM, Muzi M, Swanson KR, et al. Regional hypoxia in glioblastoma multiforme quantified with [18F]fluoromisonidazole positron emission tomography before radiotherapy: correlation with time to progression and survival. Clin Cancer Res. 2008;14:2623–30.

29. Swanson KR, Chakraborty G, Wang CH, et al. Complementary but distinct roles for MRI and 18F-fluoromisonidazole PET in the assessment of human glioblastomas. J Nucl Med. 2009;50:36–44.

30. Szeto MD, Chakraborty G, Hadley J, et al. Quantitative metrics of net proliferation and invasion link biological aggressiveness assessed by MRI with hypoxia assessed by FMISO-PET in newly diagnosed glioblastomas. Cancer Res. 2009;69:4502–9.

31. Kawai N, Maeda Y, Kudomi N, et al. Correlation of biological aggressiveness assessed by 11C-methionine PET and hypoxic burden assessed by 18F-fluoromisonidazole PET in newly diagnosed glioblastoma. Eur J Nucl Med Mol Imaging. 2011;38:441–50.

32. Yamamoto Y, Maeda Y, Kawai N, et al. Hypoxia assessed by 18F-fluoromisonidazole positron emission tomography in newly diagnosed gliomas. Nucl Med Commun. 2012;33:621–5.

33. Grunbaum Z, Freauff SJ, Krohn KA, Wilbur DS, Magee S, Rasey JS. Synthesis and characterization of congeners of misonidazole for imaging hypoxia. J Nucl Med. 1987;28:68–75.

34. Thorwarth D, Eschmann SM, Paulsen F, Alber M. A kinetic model for dynamic [18F]-Fmiso PET data to analyse tumour hypoxia. Phys Med Biol. 2005;50:2209–24.

35. Oh SJ, Chi DY, Mosdzianowski C, et al. Fully automated synthesis of [18F]fluoromisonidazole using a conventional [18F]FDG module. Nucl Med Biol. 2005;32:899–905.

36. Tang G, Wang M, Tang X, Gan M, Luo L. Fully automated one-pot synthesis of [18F]fluoromisonidazole. Nucl Med Biol. 2005;32:553–8.

37. Minoshima S, Frey KA, Koeppe RA, Foster NL, Kuhl DE. A diagnostic approach in Alzheimer's disease using three-dimensional stereotactic surface projections of fluorine-18-FDG PET. J Nucl Med. 1995;36:1238–48.
38. Minoshima S, Koeppe RA, Frey KA, Kuhl DE. Anatomic standardization: linear scaling and nonlinear warping of functional brain images. J Nucl Med. 1994;35:1528–37.
39. Kracht LW, Miletic H, Busch S, et al. Delineation of brain tumor extent with [11C]L-methionine positron emission tomography: local comparison with stereotactic histopathology. Clin Cancer Res. 2004;10:7163–70.
40. Galldiks N, Ullrich R, Schroeter M, Fink GR, Jacobs AH, Kracht LW. Volumetry of [(11)C]-methionine PET uptake and MRI contrast enhancement in patients with recurrent glioblastoma multiforme. Eur J Nucl Med Mol Imaging. 2010;37:84–92.
41. Lee ST, Scott AM. Hypoxia positron emission tomography imaging with 18f-fluoromiso-nidazole. Semin Nucl Med. 2007;37:451–61.
42. Collingridge DR, Piepmeier JM, Rockwell S, Knisely JP. Polarographic measurements of oxygen tension in human glioma and surrounding peritumoural brain tissue. Radiother Oncol. 1999;53:127–31.
43. Koch CJ, Evans SM. Non-invasive PET and SPECT imaging of tissue hypoxia using isotopi-cally labeled 2-nitroimidazoles. Adv Exp Med Biol. 2003;510:285–92.
44. Rasey JS, Nelson NJ, Chin L, Evans ML, Grunbaum Z. Characteristics of the binding of labeled fluoromisonidazole in cells in vitro. Radiat Res. 1990;122:301–8.
45. Kato T, Shinoda J, Oka N, et al. Analysis of 11C-methionine uptake in low-grade gliomas and correlation with proliferative activity. AJNR Am J Neuroradiol. 2008;29:1867–71.
46. Manabe O, Hattori N, Yamaguchi S, et al. Oligodendroglial component complicates the prediction of tumour grading with metabolic imaging. Eur J Nucl Med Mol Imaging. 2015;42:896–904.
47. Yamaguchi S, Terasaka S, Kobayashi H, et al. Combined use of positron emission tomography with (18)F-fluorodeoxyglucose and (11)C-methionine for preoperative evaluation of gliomas. No Shinkei Geka. 2010;38:621–8.
48. Kobayashi K, Hirata K, Yamaguchi S, et al. Prognostic value of volume-based measurements on (11)C-methionine PET in glioma patients. Eur J Nucl Med Mol Imaging. 2015;42:1071–80.
49. Kurihara H, Honda N, Kono Y, Arai Y. Radiolabelled agents for PET imaging of tumor hypoxia. Curr Med Chem. 2012;19:3282–9.
50. Sorger D, Patt M, Kumar P, et al. [18F]Fluoroazomycinarabinofuranoside (18FAZA) and [18F]Fluoromisonidazole (18FMISO): a comparative study of their selective uptake in hyp-oxic cells and PET imaging in experimental rat tumors. Nucl Med Biol. 2003;30:317–26.
51. Postema EJ, McEwan AJ, Riauka TA, et al. Initial results of hypoxia imaging using 1-alpha-D:−(5-deoxy-5-[18F]-fluoroarabinofuranosyl)-2-nitroimidazole (18F-FAZA). Eur J Nucl Med Mol Imaging. 2009;36:1565–73.
52. O'Donoghue JA, Zanzonico P, Pugachev A, et al. Assessment of regional tumor hypoxia using 18F-fluoromisonidazole and 64Cu(II)-diacetyl-bis(N4-methylthiosemicarbazone) positron emission tomography: Comparative study featuring microPET imaging, Po2 probe measure-ment, autoradiography, and fluorescent microscopy in the R3327-AT and FaDu rat tumor models. Int J Radiat Oncol Biol Phys. 2005;61:1493–502.
53. Dence CS, Ponde DE, Welch MJ, Lewis JS. Autoradiographic and small-animal PET com-parisons between (18)F-FMISO, (18)F-FDG, (18)F-FLT and the hypoxic selective (64)Cu-ATSM in a rodent model of cancer. Nucl Med Biol. 2008;35:713–20.
54. Tateishi K, Tateishi U, Sato M, et al. Application of 62Cu-diacetyl-bis (N4-methylthiosemi-carbazone) PET imaging to predict highly malignant tumor grades and hypoxia-inducible factor-1alpha expression in patients with glioma. AJNR Am J Neuroradiol. 2013;34:92–9.
55. Ziemer LS, Evans SM, Kachur AV, et al. Noninvasive imaging of tumor hypoxia in rats using the 2-nitroimidazole 18F-EF5. Eur J Nucl Med Mol Imaging. 2003;30:259–66.
56. Evans SM, Jenkins KW, Jenkins WT, et al. Imaging and analytical methods as applied to the evaluation of vasculature and hypoxia in human brain tumors. Radiat Res. 2008;170:677–90.
57. Koch CJ, Shuman AL, Jenkins WT, et al. The radiation response of cells from 9L gliosarcoma tumours is correlated with [F18]-EF5 uptake. Int J Radiat Biol. 2009;85:1137–47.

Chapter 19
Evolution and Protection of Cerebral Infarction Evaluated by PET and SPECT

Eku Shimosegawa

Abstract Since cerebral infarction results from a reduction of cerebral blood flow (CBF) by the occlusion or stenosis of carotid or intracranial arteries, CBF is a primary parameter to predict of ischemic brain injury. Single-photon emission tomography (SPECT) and positron emission tomography (PET) contributed to evaluate loss of cerebral autoregulation, uncoupling state between CBF and brain metabolism, and ischemic penumbra. Measurement of CBF and oxygen metabolism by ^{15}O PET revealed the process of infarct growth in hyperacute stage of cerebral infarction and areas with depressed oxygen metabolism, but normal water diffusion in magnetic resonance imaging (MRI) was termed as "metabolic penumbra." Recently, some researchers shed light on the role of glial cells in the energy metabolism of the brain and ^{11}C-acetate PET and demonstrated that astrocytic energy metabolism in TCA cycle was protective against ischemia. SPECT and PET studies for secondary reaction after ischemia (i.e., selective neuronal loss by ^{123}I-iomazenil SPECT and ^{11}C-flumazenil PET, tissue hypoxia by ^{18}F-FMISO PET, and neuroinflammation by TSPO-PET) are expected as new biomarkers. Combining these imaging biomarkers with classical CBF measurement may contribute to develop innovative drugs for pharmacological neuroprotection in the therapy of cerebral infarction.

Keywords Cerebral infarction • SPECT • PET • Hypoxia • TSPO-PET

19.1 Introduction

Cerebral infarction results from a reduction in cerebral blood flow (CBF) arising from the occlusion or stenosis of carotid or intracranial arteries, and the progression of this event typically ends with the necrosis of various brain tissue components, including neurons. Since tissue damage varies according to the severity of brain

E. Shimosegawa, MD, PhD (✉)
Department of Molecular Imaging in Medicine, Graduate School of Medicine,
Osaka University, 2-2 Yamadaoka, Suita, Osaka 565-0871, Japan
e-mail: eku@mi.med.osaka-u.ac.jp

© The Author(s) 2016
Y. Kuge et al. (eds.), *Perspectives on Nuclear Medicine for Molecular Diagnosis and Integrated Therapy*, DOI 10.1007/978-4-431-55894-1_19

ischemia, CBF is a primary parameter for predicting the extent of ischemic brain injury.

Positron emission tomography (PET) and single-photon emission computed tomography (SPECT) have contributed to the elucidation of the disease process responsible for brain ischemia from an acute to chronic stage. PET studies have mainly measured CBF and oxygen metabolism but have been expanded to include the detection of neuronal loss, tissue hypoxia, and neuroinflammation. Quantitative ^{15}O PET measurements can provide information on CBF, the cerebral metabolic rate of oxygen ($CMRO_2$), the cerebral blood volume (CBV), and the oxygen extraction fraction (OEF), and these parameters enable impaired cerebral autoregulation and the uncoupling of perfusion and metabolism to be diagnosed based on absolute values. The SPECT studies can visualize the magnitude and extent of ischemia in a clinical setting. Neurons are more vulnerable than other cell groups in the brain, and selective neuronal loss sometimes occurs in patients with mild to moderate brain ischemia. PET and SPECT are advantageous for demonstrating this type of brain injury, which cannot be visualized by comparing computed tomography (CT) and magnetic resonance imaging (MRI) findings. PET imaging of tissue hypoxia is expected to distinguish permanent and temporal ischemic areas surrounding the ischemic core. Translocator protein (TSPO) PET can represent neuroinflammation in areas with evolving infarcts and may become a biomarker for neuroprotective therapy. Recently, important roles of astrocytes in the energy metabolism of the brain have been reported. The imaging of astrocytes using ^{11}C-acetate PET may provide a sensitive marker for evaluating glial metabolism in the ischemic brain. The purpose of using these imaging probes depends on the course or stage of

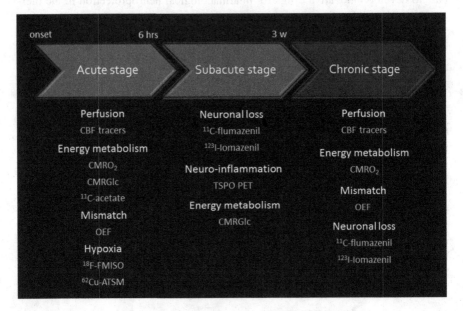

Fig. 19.1 Time course of infarct evolution and related PET/SPECT imaging

cerebral infarction (Fig. 19.1). In this chapter, we introduce the use of PET and SPECT imaging in studies to clarify the process of cerebral infarction.

19.2 Perfusion and Oxygen Metabolism in Brain Ischemia

CBF is a key parameter of ischemic brain damage that can be quantitatively measured using PET and SPECT. A decrease in the cerebral perfusion pressure (CPP) induces primary damage to the supply of oxygen and energy substance to the brain. Protective mechanisms against reductions in the CPP can be evaluated using PET and SPECT. The first mechanism is "cerebral autoregulation," the origin of which is cardiac pump function. CBF is constant within a mean arterial blood pressure (MABP) range of 60–160 mmHg [1]. To maintain a constant CBF, cerebral precapillary arterioles can dilate when the CPP decreases and can constrict when the CPP increases. Although this mechanism of dilation and constriction for cerebral autoregulation remains unclear, recent studies have indicated that CBF control is initiated in the cerebral capillaries, where pericytes can constrict capillaries in response to the effect of noradrenaline [2]. Cerebral autoregulation is disturbed by brain ischemia [3], and its capacity can be estimated using the cerebral vasoreactivity (CVR) to the change in the arterial partial pressure of carbon dioxide ($PaCO_2$). In SPECT studies, acetazolamide, which is another vasodilating agent, is used to test CVR. A reduced CVR in patients with steno-occlusive carotid artery disease is a major predictor of stroke recurrence [4, 5].

By combining this information with data on CBF and oxygen metabolism measured using ^{15}O PET, we can evaluate other protective states against CPP reduction (Fig. 19.2). When cerebral autoregulation is functioning well, CBF remains normal and the CBV increases, indicating the dilatation of collateral vessels. When the CPP is reduced beyond the point of compensation by vasodilatation, the cerebral autoregulation is exhausted and the CBF begins to decrease.

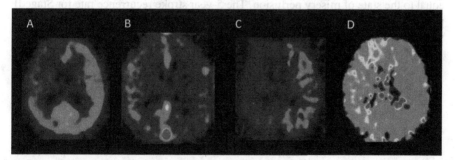

Fig. 19.2 ^{15}O PET images in a patient with right carotid and MCA occlusion. PET images of (a) CBF, (b) CBV, (c) CPP, and (d) OEF. The CPP images were created by dividing CBF and CBV. The area with a severe CPP reduction corresponded to the area with an elevated OEF (misery perfusion)

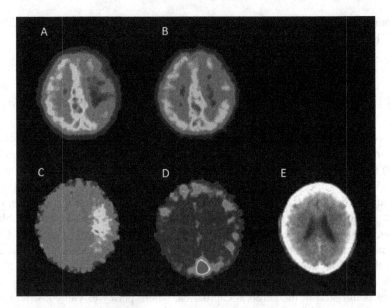

Fig. 19.3 Misery perfusion in a patient with acute left MCA occlusion. PET images of (**a**) CBF, (**b**) CMRO$_2$, (**c**) OEF, and (**d**) CBV examined on the day of stroke onset. The CBF in the left MCA territory reduced, whereas the CMRO$_2$ in the corresponding area was relatively preserved. The OEF was elevated in the same area, indicating an uncoupled state between perfusion and oxygen metabolism (misery perfusion). A CT image obtained on the same day (**e**) did not show any morphological changes

When CMRO$_2$ is preserved, then the OEF starts to increase. Such increases in the OEF are known as "misery perfusion" and can be observed during the acute stage of cerebral infarction (Fig. 19.3). In the chronic stage of cerebral infarction, misery perfusion in patients with unilateral carotid artery occlusion suggests a high probability of stroke recurrence [6–8]. Powers et al. classified the severity of cerebral ischemia from Stage 0 to Stage II according to CBF, CBV, and OEF [9]. Stage II is equal to the state of misery perfusion. The 5-year stroke recurrence rate for Stage II patients with unilateral steno-occlusive internal carotid artery (ICA) was 70 %, whereas it was 20 % for Stage 0 and I patients [8].

19.3 Infarct Growth in Acute Cerebral Infarction

The ischemic threshold of CBF has been thoroughly evaluated in both experimental studies and clinical studies. Symon and colleagues revealed a relationship between CBF, neurological deficits, and tissue damage in baboon models of cerebral ische-mia [10]. They showed that the electric activity of somatosensory evoked potentials in cerebral tissue was preserved at a CBF above 20 mL/100 g/min (40 % of normal level), whereas it was impaired when the CBF decreased to 10–20 mL/100 g/min.

Although this impaired electric activity was reversible by recirculation, irreversible damage resulting from an elevated extracellular potassium concentration and subsequent cell death occurred when the CBF was reduced to less than 6–10 mL/100 g/min. Astrup, Siesjo, and Symon defined the ischemic penumbra as brain tissue with CBF thresholds between electric (20 mL/100 g/min) and membrane failure (6–10 mL/100 g/min) [11]. In a baboon model, Jones et al. found that a longer period of ischemia was associated with a higher threshold for membrane failure [12]. Their studies indicated that the ischemic penumbra should be restored as early as possible to reduce the volume of cerebral infarction. Clinical SPECT studies have demonstrated the validity of evaluating the ischemic threshold during the acute stage of infarction. Shimosegawa et al. evaluated SPECT images within 6 h of onset in ischemic stroke patients and revealed that a CBF of less than 30–50 % of that in unaffected brain regions was capable of inducing cerebral infarction [13] (Fig. 19.4). When the CBF was less than 20 % of that in the unaffected hemisphere, the probability of hemorrhagic infarction after recanalization therapy increased [14].

Although the CBF threshold has been established in both experimental and clinical studies, the metabolic threshold and its relation to the development of infarction has not yet been clarified. In a ^{15}O PET study of patients with cerebral infarction where imaging was performed within 6 h of onset, Shimosegawa et al. demonstrated that infarct growth occurred in brain lesions with a depressed $CMRO_2$ but normal water diffusion on diffusion-weighted imaging (DWI) [15] (Fig. 19.5). Peri-infarct areas with a $CMRO_2$ of less than 45–62 % of that in unaffected brain regions on the initial ^{15}O PET showed volume expansion of the brain infarction at 3 days after onset, and they named this phenomenon "metabolic penumbra." The normal diffusion in these areas indicated that adenosine triphosphate (ATP) synthesis was still preserved to a degree sufficient to maintain an

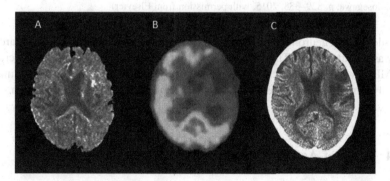

Fig. 19.4 Prediction of cerebral infarction by acute CBF-SPECT. A diffusion-weighted MR image obtained at 1.3 h after onset (**a**) demonstrated only a small lesion in the frontal lobe. A ^{99m}HMPAO-SPECT image obtained at 2.3 h after onset (**b**) showed a broad reduction in CBF in the left cerebral hemisphere. A CBF reduction of more than 50 %, compared with the contralateral region, was observed in the left frontal lobe, and this area progressed into a complete infarction visible on a CT image obtained 4 days after onset (**c**)

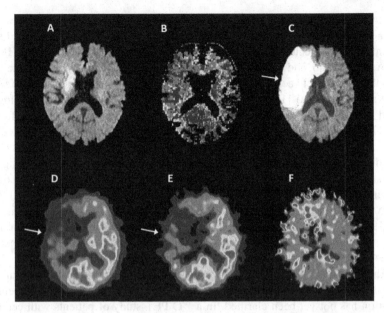

Fig. 19.5 Metabolic penumbra in acute brain infarction. (**a**) DWI of MRI obtained 4 h after onset, (**b**) perfusion-weighted image (PWI) obtained 4 h after onset, (**c**) DWI obtained 3 days after onset, (**d**) CBF obtained 3 h after onset, (**e**) CMRO$_2$ obtained 3 h after onset, and (**f**) OEF obtained 3 h of onset in a patient with right ICA embolic occlusion. An MRI examination indicated PWI–DWI mismatch in the territory of the right ICA. DWI on day 3 indicated an evolution of the infarction within the mismatch. The initial PET examination indicated that the PWI–DWI mismatch lesion exhibited reductions in CBF and CMRO$_2$ associated with misery perfusion (increased OEF, *white arrow*). The PWI–DWI mismatch corresponded to suppressed energy metabolism that was still higher than the threshold for ion pump failure (Reprinted from Brain Mapping: An Encyclopedic Reference, Vol. 3/1st edition, Arthur W. Toga (Editor in Chief), Hemodynamic and Metabolic Disturbances in Acute Cerebral Infarction (title)/Clinical Brain Mapping (chapter), written by E. Shimosegawa, p. 829–838, 2015, with permission from Elsevier)

ATP-dependent neuronal membrane ion pump in the area of the evolving infarct as early as 6 h after onset. Therefore, a metabolic penumbra with a moderate decrease in CMRO$_2$ would be a critical treatment target, using early reperfusion and pharmacological neuroprotection to reduce the volume expansion of the brain infarction.

19.4 Role of Astrocytic Function in Brain Ischemia

Recently, some researchers have shed light on the role of glial cells in energy metabolism in the brain. Glutamate is a major excitatory neurotransmitter of the brain, and glutamate in the synaptic cleft is removed by astrocytes surrounding glutaminergic synapses. The removed glutamate is converted into glutamine in astrocytes by glutamine synthetase. Glutamine is released by astrocytes and taken up by neuronal terminals, where it is enzymatically reconverted to glutamate and stored in the neurotransmitter pool for the next transmission. This process is called "glutamate-glutamine cycle" and requires ATP [16]. Furthermore, astrocytes play an important role in glycolysis in the brain. Activation by the glutamate transporter on the astrocytic membrane stimulates glucose uptake into astrocytes. This glucose is processed glycolytically, resulting in the release of lactate as an energy substrate for neurons. Lactate produced by this process is transferred to neurons for oxidation (the astrocyte-neuron lactate shuttle: ANLS) [17]. This lactate produces two ATP molecules, which contribute to the Na-K ion pump function and the synthesis of glutamine from glutamate. In ischemic brain where ATP synthesis is restricted, the conversion of glutamate in the synaptic cleft is disturbed. Continuous stimulation by glutamate induces an influx of Ca^{2+} ion, resulting in anoxic depolarization, and leads to inflammation and apoptosis. Therefore, the glutamate-glutamine cycle and ANLS are deeply related to astrocytic function and plays a critical role in the evolution from penumbra to infarction.

For the specific imaging of astrocyte, acetate is expected to be useful as a selective marker of astrocytic energy metabolism [18, 19]. ^{14}C-acetate is rapidly incorporated into glutamine via glutamate by glutamine synthetase localized in astrocytic cells [20]. Hosoi et al. demonstrated that ^{14}C-acetate uptake is dramatically decreased in a 3-min ischemia and reperfusion model, indicating that the metabolic and functional impairment of astrocytes continues after the restoration of CBF [21]. ^{11}C-labeled acetate could be a promising PET tracer for the evaluation of astrocytic metabolism in human studies (Fig. 19.6).

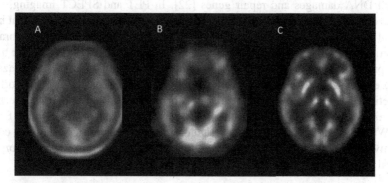

Fig. 19.6 Qualitative and quantitative ^{11}C-acetate PET imaging for astrocytic energy metabolism. (**a**) An averaged ^{11}C-acetate PET image (from 0 to 40 min) and (**b**) an averaged Kmono image in a healthy volunteer. The energy metabolism evaluated using the Kmono image was different from the normal oxygen metabolism evaluated using the $CMRO_2$ image (**c**)

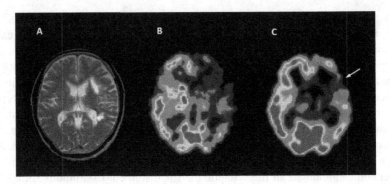

Fig. 19.7 Selective neuronal loss: (**a**) T_2-weighted image (T_2WI) in a patient with subcortical infarction of the left putamen 1.5 months after onset, (**b**) CBF image of the corresponding slice obtained by ^{123}I-IMP SPECT, and (**c**) ^{123}I-iomazenil SPECT image of the corresponding slice. The MR image showed no obvious lesion in the left cortical area, whereas ^{123}I-iomazenil SPECT demonstrated a decrease in accumulation (*white arrow*), indicating selective neuronal loss. The CBF reduction extended beyond the cortical areas of ^{123}I-iomazenil reduction (Reprinted from Brain Mapping: An Encyclopedic Reference, Vol. 3/1st edition, Arthur W. Toga (Editor in Chief), Hemodynamic and Metabolic Disturbances in Acute Cerebral Infarction (title)/Clinical Brain Mapping (chapter), written by E. Shimosegawa, p. 829–838, 2015, with permission from Elsevier)

19.5   Selective Neuronal Loss in Ischemic Brain Injury

Tissue vulnerability differs among neurons, glial cells, and blood vessels. Selective neuronal necrosis is known to occur in neuron-specific ischemic injury, where other cell components are preserved, and is associated with the expression of apoptosis-related DNA damages and repair genes [22]. In PET and SPECT imaging, ^{11}C-flumazenil and ^{123}I-iomazenil are considered to be neuron-specific tracers that bind central benzodiazepine receptors that are specifically localized on the membranes of cortical neurons. Preserved ^{11}C-flumazenil accumulation in acute ischemic brain can predict the probability of surviving an infarct [23, 24]. Hatazawa et al. examined ^{123}I-iomazenil SPECT in patients with cortical and subcortical infarction. They reported a patient with global aphasia who had a purely subcortical infarction and significantly diminished ^{123}I-iomazenil uptake in CT-negative Broca and Wernicke areas [25]. This result indicated that ^{123}I-iomazenil SPECT could sensitively detect lesions responsible for clinical symptoms, compared with morphological examinations (Fig. 19.7).

19.6   Detection of Tissue Hypoxia

Tissue hypoxia can be visualized using ^{18}F-labeled nitroimidazole derivatives or [62/64]Cu-labeled lipophilic chelate compounds. ^{18}F-fluoromisonidazole (^{18}F-FMISO) PET is a representative hypoxic marker. Under hypoxic conditions, ^{18}F-FMISO passively diffuses into cells and is reduced by nitroreductase enzymes and trapped by intracellular molecules. The retention of ^{18}F-FMISO is inversely proportional to the tissue partial pressure of O_2. Takasawa et al. revealed that the selective accumulation of ^{18}F-FMISO was found in permanent and temporal ischemic areas surrounding the ischemic core [26]. They demonstrated that ^{18}F-FMISO uptake in the ischemic brain was only elevated during the early phase of middle cerebral artery (MCA) occlusion. After early reperfusion, no demonstrable tracer retention was observed. In patients with an acute MCA territory stroke, Markus et al. reported that ^{18}F-FMISO PET showed the temporal evolution of tissue hypoxia [27]. A higher hypoxic volume was observed in the core of the infarct within 6 h of onset, and the location moved to the periphery or external to the infarct at later time points. They also showed that tissue without ^{18}F-FMISO uptake within the final infarct was presumed to have infarcted by the time of the acute ^{18}F-FMISO PET. These experimental and clinical results are very interesting because they suggested that ^{18}F-FMISO uptake changes continuously during the course of brain infarction. Since ^{18}F-FMISO PET is unable to discriminate between complete infarcted area and non-hypoxic viable tissue during the acute stage of infarction, the timing of the PET examination is likely to be critical for diagnosing whether the tissue is salvageable.

19.7 Imaging of Neuroinflammation

In focal brain ischemia, inflammatory reactions mainly occur in the peri-infarct area and lead to an overexpression of peripheral benzodiazepine receptors (PBR)/18-kDa TSPO on the membrane of activated microglia, macrophages, and activated astrocytes. Several PET tracers that specifically bind to TSPO have been developed as biomarkers of neuroinflammation. Imaizumi et al. demonstrated that ^{11}C-PBR28 accumulated in the peri-infarct lesions of a rat ischemia model, indicating that neuroinflammation does not occur in the ischemic core but in penumbral lesions [28]. In our preclinical study using a temporary MCA occlusion model, ^{11}C-DPA-713 uptake increased in the area surrounding the infarct core after 4 days of ischemia, where the expression of microglia/macrophages was positive using CD11b immunostaining (Fig. 19.8). In an impressive study, Martín et al. reported that ^{18}F-DPA-714 uptake decreased at 7 days after cerebral ischemia in rats treated with minocycline, compared with saline-treated animals [29]. Whether the increased regional microglia/macrophage activation visualized by TSPO PET is a good biomarker remains controversial. TSPO molecular imaging, however, might have diagnostic potential for assessing therapeutic strategies, such as the use of neuroprotective or anti-inflammatory drugs during the acute or subacute stage of cerebral infarction.

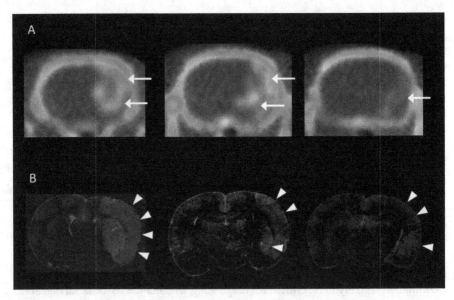

Fig. 19.8 TSPO PET image of rat ischemic model. (**a**) ^{11}C-DPA713 PET and (**b**) the corresponding CD11b immunostaining image. ^{11}C-DPA713 accumulated in the peripheral region of the ischemic core at 4 days after 60 min of MCA occlusion and reperfusion (*white arrows*). The CD11b-positive findings agreed with the uptake of ^{11}C-DPA713 (*white arrow* heads), indicating that macrophages/microglia were activated by neuroinflammation after brain ischemia

19.8 Summary

Measurements of hemodynamic and metabolic disturbances using PET and SPECT have been utilized to study the acute and chronic stages of cerebral infarction. CBF, $CMRO_2$, CBV, OEF, and CVR are basic parameters for estimating CPP reduction. An acute metabolic penumbra (decreased $CMRO_2$ in peri-infarct area on initial PET) and misery perfusion (areas with decreased CBF with maintained $CMRO_2$ in ischemic brain) during the acute and chronic stages are indicators of evolving infarction. Astrocytes have a protective role against cerebral infarction by reducing the glutamate concentration during ischemia, and ^{11}C-acetate PET may provide information regarding glial cell function. Neuron-specific imaging can only be performed using PET and SPECT, and it would be useful to collate the clinical symptoms with neuronal damage. PET tracers for tissue hypoxia and neuro-inflammation have been developed and are promising biomarkers for detecting infarct growth and salvageable tissue and are expected to become useful as probes in future therapeutic interventions.

References

1. Paulson OB, Strandgaard S, Edvinsson L. Cerebral autoregulation. Cerebrovasc Brain Metab Rev. 1990;2:161–92.
2. Peppiatt CM, Howarth C, Mobbs P, Attwell D. Bidirectional control of CNS capillary diameter by pericytes. Nature. 2006;443:700–4.
3. Lassen NA. The luxury perfusion syndrome and its possible relation to acute metabolic acidosis localized within the brain. Lancet. 1966;2:1113–5.
4. Kuroda S, Houkin K, Kamiyama H, Mitsumori K, Iwasaki Y, Abe H. Long-term prognosis of medically treated patients with internal carotid or middle cerebral artery occlusion: can acetazolamide test predict it? Stroke. 2001;32:2110–6.
5. Ogasawara K, Ogawa A, Yoshimoto T. Cerebrovascular reactivity to acetazolamide and outcome in patients with symptomatic internal carotid or middle cerebral artery occlusion: a xenon-133 single-photon emission computed tomography study. Stroke. 2002;33:1857–62.
6. Yamauchi H, Fukuyama H, Nagahama Y, Nabatame H, Nakamura K, Yamamoto Y, et al. Evidence of misery perfusion and risk for recurrent stroke in major cerebral arterial occlusive diseases from PET. J Neurol Neurosurg Psychiatry. 1996;61:18–25.
7. Grubb Jr RL, Derdeyn CP, Fritsch SM, Carpenter DA, Yundt KD, Videen TO, et al. Importance of hemodynamic factors in the prognosis of symptomatic carotid occlusion. JAMA. 1998;280:1055–60.
8. Yamauchi H, Fukuyama H, Nagahama Y, Nabatame H, Ueno M, Nishizawa S, et al. Significance of increased oxygen extraction fraction in five-year prognosis of major cerebral arterial occlusive diseases. J Nucl Med. 1999;40:1992–8.
9. Powers WJ, Grubb Jr RL, Raichle ME. Physiological responses to focal cerebral ischemia in humans. Ann Neurol. 1984;16:546–52.
10. Symon L, Pasztor E, Branston NM. The distribution and density of reduced cerebral blood flow following acute middle cerebral artery occlusion: an experimental study by the technique of hydrogen clearance in baboons. Stroke. 1975;6:476–81.
11. Astrup J, Siesjo BK, Symon L. Thresholds in cerebral ischemia- the ischemic penumbra. Stroke. 1981;12:723–5.
12. Jones TH, Morawetz RB, Crowell RM, Marcoux FW, FitzGibbon SJ, DeGirolami U, et al. Thresholds of focal cerebral ischemia in awake monkeys. J Neurosurg. 1981;54:583–5.
13. Shimosegawa E, Hatazawa J, Inugami A, Fujita H, Ogawa T, Aizawa Y, et al. Cerebral infarction within six hours of onset: prediction of complete infarction with technetium-99m-HMPAO SPECT. J Nucl Med. 1994;35:1097–103.
14. Ueda T, Hatakeyama T, Kumon Y, Sasaki S, Uraoka T. Evaluation of risk of hemorrhagic transformation in local intra-arterial thrombolysis in acute ischemic stroke by initial SPECT. Stroke. 1994;25:298–303.
15. Shimosegawa E, Hatazawa J, Ibaraki M, Toyoshima H, Suzuki A. Metabolic penumbra in acute brain infarction: a correlation with infarct growth. Ann Neurol. 2005;57:495–504.

16. Dienel GA, Cruz NF. Astrocyte activation in working brain: energy supplied by minor substrates. Neurochem Int. 2006;48:568–95.
17. Pellerin L, Magistretti P. Sweet sixteen for ANLS. J Cereb Blood Flow Metab. 2012;32: 1152–66.
18. Muir D, Berl S, Clarke DD. Acetate and fluoroacetate as possible markers for glial metabolism in vivo. Brain Res. 1986;380:336–40.
19. Cerdan S, Kunnecke B, Seelig J. Cerebral metabolism of [1,2-[13]C2]acetate as detected by in vivo and in vitro ^{13}C NMR. J Biol Chem. 1990;265:12916–26.
20. Martinez Hernandez A, Bell KP, Norenberg MD. Glutamine synthetase: glial localization in brain. Science. 1977;195:1356–8.
21. Hosoi R, Kashiwagi Y, Tokumura M, Abe K, Hatazawa J, Inoue O. Sensitive reduction in 14C-acetate uptake in a short-term ischemic rat brain. J Stroke Cerebrovasc Dis. 2007;16: 77–81.
22. Nedergaard M. Neuronal injury in the infarct border: a neuropathological study in the rat. Acta Neuropath (Berl). 1987;73:267–74.
23. Heiss WD, Kracht LW, Thiel A, Grond M, Pawlik G. Penumbral probability thresholds of cortical flumazenil binding and blood flow predicting tissue outcome in patients with cerebral ischaemia. Brain. 2001;124:20–9.
24. Guadagno JV, Jones PS, Aigbirhio FI, Wang D, Fryer TD, Day DJ, et al. Selective neuronal loss in rescued penumbra relates to initial hypoperfusion. Brain. 2008;131:2666–78.
25. Hatazawa J, Satoh T, Shimosegawa E, Okudera T, Inugami A, Ogawa T, et al. Evaluation of cerebral infarction with iodine 123-iomazenil SPECT. J Nucl Med. 1995;36:2154–61.
26. Takasawa M, Beech JS, Fryer TD, Hong YT, Hughes JL, Igase K, et al. Imaging of brain hypoxia in permanent and temporary middle cerebral artery occlusion in the rat using ^{18}F-fluoromisonidazole and positron emission tomography: a pilot study. J Cereb Blood Flow Metab. 2007;27: 679–89.
27. Markus R, Reutens DC, Kazui S, Read S, Wright P, Chambers BR, et al. Topography and temporal evolution of hypoxic viable tissue identified by ^{18}F-fluoromisonidazole positron emission tomography in humans after ischemic stroke. Stroke. 2003;34:2646–52.
28. Imaizumi M, Kim HJ, Zoghbi SS, Briard E, Hong J, Musachio JL, et al. PET imaging with [11C]PBR28 can localize and quantify upregulated peripheral benzodiazepine receptors associated with cerebral ischemia in rat. Neurosci Lett. 2007;411:200–5.
29. Martín A, Boisgard R, Kassiou M, Dollé F, Tavitian B. Reduced PBR/TSPO expression after minocycline treatment in a rat model of focal cerebral ischemia: a PET study using [^{18}F]DPA-714. Mol Imaging Biol. 2010;13:10–5.

Chapter 20
Brain Development and Aging Using Large Brain MRI Database

Yasuyuki Taki

Abstract Now we confront a super aging society in Japan. In the situation, it is important to preserve our cognitive function for entire life by preventing us from pathological brain aging. To perform the aim, we have built a large brain magnetic resonance imaging (MRI) database from around 3,000 subjects aged from 5 to 80 in order to reveal how brain develops and ages. We have also collected several cognitive functions, lifestyle such as eating and sleeping habits, and genetic data. Using the database, we have revealed normal brain development and aging and also have revealed what factors affect brain development and aging. For example, sleep duration is significantly associated with the gray matter volume of the bilateral hippocampi. In addition, there were significant negative correlation between alcohol drinking and gray matter volume of the frontoparietal region and body mass index and gray matter volume of the hippocampus in cross-sectional analysis. In addition, having intellectual curiosity showed significant negative correlation with regional gray matter volume decline rate in the temporoparietal region. These findings help understanding the mechanism of brain development and aging as well as performing differential diagnosis or diagnosis at an early stage of several diseases/disorders such as autism and Alzheimer's disease.

Keywords Brain development • Brain aging • Magnetic resonance imaging • Database • Preventive medicine • Normal subject

Y. Taki (✉)
Department of Nuclear Medicine & Radiology, Institute of Development, Aging and Cancer, Tohoku University, 4-1 Seiryo-cho, Aoba-ku, 980-8575 Sendai, Japan

Division of Medical Neuroimage Analysis, Department of Community Medical Supports, Tohoku Medical Megabank Organization, Tohoku University, 4-1 Seiryo-cho, Aoba-ku, 980-8575 Sendai, Japan

Division of Developmental Cognitive Neuroscience, Institute of Development, Aging and Cancer, Tohoku University, 4-1 Seiryo-cho, Aoba-ku, 980-8575 Sendai, Japan
e-mail: ytaki@idac.tohoku.ac.jp

© The Author(s) 2016 263
Y. Kuge et al. (eds.), *Perspectives on Nuclear Medicine for Molecular Diagnosis and Integrated Therapy*, DOI 10.1007/978-4-431-55894-1_20

20.1   Introduction

Now we confront a super aging society in Japan. In the situation, it is important to preserve our cognitive function for entire life by preventing us from pathological brain aging. Recently, the importance of human neuroimaging database was recognized greatly. The normal brain structure and function database can be used as the references not only for neuroimaging study for humans but also for early diagnosis and computer-aided automated diagnosis of the brain diseases. The most remarkable recently developed method for brain image analysis is voxel-based morphometry (VBM). It includes anatomical standardization of the brain to a standard brain, brain tissue segmentation and finally voxel-based statistical analysis based on general linear model. This technique enables us to extract brain regions which show correlations between tissue volume and variables, such as age, sex, and other subject's characteristics. We can analyze not only age-related normal changes but also diseased brain, such as dementia and schizophrenia. It has been believed that functional imaging precede structural imaging to detect early pathological findings of the diseases. However, recent development of high-resolution structural imaging and sophisticated analytical technique enable us to detect the brain disease at very early stage. Now we have collected over 3,000 brain MRI of healthy Japanese aged from 5 to 80 and constructed an MRI database together with their characteristics such as age, sex, lifestyle information, blood pressure, present and past disease history, and cognitive functions. This is a largest brain MRI database in Japan and one of the largest one in the world.

20.2   Imaging Studies of Brain Development

20.2.1   Correlation Between Gray Matter Density-Adjusted Brain Perfusion and Age Using Brain MR Images of 202 Healthy Children

In understanding brain aging, the knowledge of brain maturation is very important, for the relationship between brain maturation and brain aging is regarding as a "mirror pattern." In detail, brain regions that mature earlier such as occipital regions are robust in brain aging, whereas brain regions that mature rather late such as prefrontal regions are vulnerable for aging. Brain development continues through childhood and adolescence. Recently, it has been revealed that human brain development is a structurally and functionally nonlinear process. However, despite this growing wealth of knowledge about maturational changes in brain structure in children, the trajectory of brain perfusion with age in healthy children is not yet well documented.

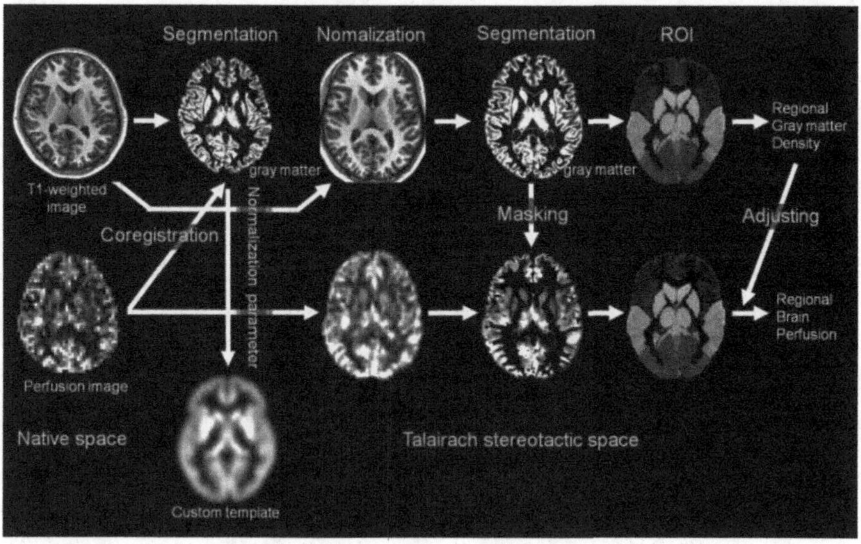

Fig. 20.1 Schematic of the image analysis

Recently, arterial spin-labeling (ASL) perfusion magnetic resonance imaging (MRI) has been developed for evaluating brain perfusion. We examined the correlation between brain perfusion and age using pulsed ASL MRI in a large number of healthy children.

We collected data on brain structural and ASL perfusion MRI in 202 healthy children aged 5–18 years. Structural MRI data were segmented and normalized, applying a voxel-based morphometric analysis. Perfusion MRI was normalized using the normalization parameter of the corresponding structural MRI. We calculated brain perfusion with an adjustment for gray matter density (BP-GMD) by dividing normalized ASL MRI by normalized gray matter segments in 22 regions. Next, we analyzed the correlation between BP-GMD and age in each region by estimating linear, quadratic, and cubic polynomial functions, using the Akaike information criterion (Fig. 20.1).

As a result, the correlation between BP-GMD and age showed an inverted U shape followed by a U-shaped trajectory in most regions [1–3]. In addition, age at which BP-GMD was highest was different among the lobes and gray matter regions, and the BP-GMD association with age increased from the occipital to the frontal lobe via the temporal and parietal lobes.

In the frontal lobe, all gray matter regions showed an inverted U-shaped trajectory for the correlation between BP-GMD and age, and the best fit was a negative quadratic or positive cubic polynomial function. The estimated age at which BP-GMD was highest was earlier in the precentral gyrus, cingulate gyrus, and anterior cingulate cortex than in the superior, middle, and inferior frontal gyri (Fig. 20.2).

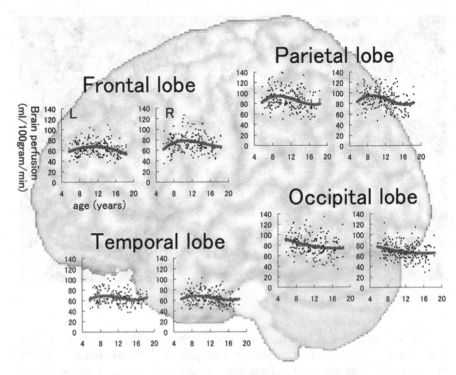

Fig. 20.2 Correlation between brain perfusion, adjusted for gray matter density, and age in the frontal lobe, parietal lobe, occipital lobe, and temporal lobe in each hemisphere

We demonstrated a correlation between BP-GMD and age using ASL brain perfusion MRI in a large number of healthy children over a wide age range. As a result, the trajectory of the correlation between BP-GMD and age showed an inverted U-shaped second-order polynomial function in most regions in the frontal lobe, a third-order polynomial function in the parietal and temporal lobes, and a U-shaped second-order and negative linear correlation in the occipital lobe. Our results indicate that higher-order association cortices mature after the lower-order cortices in terms of brain perfusion. As a result, the trajectory of the correlation between BP-GMD and age showed an inverted U shape followed by a U-shaped trajectory in most regions. In addition, the age at which BP-GMD was highest was different among the lobes and gray matter regions, showing a progression from the occipital lobe to the frontal lobe, via the temporal and parietal lobes. Our results indicate that higher-order association cortices mature after the lower-order cortices mature. This may help not only clarify the mechanisms of normal brain maturation from the viewpoint of brain perfusion but also distinguish normal from developmental disorders that show abnormal brain perfusion patterns.

20.2.2 Correlation Between Sleep Duration and Gray Matter Volume Using Brain MR Images of 290 Healthy Children

Sleep is essential for living beings, and sleep loss has been shown to affect hippocampal structure and function in rats by inhibiting cell proliferation and neurogenesis in this region of the brain. We aimed to analyze the correlation between sleep duration and the hippocampal volume using brain magnetic resonance images of 290 healthy children aged 5–18 years. We examined the volume of gray matter, white matter, and the cerebrospinal fluid (CSF) space in the brain using a fully automated and established neuroimaging technique, voxel-based morphometry, which enabled global analysis of brain structure without bias toward any specific brain region while permitting the identification of potential differences or abnormalities in brain structures. We found that the regional gray matter volume of the bilateral hippocampal body was significantly positively correlated with sleep duration during weekdays after adjusting for age, sex, and intracranial volume [4]. Our results indicated that sleep duration affects the hippocampal regional gray matter volume of healthy children. These findings advance our understanding of the importance of sleep habits in the daily lives of healthy children.

20.3 Imaging Studies of Brain Aging

20.3.1 Correlation Between Baseline Regional Gray Matter Volume and Global Gray Matter Volume Decline Rate

Evaluating whole-brain or global gray matter volume decline rate is important in distinguishing neurodegenerative diseases from normal aging and in anticipating cognitive decline over a given period in non-demented subjects. Whether a significant negative correlation exists between baseline regional gray matter volume of several regions and global gray matter volume decline in the subsequent time period in healthy subjects has not yet been clarified. Therefore, we analyzed the correlation between baseline regional gray matter volumes and the rate of global gray matter volume decline in the period following baseline using magnetic resonance images of the brains of 381 healthy subjects by applying a longitudinal design over 6 years using voxel-based morphometry.

All subjects were Japanese individuals recruited from our previous brain-imaging project. We selected participants who had lived in Sendai City at the time of the previous study, whose collected data had no missing values and who had no serious medical problems from an initial 1604 eligible persons. All participants were screened with a mail-in health questionnaire and underwent telephone and personal interviews. Persons who reported a history of any malignant tumor, head trauma with loss of consciousness for >5 min, cerebrovascular disease, epilepsy, any psychiatric disease, or claustrophobia were excluded from the study. All subjects were screened for dementia using the Mini-Mental State Examination (MMSE). An experienced neuroradiologist examined the MR scans for any tumors and cerebrovascular disease. The final sample consisted of 381 participants (40.1 % of the eligible cohort: 158 men, 223 women). All images were collected using the same 0.5 T MR scanner, including baseline images using MP-RAGE pulse sequences. After the image acquisition, all MR images were analyzed using statistical parametric mapping 2 in Matlab. We calculated gray matter volume and white matter volume using fully automated techniques. To normalize the head size of each subject, we defined the gray matter ratio (GMR) as the percentage of gray matter volume divided by the intracranial volume. Next, to reveal the annualized rate of change in GMR with age, we determined the annual percentage change in GMR (APC_{GMR}) for each subject. We determined regional gray matter volume using voxel-based morphometry. To investigate the correlation between baseline regional gray matter volume and APC_{GMR}, we performed a multiple regression analysis with age, gender, intracranial volume, and APC_{GMR} as independent valuables and baseline regional gray matter volume as a dependent valuable. We used the random field theory method to correct for the Familywise Error Rate (FWE); any resulting P-value less than 0.05 was considered significant. Next, we tested whether the gray matter regional volume that showed the significant negative correlation with APC_{GMR} at baseline could predict whether the APC_{GMR} was above or below the APC_{GMR} mean by applying a standard (not stepwise) linear discriminant analysis in SPSS11.5. For the discriminant analysis, we used the mean gray matter volume over a cluster in each region, and the regional gray matter volume as defined by multiple regression analysis. We set the significance level at $P < 0.05$.

As a result, the gray matter regions showing significant negative correlation with APC_{GMR} adjusted for age, gender, and intracranial volume are shown in Fig. 20.1. Baseline regional gray matter volumes of the right PCC/precuneus and the left hippocampus showed significant negative correlations with APC_{GMR} after adjusting for age, gender, and intracranial volume (right PCC/precuneus, $t = 5.42$, $P = 0.020$; left hippocampus, $t = 5.29$, $P = 0.035$) [1]. Therefore, we used the gray matter regions of the right PCC/precuneus and the left hippocampus in the next discriminant analysis. Baseline regional gray matter volume of both the right PCC/precuneus and the left hippocampus significantly distinguished whether APC_{GMR} was above or below the APC_{GMR} mean. The F-value, p-value, and discriminant function coefficient were 13.51, <0.001, and 0.833 in the right PCC/precuneus and 5.71, 0.017, and 0.350 in the left hippocampus, respectively. Overall, 58.4 % of the APC_{GMR} (55.8 % of APC_{GMR} below the mean of APC_{GMR} and 60.9 % of APC_{GMR} above the mean of APC_{GMR}) was correctly distinguished using the discriminant function (Fig. 20.3).

This study provides the first longitudinal findings showing that baseline regional gray matter volumes in the right PCC/precuneus and the left hippocampus show a significant negative correlation with the rate of global gray matter volume decline

Fig. 20.3 Gray matter regions showing significant negative correlations with annual percent change of the gray matter ratio (APC$_{GMR}$) adjusted for age, gender, and intracranial volume

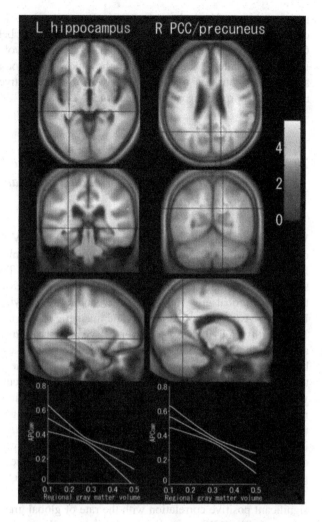

in the following period, as represented by APC$_{GMR}$, adjusting for age, gender, and intracranial volume. In addition, baseline regional gray matter volumes of both the right PCC/precuneus and the left hippocampus significantly distinguished whether the APC$_{GMR}$ was above or below the APC$_{GMR}$ mean. These results indicate that subjects who had smaller baseline regional gray matter volumes in those regions showed higher rate of global gray matter volume decline in the following period.

In summary, using a longitudinal design over 6 years in 381 community-dwelling healthy individuals, we examined the correlation between baseline regional gray matter volume and the rate of global gray matter volume decline in the following period. We found a significant negative correlation between APC$_{GMR}$ and the baseline regional gray matter volumes of the right PCC/precunei and the left hippocampus after adjusting for age and gender. In addition, baseline regional gray matter volume of both the right PCC/precuneus and the left hippocampus significantly distinguished whether the APC_{GMR} was above or below the APC_{GMR} mean. Our results suggest that baseline regional gray matter volume predicts the rate of global gray matter volume decline in the following period in healthy subjects. Our study may contribute to distinguishing neurodegenerative diseases from normal aging and to predicting cognitive decline.

20.3.2   Correlation Between Degree of White Matter Hyperintensities and Global Gray Matter Volume Decline Rate

Whether the degree of white matter hyperintensities (WMHs) shows a significant correlation with the rate of global gray matter volume decline over a period following initial baseline measurement remains unclear. The purpose of the present study was to reveal the relationship between the degree of WMHs at baseline and the rate of global gray matter volume decline by applying a longitudinal design. Using a 6-year longitudinal design and magnetic resonance images of the brains of 160 healthy individuals aged over 50 years and living in the community, we analyzed the correlation between degree of WMHs using Fazekas scaling at baseline and rate of global gray matter volume decline 6 years later. To obtain the rate of global gray matter volume decline, we calculated global gray matter volume and intracranial volume at baseline and at follow-up using a fully automated method. As a result, the annual percentage change in the gray matter ratio (GMR, APC_{GMR}), in which GMR represents the percentage of gray matter volume in the intracranial volume, showed a significant positive correlation with the degree of deep WMHs and periventricular WMHs at baseline, after adjusting for age, gender, present history of hypertension, and diabetes mellitus [2].

The degree of WMHs, both DWMH and PVWMH, at baseline showed a significant positive correlation with the rate of global gray matter volume decline, represented by APC_{GMR}, adjusting for age, gender, and present history of hypertension and diabetes mellitus in healthy subjects using longitudinal analysis. To our knowledge, we are the first to show the correlation between the degree of WMHs at baseline and the rate of subsequent global gray matter volume decline in healthy elderly individuals. Our result is partially consistent with recent studies that showed a significant positive correlation between the degree or load of WMHs and decreases in gray matter volume in healthy elderly people, although those studies were conducted using cross-sectional design. However, another recent study using longitudinal analysis has shown that WMH is not a predictor of brain atrophy rate in elderly subjects. The inconsistency between the findings of the recent study and the present study may have arisen from differences in the volume that was measured. In the present study, we focused on the rate of decline of gray matter volume, not whole-brain volume, because gray matter volume is significantly correlated with several cognitive functions. Our results suggest that the rate of global gray matter volume decline could be predicted using the degree of WMHs at baseline, evaluated by simple visual scaling.

In summary, using a longitudinal design over 6 years in 160 community-dwelling healthy individuals, the degree of WMHs was measured at baseline, and the rate of global gray matter volume decline was obtained. As a result, APC_{GMR} showed a significant positive correlation with the degree of deep WMHs and periventricular WMHs at baseline adjusting for age, gender, and present history of hypertension and diabetes mellitus. Our results suggest that degree of WMHs at baseline predicts the rate of subsequent gray matter volume decline and also suggests that simple visual scaling of WMHs could contribute to the prediction of the rate of global gray matter volume decline.

20.3.3 Risk Factors for Brain Volume Decrease

20.3.3.1 Alcohol Drinking

We also tested the correlation between gray matter ratio and lifetime alcohol intake. There was a strong negative correlation between the log-transformed lifetime alcohol intake and the gray matter ratio [5]. Figure 20.4 shows the gray matter regions that had a significant negative correlation between the lifetime alcohol intake and the regional gray matter volume. The gray matter volume of the bilateral middle frontal gyri showed a significant negative correlation with the log-transformed lifetime alcohol intake.

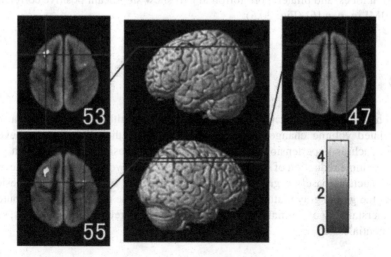

Fig. 20.4 Brain regions that showed negative correction between gray matter volume and lifetime alcohol intake

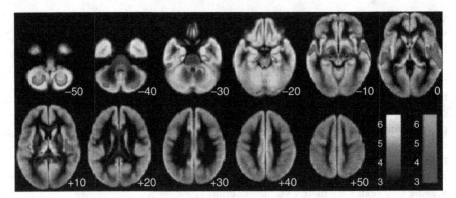

Fig. 20.5 T brain regions that showed correlations between gray matter volume and body mass index (BMI). *Red* and *blue color* indicated negative and positive correlations, respectively

20.3.3.2 Obesity

We tested correlation between gray matter ratio and obesity. As an indicator for obesity, body mass index (BMI) was used. Volumetric analysis revealed that there are significant negative correlations between BMI and the gray matter ratio, which represents the percentage of gray matter volume in the intracranial volume, in men ($p < 0.001$, adjusting for age, systolic blood pressure, and lifetime alcohol intake), whereas not in women. VBM revealed that regional gray matter volumes of the bilateral medial temporal lobe, occipital lobe, frontal lobe, and anterior lobe of the cerebellum show significant negative correlation with BMI, and those of the posterior lobe of the cerebellum, perisylvian regions of the bilateral frontal and temporal lobes, and bilateral orbitofrontal gyri show significant positive correlation with BMI in men [6] (Fig. 20.5).

20.4 Conclusion

We constructed a large-scale brain MRI database for healthy Japanese and clarified age-related volume changes of the human brain and their risk factors. Several factors such as hypertension, alcohol drinking, and obesity are related with gray matter volume reduction of several regions. In addition, we have shown that several factors such as baseline gray matter volume structure and white matter lesions predict the global gray matter volume decline rate. These results may contribute to the understanding of normal brain aging, as well as age-related brain diseases, such as dementia.

References

1. Taki Y, Hashizume H, Sassa Y, Takeuchi H, Wu K, Asano M, Asano K, Fukuda H, Kawashima R. Correlation between gray matter density-adjusted brain perfusion and age using brain MR images of 202 healthy children. Hum Brain Mapp. 2011;32:1973–85.
2. Taki Y, Kinomura S, Sato K, Goto R, Wu K, Kawashima R, Fukuda H. Correlation between baseline regional gray matter volume and global gray matter volume decline rate. Neuroimage. 2011;54:743–9.
3. Taki Y, Kinomura S, Sato K, Goto R, Wu K, Kawashima R, Fukuda H. Correlation between degree of white matter hyperintensities and global gray matter volume decline rate. Neuroradiology. 2011;53:397–403.
4. Taki Y, Thyreau B, Hashizume H, Sassa Y, Takeuchi H, Wu K, Kotozaki Y, Nouchi R, Asano M, Asano K, Fukuda H, Kawashima R. Sleep duration during weekdays affects hippocampal gray matter volume in healthy children. NeuroImage. 2012;60:471–5.
5. Taki Y, Kinomura S, Sato K, Goto R, Inoue K, Okada K, Ono S, Kawashima R, Fukuda H. Both global gray matter volume and regional gray matter volume negatively correlate with lifetime alcohol intake in non-alcohol-dependent Japanese men. A volumetric analysis and a voxel-based morphometry. Alcoholism Clin Exp Res. 2006;30:1045–50.
6. Taki Y, Kinomura S, Sato K, Inoue K, Goto R, Okada K, Uchida S, Kawashima R, Fukuda H. Relationship between body mass index and gray matter volumes in 1428 healthy individuals. Obes Res. 2008;16:119–24.

Part V
Oncology

Chapter 21
Back to the Future: Nuclear Medicine Rediscovers Its Therapeutic Roots

Rodney J. Hicks

Abstract Before the advent of diagnostic imaging, nuclear medicine was a treatment modality. The first therapeutic application of radioisotopes was almost contemporaneous with the discovery of radioactivity. P-32 became one of the first effective therapies for a range of malignant blood disorders; I-131 was established as the benchmark for the treatment of metastatic thyroid cancer; Sr-89 was recognised to provide palliative benefit in advanced prostate cancer. The development of tomographic imaging with SPECT and PET, further enhanced by hybrid CT or MRI devices, has recently focussed the speciality of nuclear medicine on the diagnostic use of isotopes. Against this trend there has been renewed awareness on the ability of radiotracers to identify potential therapeutic targets and to use this information to select patients for and to monitor the efficacy of targeted therapies using radioisotopes. This process has been termed "theranostics". A significant factor in the rebirth of therapeutic nuclear medicine has been the development of peptides labelled with Ga-68 and Lu-177. Ga-68 DOTA-octreotate PET/CT and Lu-177 DOTA-octreotate peptide receptor radionuclide therapy (PRRT) provides the modern prototype of the theranostic paradigm. Experience with PRRT has, however, emphasised the need for a more rigorous scientific approach to radionuclide therapy. The future holds promise of wide range of therapeutic options based on diagnostic/therapeutic pairs including I-124/I-131 and Cu-64/Cu-67. Quantitative SPECT/CT and PET/CT will be key platform technologies for planning and monitoring such therapy and will realise the true promise of molecular imaging in characterising rather than just finding disease.

R.J. Hicks, MB BS (Hons), MD, FRACP (✉)
Cancer Imaging, The Peter MacCallum Cancer Centre, St Andrew's Place East, Melbourne, VIC 3002, Australia

Neuroendocrine Service, The Peter MacCallum Cancer Centre, Melbourne, Australia

Department of Medicine, St Vincent's Hospital, Fitzroy, VIC, Australia

Department of Radiology, Royal Melbourne Hospital, Parkville, VIC, Australia

Molecular Imaging and Targeted Therapeutics Laboratory, The Sir Peter MacCallum Department of Oncology, The University of Melbourne, Parkville, Australia
e-mail: rod.hicks@petermac.org

© The Author(s) 2016
Y. Kuge et al. (eds.), *Perspectives on Nuclear Medicine for Molecular Diagnosis and Integrated Therapy*, DOI 10.1007/978-4-431-55894-1_21

Keywords Positron emission tomography • Radionuclide therapy • Theranostics • Peptide receptor • Neuroendocrine tumour

21.1 Introduction

Many current practitioners working in nuclear medicine are unaware of its rich history as a therapeutic modality. For interested readers, a delightful series of anecdotes and historical vignettes are contained in Marshall Brucer's "A Chronology of Nuclear Medicine" (Publisher: Robert R Butaine (September 1990) ISBN-10: 096256740X, ISBN-13: 978–0962567407). To summarise this fascinating tale of discovery, serendipity and human sacrifice are beyond the scope of this paper but I will try to cover its key events in order to provide a background to current advances in nuclear medicine practice that I believe will be fundamental to its future evolution.

21.2 Radioisotopes Become Therapeutic Tools

Shortly after the discovery of radioactivity in naturally occurring elements by Henri Becquerel in 1896 and the subsequent isolation of radium by Marie and Pierre Curie in 1898, Pierre Curie became aware of the potential of radioactive elements to damage cells, when he himself sustained a very slow healing radiation ulcer on his chest after carrying a sample of radium to a lecture at the Sorbonne in Paris. Louis Pasteur opined that chance favours the prepared mind. In this case, this simultaneously unfortunate but fortuitous event led Pierre Curie to ponder whether radium might have potential therapeutic application in the treatment of malignant skin lesions. In a seminal example of translational research, he discussed this with a medical colleague, Henri-Alexandre Danlos, who successfully treated patients with aggressive squamous cell and basal cell cancers. This quickly led to the dissemination of radium throughout the world for treatment, first of skin cancers and, later, of all manner of malignancies. Intra-tumoural administration of radium was a forerunner of modern brachytherapy. However, it soon became clear that despite, at times, dramatic therapeutic effects, this treatment, particularly when administered systemically, could have significant side effects, including death but, particularly, haematological disorders and, in the case of radium, osteosarcoma. Marie Curie herself died of aplastic anaemia. Although this has been attributed to her exposure to radioisotopes, she also would have received substantial radiation while using unshielded X-rays while operating a field ambulance service in World War 1.

The development of the cyclotron by Ernest O. Lawrence provided a range of new isotopes [1]. One of these, P-32, was found to suppress blood counts, and again in a serendipitous manner, Lawrence's brother was a haematologist and decided to try this agent for the treatment of a patient. This patient was, in fact, a medical student, with chronic myeloid leukaemia. The dramatic benefit from this treatment led to its use in a range of other blood malignancies. P-32 remains a useful treatment for myeloproliferative syndromes, especially in the elderly who tolerate chemotherapy poorly. In studying calcium metabolism using Sr-89, a Belgian by the name of Charles Pecher believed he had discovered a cure for metastatic prostate cancer following dramatic and complete pain relief in a patient suffering from advanced stages of this disease. Although this discovery was lost for a period of time due to a combination of the untimely death by suicide of Pecher and suppression of information about the American nuclear weapons program, it was "rediscovered" in the 1970s and was the first of a range of bone-seeking radiopharmaceuticals that came into widespread use in the 1980s and 1990s [2]. In studying thyroid function using I-130 in the 1930s, the development of hypothyroidism was recognised and leveraged for the treatment of thyrotoxicosis. Subsequently, Glenn Seaborg and John Livingood made I-131 and Sam Seidlin applied it to the treatment of metastatic thyroid cancer in the 1940s [3]. It has since become an integral part of the management of thyroid cancer. The ability to iodinate biologically relevant molecules was translated into other therapies including I-131 metaiodobenzylguanidine. I was privileged to be trained in therapeutic nuclear medicine at the University of Michigan by the some of the pioneers of this therapy, James Sisson and Brahm Shapiro [4]. This treatment remains an important therapeutic option for the treatment of metastatic phaeochromocytoma and paraganglioma and also in refractory neuroblastoma [5]. While these therapeutic techniques have continued to be used by nuclear medicine physicians, with the exception of I-131 therapy of thyroid cancer, they are often seen as the treatment of last resort after surgery, chemotherapy, targeted agents and radiotherapy have failed.

21.3   The Rise and Rise of Imaging

In evaluating the uptake and retention of I-131 in thyroid cancer metastases, Sam Seidlin used a Geiger-Muller counter since nuclear imaging hadn't been conceived. It wasn't until the advent of the rectilinear scanner, conceived by Benedict Cassen, that it became possible to image the internal distribution of radiopharmaceuticals. In the first of many seminal contributions to the field of nuclear medicine, David Kuhl combined photographic film to the rectilinear scanner to create the photoscanner [6]. He subsequently developed the principles of tomographic imaging while being a resident in the Radiology Department of the University of Pennsylvania [7]. Using an Am-245 source, he created the first transmission scan, a forerunner of X-ray computed tomography [8], and also performed emission tomography, the forerunner of single-photon emission computed tomography (SPECT) [9]. Gordon Brownell developed coincidence detection to acquire multiplanar images from positron-emitting radionuclides, and Michael Phelps and Ed Hoffman adopted this approach and combined it with the tomographic method developed by Kuhl to create positron emission tomography (PET). The first human scanner was released in 1976 [10]. The real revolution in PET came with the development of the glucose analogue F-18 fluorodeoxyglucose (FDG) [11]. It was both fortunate and tragic that FDG was one of the first PET tracers to become available. Its excellent performance for evaluating diseases of the heart [12] and brain [13] and more recently cancer has stifled the clinical application of other PET tracers. Even its lack of specificity in whole-body imaging mode has found application for the imaging of infection and inflammation.

Throughout the world FDG PET/CT has become the dominant molecular imaging technique for evaluating cancer with demonstrated effectiveness in diagnosis, staging, therapeutic response assessment and restaging. Further, it provides information of about the biological aggressiveness of tumours. With the addition of anatomical landmarks from CT, some see FDG as the ideal "contrast agent" for cancer detection and has encouraged many to consider nuclear medicine as a diagnostic imaging technique that should be integrated into radiology. This view has been strengthened by the development of hybrid PET-MRI scanners, which have a particular strength in localisation of disease sites.

The wider availability of PET/CT scanners has, however, made positron-emitting radiopharmaceuticals that were developed and used in the era of rectilinear scanners but which fell out of favour with the introduction of the gamma camera, attractive again. F-18 sodium fluoride (NaF) was formerly a widely used agent for bone scanning but was replaced by Tc-99 m bisphosphonates in routine nuclear medicine practice as the gamma camera replaced rectilinear scanners. NaF PET/CT is, however, clearly superior to Tc-99 m MDP SPECT/CT in terms of spatial and contrast resolution, enhancing both sensitivity and specificity [14]. Gallium-68 is another example of an old radionuclide being seen in a new light and will be addressed later.

The major focus of much PET radiopharmaceutical development has, however, been on compounds labelled with fluorine-18. This is a radionuclide that is easily produced in small cyclotrons in abundant quantities after a relatively short period of target irradiation. Its physical half-life is attractive both for distribution and imaging. In my own department we chose to establish fluorinated PET tracers in addressing areas in which FDG has demonstrable weaknesses and the alternative SPECT agents are also suboptimal. As a result, the amino acid analogue, F-18 fluoro-ethyl-tyrosine (FET), which has low uptake in normal brain tissue but enhanced transport into brain tumours, has replaced both FDG PET and Tl-201 SPECT brain tumour imaging in our facility [15], as it has in many other centres [16]. Similarly, the proliferation tracer, F-18 fluorothymidine (FLT) provides a conceptually more robust evaluation of the status of bone marrow function than does a range of techniques previously used to assess this using a gamma camera. Whereas we previously utilised either radiolabelled white blood cells or Tc-99 m antimony colloid scanning, we now exclusively use FLT to assess bone marrow reserves [17] or to assess unexplained cytopaenias. Preliminary data suggests a potential role of this agent for assessing leukaemias [18]. Similarly, agents such as F-18 fluoro-methyl-choline (FCH) have also found a clinical role in the evaluation of cancers that tend to have low uptake of the conventional oncological PET tracer,

Table 21.1 Fluorinated tracers used clinically at the Peter MacCallum Cancer Centre

Agent	Abbreviation	Process	Clinical use
[18]F-fluoro-deoxyglucose	FDG	Glycolytic metabolism	Most cancers
			Neutropaenic sepsis
[18]F-fluoro-thymidine	FLT	Cell proliferation	Marrow status
			Tumour proliferation
[18]F-sodium fluoride	NaF	Bone formation	Prostate cancer, breast cancer, osteosarcoma etc.
[18]F-fluoro-methyl-choline	FCH	Membrane synthesis	Prostate cancer, lobular breast cancer
[18]F-fluoro-ethyl-tyrosine	FET	Amino acid transport	Brain tumours
[18]F-fluoro-azomycin-aribinoside	FAZA	Hypoxia	Assessment for hypoxia cytotoxins

FDG [19]. Prostate cancer and lobular breast cancer are notable examples [20]. Table 21.1 provides a list of fluorinated agents routinely used in my department for oncological indications. We have a range of other F-18-labelled agents that are still being evaluated in clinical trials. These include an agent with high specificity for melanin, an attractive target for imaging malignant melanoma.

Despite the attraction of F-18, there remained many aspects of oncological imaging practice that were still best served by single-photon-emitting radionuclides. This situation has more recently been addressed by development of gallium-68-based tracers. The germanium-gallium-68 generator has reintroduced a radionuclide that was first described more than 50 years ago. Providing an alternative to the technetium-99 m generator, Ga-68 provides the option of centres without immediate access to a cyclotron, or even those with access to cyclotron products, to a potentially wide array of radiotracers that can replace existing nuclear medicine techniques.

The most established of these tracers are the somatostatin analogues, which have significantly impacted the management of patients with a range of neuroendocrine tumour (NET) [21]. Where available, these Ga-68 agents have largely replaced the conventional nuclear medicine imaging technique of In-111 DTPA-octreotide scintigraphy due to a combination of significantly enhanced diagnostic accuracy, greater patient convenience and more favourable radiation dosimetry. However, there is a range of other agents that could rapidly enter into routine nuclear medicine practice. These include agents for renal scanning [22] and ventilation-perfusion imaging [23]. Table 21.2 provides a list of Ga-68-labelled agents that are used clinically in my department.

There has also been a move to replace I-131, which has unfavourable imaging and radiation dose characteristics with I-123 for SPECT/CT diagnostic imaging. We clearly preferred this agent to I-131, but when comparing it to FDG, the technical differences between the scans often limited comparison of tracer avidity, particularly for small lesions. Accordingly, we have moved to using I-124, particularly in patients likely to come to I-131-based therapy. The treatment of metastatic thyroid cancer, phaeochromocytoma/paraganglioma, neuroblastoma and

Table 21.2 Gallium-68 tracers used clinically at the Peter MacCallum Cancer Centre

Agent	Abbreviation	Process	Clinical use
68Ga-DOTA-octreotate	GaTate	SSTR	NET
			Phaeo/PGL
68Ga-DOTA-exendin-4	Ga-GLP-1	GLP-1 receptor	Insulinoma/MTC
68Ga-nano-aerosol	Galligas	Ventilation	VQ scanning
68Ga-macro-aggregated albumin	Ga-MAA	Lung perfusion	VQ scanning
68Ga-EDTA	Ga-EDTA	Renal filtration	Renal scanning
68Ga-HBED-PSMA	Ga-PSMA	PSMA cell surface expression	Prostate cancer
			Renal cancer
68Ga-nano-colloid	Ga-colloid	Phagocytosis	SLN imaging
68Ga-tropolone	Ga-RBC	Blood products	Blood pool imaging

SSTR somatostatin receptor, *NET* neuroendocrine tumour, *Phaeo/PGL* phaeochromocytoma/paraganglioma, *SNL* sentinel lymph node, *RBC* red blood cell

Table 21.3 Iodine-124 tracers used clinically at the Peter MacCallum Cancer Centre

Agent	Abbreviation	Process	Clinical use
124I-iodide	I-124	NaI symporter	Thyroid cancer
124I-meta-iodo-benzylguanidine	I-124 MIBG	Catecholamine transporter	Phaeo/PGL
			Neuroblastoma

Phaeo/PGL phaeochromocytoma/paraganglioma

lymphoma with iodinated products has opened the way for the "theranostic" application of I-124-labelled tracers. Table 21.3 provides a list of I-124 compounds used clinically in my department.

In addition to these tracers, we are involved in developing further agents for clinical PET scanning or validating agents that have been developed elsewhere. These include agents labelled with Cu-64 and Zr-89. These agents will play, we believe, an important role in further advancing the safety and efficacy of radionuclide therapy as well as putting it on a solid scientific footing. Table 21.4 provides a list of agents that are being evaluated prior to moving into routine clinical use.

This catalogue of tracers is not limited by opportunities for further relevant clinical applications but rather by the challenges posed by producing such a large array of tracers in an academic department, particularly in the context of increasingly stringent requirements for product to comply with good manufacturing practice (GMP). We have partly overcome these issues by partnering with a commercial supplier of PET tracers who have helped to transition tracers from the research domain into routine clinical practice by producing and distributing GMP-certified agents more widely. By achieving economies of scale not feasible in a hospital-based radiopharmacy, tracers like FLT, FET and NaF are now readily available to other PET facilities in our region. As experience with these tracers has grown, the role of PET has become ever more enthusiastically embraced by medical

Table 21.4 Other tracers being evaluated at the Peter MacCallum Cancer Centre

Agent	Abbreviation	Process	Clinical use
^{18}F-Fluoronicotinamide	MEL-50	Melanin	Melanoma
^{64}Cu-SAT-octreotate	CuSARTATE	SSTR	NET
^{79}Zr-trastuzumab	Zr-CEPTIN	HER-2 receptor	Breast cancer
^{124}I-metomidate	I-124 rituxan	Cortisol synthesis	Adrenocortical cancer

SSTR somatostatin receptor, NET neuroendocrine tumour

and radiation oncologists as well as by surgeons. There are, in many countries, impediments to dissemination of these techniques as a result of health technology assessment regimes that require a significantly higher level of evidence than existed for older technologies prior to allowing their use and, particularly, reimbursing their cost. Notwithstanding these limitations, it seems inevitable that hybrid PET devices will become the preferred diagnostic imaging technique in cancer at least [24].

21.4   The Slow Rebirth of Radionuclide Therapy

Many hoped that small-molecule kinase inhibitors that target specific mutations in cancer cells would be the final solution in cancer therapy. The dramatic metabolic responses seen in gastrointestinal stromal tumours (GISTs) provided great excitement, as this was a disease previously without effective therapies. The use of BRAF inhibitors to combat the most common mutation in malignant melanoma was similarly ground-breaking and again accompanied by marked and early metabolic response in FDG PET [25]. However, it has become very clear that resistance to such agents develops almost universally, sometimes after only a brief response. This resistance arises due to genomic heterogeneity and evolution of tumours under the selective pressure of signal transduction blockade. If cells lack the specific therapeutic target or develop a means of bypassing its role in promoting tumour growth, the therapy ceases to work. Similarly, if delivery of the drug to the tumour is impaired, inadequate drug levels may allow cells to survive. While radionuclide therapy also relies on target expression, it is possible to measure the expression of any given target in individual lesions serially over time and on a whole-body scale. Thus, the task of selecting patients for radionuclide therapy and predicting which lesions will respond, and those that are unlikely to, is significantly easier than it is for targeted therapies where treatment selection is typically made on the basis of a tiny piece of biopsy material, which is assumed to be representative of all sites of disease. Furthermore, unlike drugs that require each cell to express the target, the particle range of many therapeutic isotopes means that a cell with high uptake can lethally irradiate nearby cancer cells that might themselves either lack the target or take up insufficient of the agent to have a direct toxic effect. The recognition of microscopic tissue heterogeneity within tumours provides a strong rational basis for radionuclide therapy with crossfire effect overcoming spatial heterogeneity of target expression, at least at the microscopic scale.

While the old war horses, I-131 and Y-90, remain important therapeutic radionuclides, the renaissance of radionuclide therapy has been driven y the development of Lu-177. The physical characteristics of this isotope make it highly attractive for therapy. Although it has sufficient gamma emissions to allow reasonably highly-quality post-therapy imaging, they are not so abundant to pose a major external radiation hazard allowing treatment to usually be performed on an outpatient basis. The decay rate delivers radiation over several weeks but the beta-particle range of only 1–2 mm means that relatively little radiation is delivered to normal cells close to tumour deposits. This is especially beneficial for treating patients with rather heavy infiltration of the liver or bone marrow. Recent studies have also indicated the potential of alpha-particle-emitting radionuclides such as Ra-223 [26], which deliver radiation over only a few cell diameters.

Lu-177 DOTA-octreotate (LuTate) has revolutionised our treatment of NET. Building on the pioneering work of the Erasmus Medical Center in Rotterdam, Holland, we added radiosensitising chemotherapy to the therapeutic regimen [27] and have achieved excellent progression-free and overall survival rates even in patients who would be considered to have a poor prognosis based on the presence of high FDG avidity [28]. The key to achieving such outcomes has, however, been ensuring that there are no lesions with FDG uptake that lack sufficient somatostatin receptor to deliver effective radiation [29]. Again, this reflects a cogent example of the theranostic paradigm wherein personalised selection of treatment can be based on "if you can see it, you can treat it".

Another example of this approach has been the development of PSMA-binding ligands that are labelled with either I-131 [30] or Lu-177 [31]. Although preliminary, the results look impressive in patients with advanced castrate-resistant prostate cancer. As is often the case, the patients referred for such trials have often been heavily pretreated with several lines of therapy and have large burdens of disease. Our own "compassionate use" eligibility criteria similarly allowed treatment of patients who would almost certainly be ineligible for most industry-sponsored trials of novel chemotherapy or targeted agents.

Herein lies a major future issue for nuclear medicine. We see patients who are often at death's door; we usually referred them only when another oncologist has effectively abandoned the patient's care for lack of any other options and has little incentive to ever see the patient again. We see the wonderful benefit that some, indeed many, patients derive, but this is usually reported in case series that lack rigorous prospective design, defined eligibility criteria or standardised response and toxicity assessment. Accordingly, the medical community often view these trials as being flawed at best and anecdotal at worst.

If we are going to have radionuclide therapy assume the respectability it deserves as a cancer therapy, we need to adopt the trial methodology used by drug companies and stick to clearly defined protocols. There are certainly encouraging moves in this direction with both industry-funded and cooperative group trials being developed that integrate radionuclide therapy.

21.5   Long-Lived PET Isotopes with Therapeutic Pairs Provide the Vehicle for Improved Radionuclide Therapy Selection and Planning

One of the major impediments to establishing a scientific foundation for radionuclide therapy has been the inability to both predict and verify the radiation dose delivered to both tumour and normal tissues. Although planar imaging has been able to provide estimates of radiation to normal organs, the development of three-dimensional and quantitative capability of hybrid scanners have made it possible to use PET/CT to perform predictive dosimetry while quantitative SPECT/CT is being refined to allow dose verification.

My group has established methods for quantitative Lu-177 SPECT/CT [32]. This has taught us that while uptake of GaTate on pretreatment PET/CT provides a reasonable estimate of what radiation will be delivered to tumour deposits, it is clear that clearance kinetics of normal organs, particularly the kidneys, varies considerably between patients and cannot be adequately modelled using short-lived tracers. This is where longer-lived PET radionuclides will play an important role. For predictive dosimetry of I-131 agents, I-124 provides the ideal combination of a reasonably comparable physical half-life and excellent imaging characteristics. Cu-64 provides an interesting opportunity for predictive dosimetry of its therapeutic pair Cu-67 but could also be used as a PET surrogate for Lu-177 [33]. Zr-89 and Y-90 provide another interesting combination with respect to radioimmunotherapies.

In the future, the theranostic paradigm will hopefully change from a rather empiric approach of "see it, guess an administered activity and treat it in hope" to one that could be characterised as "see it, measure it, predict and verify therapeutic radiation delivery within tolerance of normal tissues". As is often the case, the past can teach us useful lessons.

References

1. Seaborg GT, Lawrence EO. Physicist, engineer, statesman of science. Science. 1958;128 (3332):1123–4. doi:10.1126/science.128.3332.1123.
2. Robinson RG, Blake GM, Preston DF, McEwan AJ, Spicer JA, Martin NL, et al. Strontium-89: treatment results and kinetics in patients with painful metastatic prostate and breast cancer in bone. Radiographics. 1989;9(2):271–81. doi:10.1148/radiographics.9.2.2467331.

3. Seidlin SM, Marinelli LD, Oshry E. Radioactive iodine therapy; effect on functioning metastases of adenocarcinoma of the thyroid. J Am Med Assoc. 1946;132(14):838–47.

4. Shapiro B, Sisson JC, Eyre P, Copp JE, Dmuchowski C, Beierwaltes WH. 131I-MIBG–a new agent in diagnosis and treatment of pheochromocytoma. Cardiology. 1985;72 Suppl 1:137–42.

5. Shulkin BL, Shapiro B. Current concepts on the diagnostic use of MIBG in children. J Nucl Med. 1998;39(4):679–88.

6. Kuhl DE, Chamberlain RH, Hale J, Gorson RO. A high-contrast photographic recorder for scintillation counter scanning. Radiology. 1956;66(5):730–9.

7. Kuhl DE, Edwards RQ. Cylindrical and section radioisotope scanning of the liver and brain. Radiology. 1964;83:926–36.

8. Kuhl DE, Hale J, Eaton WL. Transmission scanning: a useful adjunct to conventional emission scanning for accurately keying isotope deposition to radiographic anatomy. Radiology. 1966;87(2):278–84.

9. Kuhl DE, Edwards RQ, Ricci AR, Yacob RJ, Mich TJ, Alavi A. The Mark IV system for radionuclide computed tomography of the brain. Radiology. 1976;121(2):405–13.

10. Phelps ME, Hoffman EJ, Huang SC, Kuhl DE. Positron tomography: "in vivo" autoradiographic approach to measurement of cerebral hemodynamics and metabolism. Acta Neurol Scand Suppl. 1977;64:446–7.

11. Reivich M, Kuhl D, Wolf A, Greenberg J, Phelps M, Ido T, et al. Measurement of local cerebral glucose metabolism in man with 18F-2-fluoro-2-deoxy-d-glucose. Acta Neurol Scand Suppl. 1977;64:190–1.

12. Phelps ME, Hoffman EJ, Selin C, Huang SC, Robinson G, MacDonald N, et al. Investigation of [18F]2-fluoro-2-deoxyglucose for the measure of myocardial glucose metabolism. J Nucl Med. 1978;19(12):1311–9.

13. Reivich M, Kuhl D, Wolf A, Greenberg J, Phelps M, Ido T, et al. The [18F]fluorodeoxyglucose method for the measurement of local cerebral glucose utilization in man. Circ Res. 1979;44 (1):127–37.

14. Schirrmeister H, Glatting G, Hetzel J, Nussle K, Arslandemir C, Buck AK, et al. Prospective evaluation of the clinical value of planar bone scans, SPECT, and (18)F-labeled NaF PET in newly diagnosed lung cancer. J Nucl Med. 2001;42(12):1800–4.

15. Lau EW, Drummond KJ, Ware RE, Drummond E, Hogg A, Ryan G, et al. Comparative PET study using F-18 FET and F-18 FDG for the evaluation of patients with suspected brain tumour. J Clin Neurosci. 2010;17(1):43–9. doi:10.1016/j.jocn.2009.05.009.

16. Popperl G, Gotz C, Rachinger W, Gildehaus FJ, Tonn JC, Tatsch K. Value of O-(2-[18F] fluoroethyl)- L-tyrosine PET for the diagnosis of recurrent glioma. Eur J Nucl Med Mol Imaging. 2004;31(11):1464–70.

17. Campbell BA, Callahan J, Bressel M, Simoens N, Everitt S, Hofman MS, et al. Distribution atlas of proliferating bone marrow in non-small cell lung cancer patients measured by FLT-PET/CT imaging, with potential applicability in radiation therapy planning. Int J Radiat Oncol Biol Phys. 2015;92(5):1035–43. doi:10.1016/j.ijrobp.2015.04.027.

18. Buck AK, Bommer M, Juweid ME, Glatting G, Stilgenbauer S, Mottaghy FM, et al. First demonstration of leukemia imaging with the proliferation marker 18F-fluorodeoxythymidine. J Nucl Med. 2008;49(11):1756–62. doi:10.2967/jnumed.108.055335.

19. Price DT, Coleman RE, Liao RP, Robertson CN, Polascik TJ, DeGrado TR. Comparison of [18 F]fluorocholine and [18 F]fluorodeoxyglucose for positron emission tomography of androgen dependent and androgen independent prostate cancer. J Urol. 2002;168(1):273–80.

20. Beauregard JM, Williams SG, Degrado TR, Roselt P, Hicks RJ. Pilot comparison of F-fluorocholine and F-fluorodeoxyglucose PET/CT with conventional imaging in prostate cancer. J Med Imaging Radiat Oncol. 2010;54(4):325–32. doi:10.1111/j.1754-9485.2010. 02178.x.

21. Hofman MS, Kong G, Neels OC, Eu P, Hong E, Hicks RJ. High management impact of Ga-68 DOTATATE (GaTate) PET/CT for imaging neuroendocrine and other somatostatin expressing tumours. J Med Imaging Radiat Oncol. 2012;56(1):40–7. doi:10.1111/j.1754-9485.2011.02327.x.

22. Hofman M, Binns D, Johnston V, Siva S, Thompson M, Eu P, et al. 68Ga-EDTA PET/CT imaging and plasma clearance for glomerular filtration rate quantification: comparison to conventional 51Cr-EDTA. J Nucl Med. 2015;56(3):405–9. doi:10.2967/jnumed.114.147843.

23. Callahan J, Hofman MS, Siva S, Kron T, Schneider ME, Binns D, et al. High-resolution imaging of pulmonary ventilation and perfusion with 68Ga-VQ respiratory gated (4-D) PET/CT. Eur J Nucl Med Mol Imaging. 2014;41(2):343–9. doi:10.1007/s00259-013-2607-4.

24. Hicks RJ, Hofman MS. Is there still a role for SPECT-CT in oncology in the PET-CT era? Nat Rev Clin Oncol. 2012;9(12):712–20. doi:10.1038/nrclinonc.2012.188.

25. McArthur GA, Puzanov I, Amaravadi R, Ribas A, Chapman P, Kim KB, et al. Marked, homogeneous, and early [18F]fluorodeoxyglucose-positron emission tomography responses to vemurafenib in BRAF-mutant advanced melanoma. J Clin Oncol. 2012;30(14):1628–34. doi:10.1200/JCO.2011.39.1938.

26. Parker C, Nilsson S, Heinrich D, Helle SI, O'Sullivan JM, Fosså SD, et al. Alpha emitter radium-223 and survival in metastatic prostate cancer. N Engl J Med. 2013;369(3):213–23. doi:10.1056/NEJMoa1213755.

27. Kong G, Thompson M, Collins M, Herschtal A, Hofman MS, Johnston V, et al. Assessment of predictors of response and long-term survival of patients with neuroendocrine tumour treated with peptide receptor chemoradionuclide therapy (PRCRT). Eur J Nucl Med Mol Imaging. 2014;41(10):1831–44. doi:10.1007/s00259-014-2788-5.

28. Kashyap R, Hofman MS, Michael M, Kong G, Akhurst T, Eu P, et al. Favourable outcomes of (177)Lu-octreotate peptide receptor chemoradionuclide therapy in patients with FDG-avid neuroendocrine tumours. Eur J Nucl Med Mol Imaging. 2015;42(2):176–85. doi:10.1007/s00259-014-2906-4.

29. Hofman MS, Hicks RJ. Changing paradigms with molecular imaging of neuroendocrine tumors. Dis Med. 2012;14(74):71–81.

30. Zechmann CM, Afshar-Oromieh A, Armor T, Stubbs JB, Mier W, Hadaschik B, et al. Radiation dosimetry and first therapy results with a (124)I/ (131)I-labeled small molecule (MIP-1095) targeting PSMA for prostate cancer therapy. Eur J Nucl Med Mol Imaging. 2014;41(7):1280–92. doi:10.1007/s00259-014-2713-y.

31. Kratochwil C, Giesel FL, Eder M, Afshar-Oromieh A, Benešová M, Mier W, et al. [(177)Lu] Lutetium-labelled PSMA ligand-induced remission in a patient with metastatic prostate cancer. Eur J Nucl Med Mol Imaging. 2015;46(2):987–8.

32. Beauregard JM, Hofman MS, Pereira JM, Eu P, Hicks RJ. Quantitative (177)Lu SPECT (QSPECT) imaging using a commercially available SPECT/CT system. Cancer Imaging. 2011;11:56–66. doi:10.1102/1470-7330.2011.0012.

33. Paterson BM, Roselt P, Denoyer D, Cullinane C, Binns D, Noonan W, et al. PET imaging of tumours with a 64Cu labeled macrobicyclic cage amine ligand tethered to Tyr3-octreotate. Dalton Trans. 2014;43(3):1386–96. doi:10.1039/c3dt52647j.

Chapter 22
Interactive Communication Between PET Specialists and Oncologists

Huiting Che, Ying Zhang, Ying Dong, Wensheng Pan, Ling Chen,
Hong Zhang, and Mei Tian

Abstract With an increasing number of positron emission tomography (PET) facilities while a growing shortage of PET specialists in mainland China, interactive communication between PET specialists and oncologists plays a crucial role in individualized management of cancer patients and survivors. It is essential that PET specialists should be well informed by oncologists of their patients' history, current problem, treatments, and particularly, the follow-up information. Vice versa, oncologists should be advised by PET specialists on their thorough interrogation, detailed observations, as well as potential false-positive or false-negative findings – some of which might be ignored in their reports. Improving communication and coordination between PET specialists and oncologists has been linked not only to greater understanding and cooperation but also better patient management. In addition, this interactive communication is an essential element of good collaboration for multicenter clinical trials, for instance, how to make PET as an imaging biomarker to evaluate efficacy more rapidly and to increase the probability of success in a clinical trial and how to move non-FDG radiopharmaceutical forward, etc. Here, our review focuses on the conceptual framework, key features, current problems, and future perspectives on this topic.

H. Che • Y. Zhang • L. Chen • H. Zhang • M. Tian (✉)
Department of Nuclear Medicine, The Second Affiliated Hospital of Zhejiang University School of Medicine, 88 Jiefang Road, Hangzhou, Zhejiang 310009, China

Zhejiang University Medical PET Center, 88 Jiefang Road, Hangzhou, Zhejiang 310009, China

Institute of Nuclear Medicine and Molecular Imaging of Zhejiang University, Hangzhou, China

Key Laboratory of Medical Molecular Imaging of Zhejiang Province, Hangzhou, China
e-mail: meitian@zju.edu.cn

Y. Dong
Department of Oncology, The Second Affiliated Hospital of Zhejiang University School of Medicine, Hangzhou, China

W. Pan
Department of Digestive Disease, The Second Affiliated Hospital of Zhejiang University School of Medicine, Hangzhou, China

© The Author(s) 2016 289
Y. Kuge et al. (eds.), *Perspectives on Nuclear Medicine for Molecular Diagnosis and Integrated Therapy*, DOI 10.1007/978-4-431-55894-1_22

Keywords Positron emission tomography (PET) • Interdisciplinary communication • Patient care management

22.1 Introduction

With an increasing number of positron emission tomography (PET) facilities while a growing shortage of PET specialists in China, interactive communication between PET specialists and oncologists plays a crucial role in individualized management of cancer patients and survivors [1]. In most of clinical settings, cancer patients receive direct or indirect care from a multidisciplinary medical team, including PET specialists and oncologists. The interactive communication regarding patient care is extremely important for diagnostic consistency and therapeutic efficiency [2]. Usually, oncologists select their therapeutic strategy largely on patient history, laboratory tests, and imaging studies including X-ray, ultrasound (US), computed tomography (CT), magnetic resonance imaging (MRI), single photon emission computed tomography (SPECT), or hybrid imaging modalities (i.e., SPECT/CT, PET/CT, or PET/MRI) [3]. PET specialists commonly use PET/CT with ^{18}F-FDG or other radiolabeled imaging agents to evaluate the accumulation or binding activity of a particular biological target or evaluate the functional or metabolic changes after a certain kind of therapy. Among all the current commercially available PET imaging agents, ^{18}F-FDG, the most commonly and widely used in the clinic, has the highest sensitivity, specificity, or accuracy in detecting many glucose-avid cancers compared to the other conventional anatomical imaging modalities. By visualized or semiquantitative analysis of the biochemical or biophysical information on whole-body PET images, PET specialists are being able to not only provide an accurate cancer stage (pinpoint the primary and/or metastatic lesions throughout the body) but also help to select particular targeted patients for the targeted therapy [4–7]. In addition, PET is helpful to assess a specific therapeutic efficacy and detect metastasis or recurrence much earlier than the other imaging modalities in many common cancers [8–11]. Obviously, in every process of patients' management, PET specialists could provide assistance to oncologists. Therefore, a strong cooperative relationship between them can offer efficient care to the cancer patients.

22.2 Oncologists

Defined in the American Society of Clinical Oncology (ASCO), an oncologist is a physician who is specialized in treating people with cancer [12]. There are three major types of oncologists: medical, surgical, and radiation. A medical oncologist is specialized in treating cancer with chemo-, immuno-, hormonal, or targeted therapy, while a surgical oncologist is specialized in the removal of the tumor and surrounding related tissues. And a radiation oncologist is specialized in radiation therapy. Usually, these different types of oncologists need to work together in a relative late stage of cancer patient management.

22.3 PET Specialists and ^{18}F-FDG PET/CT

A PET specialist is a physician who is specialized in selecting the optimal imaging agent and acquisition protocol, interpreting PET or PET/CT images on the basis of physiological and biochemical information of the whole body and localized organs or tissues. In China, with an increasing number of PET facilities and lacking of PET specialists, most of the new PET specialists have been working as radiologists. From their point of view, PET may equal to the contrast CT or enhanced MRI. Nevertheless, they admit that PET is an important imaging approach in cancer patient management.

PET/CT technology is a novel combined method by which functional molecular information (PET) and anatomical information (CT) can be achieved simultaneously [4]. There are many radiotracers that can be used for PET/CT imaging, including ^{18}F-FDG, ^{18}F- or ^{11}C-acetate, ^{18}F- or ^{11}C-choline, etc. [13]. ^{18}F-FDG is the most widely used radiolabeled agent (or tracer) which is actively taken up and accumulated in cancer cells [4]. Since ^{18}F-FDG PET/CT can detect cancer cells at cellular and molecular levels, it is regarded as the most sensitive and specified method among current imaging modalities [14–16].

22.4 Important Roles of Oncologists and PET Specialists

Cancer is a group of disease, involving abnormal cell growth with the potential to invade or spread to other parts of the body [17]. In clinical practice, when a patient comes for unknown reasons like fever, weight loss, fatigue or elevated tumor markers, abnormal findings on US or X-ray, or in physical examinations, an experienced physician will consider "cancer" as one of her/his assumptions. If the patient has risk factors to cancer, oncologists will order specific laboratory tests and imaging examinations (including PET/CT, if available) for the patient. With patient's medical history and PET/CT images, PET specialists can provide a valuable diagnosis for oncologists. If the patient is confirmed as having cancer, the oncologist will choose an appropriate treatment for him. After the treatment, PET specialists can evaluate its efficacy with PET or PET/CT. If the treatment is effective, the patient will be followed up for a certain period of time, otherwise, the oncologists will help the patient to choose another plan. Usually, during the post-therapeutic follow-up, PET specialists can use PET or PET/CT to detect the functional or metabolic change or recurrence much earlier than other imagining modalities (Fig. 22.1).

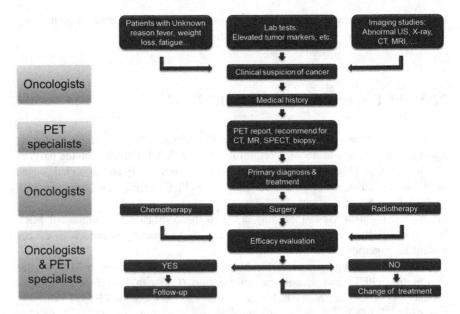

Fig. 22.1 Important roles of oncologists and PET specialists in cancer patient management

22.5 Communication Process

Communication is the process of passing information from a source to a receiver, which is classified into two models: linear and interactive. For the linear model, information is transmitted from sender to receiver via a channel without the sender receiving any feedback, i.e., PET specialist → report → oncologist → patient referring → PET specialist. While for the interactive model, it allows the sender to know that the message was received, i.e.: PET specialist ↔ oncologist. Interactive communication between PET specialists and oncologists allows these two groups to determine if the message was received and how accurately it was received.

Interactive communication is also considered as teamwork, which has the following characteristics:

1. Mutual respect and trust between team members
2. An equal voice for all members – different opinions valued
3. Resolution of conflict between team members
4. Encouragement of constructive discussion or debate
5. Ability to request and provide clarification if anything is unclear

22.6 What PET Specialists Can Do for Oncologists

PET specialists can effectively provide assistance for oncologists, such as (1) offering valuable diagnosis with important functional or metabolic information; (2) providing noninvasive overview of cancer stage; (3) monitoring therapeutic response, especially for the early stage of functional or metabolic changes after treatment; (4) follow-up and metastasis or recurrence detection; and (5) collaborating for clinical trials or other research projects.

22.6.1 Offering Valuable Diagnostic Information

A correct diagnosis is the key to suitable treatment. However, when a patient presenting nonspecific signs or symptoms (i.e., fever, tiredness, or weight loss) and when traditional imaging (i.e., X-ray, US, CT, or MRI) results are negative or controversial, PET or PET/CT could be used for an alternative diagnostic approach, and therefore, PET specialists can offer functional or metabolic diagnostic information to oncologists [18, 19].

Here is a case with unknown reason fever (Case 1):

A 71-year-old female patient who was admitted to the Department of Internal Medicine for fever with unknown reason. The fever lasted for 18 days and was treated with cefmetazole. The peak temperature reached 38.4 °C. In addition, she had a history of right hip pain 2 days prior to her fever. On her physical examination, she presented right hip tenderness without erythema, edema, or plump. On the laboratory results, tumor markers and other tests were in normal limits. She had performed Doppler ultrasound in the abdomen, lower limb arteries and deep veins, and cardiovascular and urinary systems with no remarkable findings. CT and enhanced MR in pelvic indicated a right iliac fossa abscess. In order to explore the cause to fever, she had a whole-body ^{18}F-FDG PET/CT scan. Surprisingly on PET/CT images, her ascending colon showed a hypermetabolic mass which was suspected for colon cancer (A). Therefore, she had colonoscopy that found a polypoid lesion (Is + IIc lesion) of 15-mm diameter in the ascending colon, with hyperemia and pedunculus (Fig. 22.2B). The patient and her family requested for an operation. After the operation, routine hematoxylin and eosin (HE) staining confirmed "moderately differentiated adenocarcinoma" with submucosal invasion (Fig. 22.2C).

For the suspected cancer patients with positive lab tests or imaging findings, the golden standard of diagnosis is pathological confirmation, which needs surgical resection or biopsy. Since these invasive operations might increase the risk of cancer spreading, and false-negative results may occur especially in a heterogeneous large lesion, noninvasive and sensitive imaging techniques are extremely

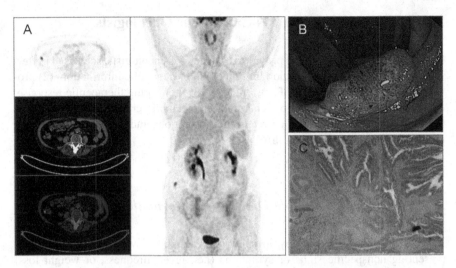

Fig. 22.2 (a) 18 F-FDG PET/CT images showed an area of intensive abnormal 18 F-FDG uptake in the ascending colon (*arrows*) with SUVmax $= 6.00(1$ h), 9.52(2 h). There was no increased ^{18}F-FDG uptake in the right lower limb. (b) Colonoscopy image. (c) Hematoxylin and eosin (HE) staining

needed. Since ^{18}F-FDG is actively accumulated in glucose-avid cancer cells, it could distinguish these cancer cells from the other noncancerous cells [4, 20]. Therefore, by using PET/CT imaging, PET specialists could offer valuable diagnostic information for oncologists.

22.6.2 Noninvasive Overview of Cancer Staging

Oncologists make treatment plan depending on various factors, for instance, a certain type of cancer, stage, gender, age, etc. Among these factors, cancer stage is the most crucial but most difficult to determine. Incorrect cancer stage will lead to poor prognosis of the patient. Underestimating the stage of the disease may lead to "positive resection margins" or unnecessary laparotomy, while overestimation of the stage may yield to ineffective treatment [21]. Although PET imaging studies are costly, it provides oncologists with important noninvasive overview of staging for making optimal choice of cancer patients.

For example, to determine the stage of non-small-cell lung cancer (NSCLC), multiple laboratory tests and imaging exams are required. Among all these examinations, high-resolution CT is currently the most frequently used in clinic. However, even if this imaging approach could provide accurate assessment of local tumor depth invasion (T), it lacks sensitivity and specificity in the assessment of

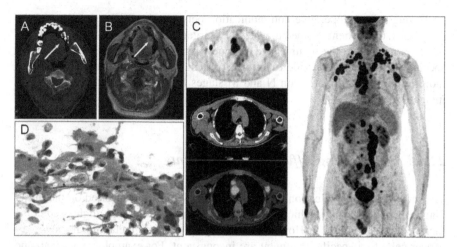

Fig. 22.3 (**a**) CT imaging detected a mass located in the left edge of the tongue (*arrow*). (**b**) MR imaging revealed a mass with long T1 and long T2 signals on the left edge of tongue, a size of 20-mm*10-mm, ill-defined margins (*arrow*). (**c**) ^{18}F-FDG PET/CT imaging showed intensive FDG uptake in the left tongue (SUVmax = 13.83), clavicle and axillary lymph nodes (SUVmax = 16.26), mediastinum (SUVmax = 17.35), ventral prostate (SUVmax = 14.40 at 1 h and SUVmax = 20.46 at 2 h post ^{18}F-FDG injection), in retroperitoneum, bottom of mesentery, and left inguinal region's lymph nodes (SUVmax = 21.47). (**d**) Fine needle aspiration confirmed for squamous cell carcinoma

regional lymph node invasion (N) and distant metastasis (M). Although PET only is not so effective in assessing T, it has great superiority in assessing N and M. Recently, hybrid PET/CT has become one of the optimal imaging technologies for lung cancer staging, and significantly improved the detectability of local and distant metastases in patients with NSCLC, and reduced both the total number of thoracotomies and the number of futile thoracotomies [5, 22–24].

Here is a case of a tongue cancer patient with distant metastases (Case 2):

A 68-year-old male patient who was admitted to the Department of Oral and Maxillofacial Surgery. The patient presented left tongue ulcer for two months; incisional biopsy confirmed the diagnosis of squamous cell carcinoma in left ventral tongue at 1 week before PET/CT scan. On physical examination, his vital signs were normal, and he presented a size of 20-mm*18-mm, firm, ill-defined, and cauliflower-like neoplasm located in the left ventral tongue with obvious tenderness, but no palpable enlarged lymph nodes were found. On laboratory workup, PSA was 196.89 ng/ml and other tests were within the normal limits. After performing the head and neck CT and MR examinations (Fig. 22.3a and b), he was intended to have a surgical operation. However, the presurgical PET/CT indicated distant metastases (Fig. 22.3c). Therefore, he was performed a fine needle aspiration in the enlarged left inguinal lymph node and confirmed the diagnosis of metastasis from the left tongue (Case 2, Fig. 22.3d). Accordingly, he was treated with chemotherapy and radiotherapy.

Through the preoperative communication between the PET specialist and the oncologist, this patient avoided unnecessary surgery and administrated optimal care plan. Namely, with the noninvasive overview on ^{18}F-FDG PET/CT images, PET specialists are able to provide functional or metabolic information on T, but also more important information on N and M stages by the whole-body or total body images [25, 26].

22.6.3 Monitoring Efficacy of Treatments

The most common evaluation of a certain therapy to cancer is based on the initial diagnosis of TNM stage, which may reveal the current status and might predict the therapeutic outcome [27]. However, the morphologic and metabolic responses of cancer cells to a specific treatment are incongruent. For example, cetuximab and other targeted therapies inhibit cancer cell growth by inhibiting the proliferation, angiogenesis, and metastatic spread and by promoting apoptosis [28–30], which should be cytostatic rather than cytotoxic [27]. However, in many cases, especially in the early-phase post-therapy, the change of cellular or biochemical function may be significant, but a measurable reduction in tumor size may not occur. Therefore, tumor size can remain relatively unchanged while tumor metabolism can be markedly reduced immediately [31].

As a result, PET specialists play an important role in offering oncologists the real-time efficacy of a specific therapy and help oncologists to make adjustment to the current therapy or change to another option.

22.6.4 Detecting Metastasis or Recurrence in Follow-Up

The chance of survival depends on the type of cancer and extent of disease at the start of treatment. However, even with the rapid development of surgical, chemo-, radio-, hormonal, and gene therapy and targeted therapies, cancers cannot be completely cured in most cases [32]. Therefore, early detection of metastasis or recurrence is clinically important and helpful for improvement of the prognosis or survival of cancer patients [33].

Here is a case of non-Hodgkin's lymphoma with recurrence detected in the follow-up PET imaging (Case 3):

A 65-year-old Chinese female was admitted to the Department of Hematology for the right back pain which lasted for 2 weeks. She was diagnosed with non-Hodgkin's lymphoma 11 years ago and had an operation followed by six cycles of postoperative chemotherapy. Recurrence was detected 6 years ago and four cycles of chemotherapy was performed. One year prior to this admission, she had severe right back pain. ^{18}F-FDG PET/CT images found enlarged lymph

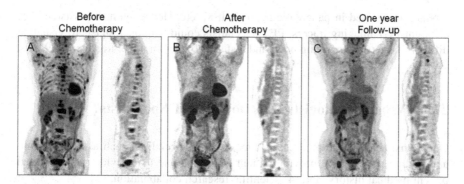

Fig. 22.4 (**a**) PET/CT showed increased FDG uptake in multiple bones, including sternum, vertebras, ribs, pelvis, etc. with maximum SUV of 6.65 in the left clavicle, 11.70 in the L1 vertebra, 5.18 in the ribs, and 5.40 in the right ilium. (**b**) PET/CT images showed normal FDG uptake in the whole body. (**c**) PET/CT images presented intensive FDG uptake in bowels with SUVmax of 5.69–10.22 in bones

nodes in the neck and multiple bones (Fig. 22.4a). After that, vertebral body biopsy confirmed diffuse large B-cell lymphoma and indicated recurrent with transformation. Therefore, the patient was performed eight cycles of chemotherapy. Immediately after the completion of chemotherapy, PET/CT showed negative FDG uptake in all lymph nodes (Fig. 22.4b). For this time, the patient felt backache again, PET/CT revealed intensive FDG uptake in bones, bowels, and cervical lymph nodes, which indicated the recurrence (Fig. 22.4c).

At present, multiple studies found that increased tumor marker level do not indicate localization of cancer. Although increasing of tumor marker levels may be the earliest indication of recurrent cancer, false-positive results may be found in some benign and physiologic conditions as well. Thus, follow-up PET/CT scans have an impact on patient management since it can provide the extended whole-body functional overview of recurrence or metastasis [11, 34, 35].

22.6.5   Research Collaborations

PET, including small-animal (or micro) PET and clinical PET, has become a requisite of cancer research in this century. The most significant advantage of PET method is that radiolabeled imaging agent (or radiotracer) could penetrate into the cell and thus make it possible to reveal the in vivo biodistribution and biochemical process of living cells [4]. Furthermore, not only limited to FDG, a glucose analogue, there are many other radiotracers, for instance, ^{11}C-choline used in prostate carcinoma [36], ^{11}C-acetate used in hepatocellular carcinoma [37],

^{13}N-ammonia used in pancreatic necrosis [38], etc. Hence, with the assistance of different PET imaging tracers, PET specialists could help oncologists to visualize different targets in the living body and test the efficacy of novel treatment [39, 40].

22.7 What Oncologists Can Do for PET Specialists?

Oncologists can also provide assistance to PET specialists, such as (1) referring appropriate patients, (2) provide patient education and (3) provide more detailed patient medical history, and (4) scientific research collaboration.

22.7.1 Referring Appropriate Patients

PET is a highly sensitive imaging method for the detection of early stage of cancer, occult recurrence, and metastasis since cancer-related metabolic abnormalities usually precede structural changes and are readily detected by PET [33]. However, if without clear clinical indication, excessive PET scanning is likely to identify harmless findings that lead to more tests, biopsy, or unnecessary surgery. Therefore, referring appropriate cancer or suspicious patients for PET imaging is the key to get better prognosis for patients.

22.7.2 Providing Detailed Medical History

FDG is not a cancer-specific agent, and false-positive findings in benign diseases may occur [41–43]. Infectious diseases (mycobacterial, fungal, bacterial infection), sarcoidosis, radiation pneumonitis, and postoperative surgical conditions have shown intense uptake, while tumors with low glycolytic activity such as adenomas, bronchoalveolar carcinomas, carcinoid tumors, low-grade lymphomas, and small-sized tumors have revealed false-negative findings on PET images.

Here is a false-positive case with tuberculosis (Case 4):

A 22-year-old Chinese male was admitted to the thoracic surgical department for right chest pain. It is a moderate and tolerable pain presented after taking a deep breath which lasted for about 1 year. He had no smoking and drinking history. On physical examination, his vital signs were normal, and he presented rough breath sounds without any other symptoms. On laboratory tests, his T-SPOT test was positive, and other tests were in normal limits, including tumor markers. He had performed X-ray and high-resolution CT in the chest. High-resolution CT indicated a 13-mm*6-mm nodule in the lateral segment of the right middle lung (Fig. 22.5b). In order to determine whether the nodule was of malignant

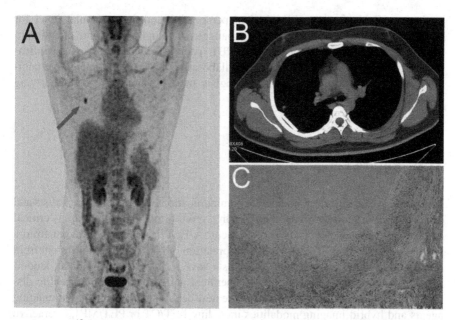

Fig. 22.5 (a) ^{18}F-FDG PET/CT images demonstrated a 12.9-mm*7.7-mm mass of intensive FDG uptake in the right middle lung (*red arrow*) with SUVmax = 5.33. (**b**) Diagnostic CT image showed a 13-mm*6-mm nodule in the lateral segment of the right middle lung. (**c**) Routine pathology of the mass revealed "chronic granulomatous inflammation"

etiology, the patient was referred for ^{18}F-FDG PET/CT imaging. On PET/CT images, a 12.9-mm*7.7-mm mass with intensive ^{18}F-FDG uptake was found in the lateral segment of the right middle lung (Fig. 22.5a). Based on the medical history (young man, nonsmoking, and moderate symptom), the PET specialist highly suspected for nonneoplastic diseases, such as tuberculosis or other inflammation despite the increased SUV value. However, the patient preferred to perform surgical resection. The pathological diagnosis verified it was inflammatory pseudotumor, tuberculosis (Fig. 22.5c).

22.7.3   Research Collaboration

PET is a functional molecular imaging technique which is based on radionuclide imaging of regional biochemistry in vivo. Biochemistry is considered the basis of diagnosis and of the planning and monitoring of treatment since the treatment of many diseases involves biochemical reactions. A number of radiolabeled PET tracers have been designed and developed to imaging the functional and biochemical process of tissues or cells which can be applied for experimental or clinical research, and can be initiated by either PET specialists or oncologists. The hybrid PET/CT not only can provide highly spatial resolution but also can reflect abnormal lesions, glucose, amino acid, nucleic acid, and gene. It is the only current imaging method available from a physiological perspective and the molecular level for quantitative evaluation of biochemical changes. Oncologists pay more attention to the efficacy of different therapies, while PET specialists focus more on the applications of various radiotracers. Through collaborative research and interactive communication, PET specialists and oncologists may explore more on underlying mechanism of cancers.

22.8 Future Perspectives

Awareness of the impact of interactive communication between PET specialists and oncologists, particularly on patient referring, monitoring, and follow-up, is critical to the proper management of cancer patient. A PET specialist is different from a conventional radiologist, and proper interpretation of a PET image is different from a radiological film reading. PET specialists have to integrate the clinical, laboratory, pathophysiological, and even biochemical understandings on a specific disease and related disease progress. With the new development of molecular imaging agents and hybrid imaging modalities including PET/CT or PET/MRI, interactive multidisciplinary communications and international collaborations become more and more important [44, 45]. In the future, interactive communication methods include, but not limited to regular specialist attendance at team meetings, telephone discussions but also shared electric archives and massive open online course (MOOC). We assume that when cloud-based medical practice is applied for the future clinical practice, interactive communication will be even more important and more related to the better patient management.

22.9 Conclusions

Interactive communication is feedback and teamwork. Awareness of the impact of interactive communication between PET specialists and oncologists is critical to the proper management of cancer patient.

References

1. *National Survey Report conducted by Chinese Society of Nuclear Medicine.* Chin J Nucl Med, 2014. 34(5): pp. 389–391.
2. Bar-Shalom R, et al. Clinical performance of PET/CT in evaluation of cancer: additional value for diagnostic Imaging and patient management. J Nucl Med. 2003;44(8):1200–9.
3. Kruse V, Van Belle S, Cocquyt V. Imaging requirements for personalized medicine: the oncologists point of view. Curr Pharm Des. 2014;20(14):2234–49.
4. Gambhir SS. Molecular imaging of cancer with positron emission tomography. Nat Rev Cancer. 2002;2(9):683–93.
5. Pieterman RM, et al. Preoperative staging of non-small-cell lung cancer with positron-emission tomography. N Engl J Med. 2000;343(4):254–61.
6. Riedl CC, et al. Retrospective analysis of 18F-FDG PET/CT for staging asymptomatic breast cancer patients younger than 40 years. J Nucl Med. 2014;55(10):1578–83.
7. Wahl RL, et al. From RECIST to PERCIST: evolving considerations for PET response criteria in solid tumors. J Nucl Med. 2009;50 Suppl 1:122S–50.
8. Bradley J, et al. Impact of FDG-PET on radiation therapy volume delineation in non-small-cell lung cancer. Int J Radiat Oncol Biol Phys. 2004;59(1):78–86.
9. Avril NE, .Weber WA. Monitoring response to treatment in patients utilizing PET. Radiol Clin North Am. 2005; 43(1): 189 – +.
10. Afshar-Oromieh A, et al. Comparison of PET imaging with a Ga-68-labelled PSMA ligand and F-18-choline-based PET/CT for the diagnosis of recurrent prostate cancer. Eur J Nucl Med Mol Imaging. 2014;41(1):11–20.
11. Marcus C, et al. F-18-FDG PET/CT and lung cancer: value of fourth and subsequent posttherapy follow-up scans for patient management. J Nucl Med. 2015;56(2):204–8.
12. Board CNE. Types of oncologists, 2013; Available from: http://www.cancer.net/navigating-cancer-care/cancer-basics/cancer-care-team/types-oncologists
13. Jadvar H. Prostate cancer: PET with F-18-FDG, F-18- or C-11-Acetate, and F-18- or C-11-Choline. J Nucl Med. 2011;52(1):81–9.
14. Nam EJ, et al. Diagnosis and staging of primary ovarian cancer: correlation between PET/CT, Doppler US, and CT or MRI. Gynecol Oncol. 2010;116(3):389–94.
15. Sosna J, et al. Blind spots at oncological CT: lessons learned from PET/CT. Cancer Imaging. 2012;12:259–68.
16. Lan BY, Kwee SA, Wong LL. Positron emission tomography in hepatobiliary and pancreatic malignancies: a review. Am J Surg. 2012;204(2):232–41.
17. Fact sheet N°297. World Health Organization. February 2014, http://www.who.int/mediacentre/factsheets/fs297/en/
18. Meller J, Sahlmann CO, Scheel AK. F-18-FDG PET and PET/CT in fever of unknown origin. J Nucl Med. 2007;48(1):35–45.
19. Hernandez-Maraver D, et al. A prospective study comparing CT, PET and PET/CT for pre-treatment clinical staging in Non-Hodgkin's and Hodgkin's lymphoma. Blood. 2009;114 (22):1508.
20. Ishimori T, Patel PV, Wahl RL. Detection of unexpected additional primary malignancies with PET/CT. J Nucl Med. 2005;46(5):752–7.
21. Seevaratnam R, et al. How useful is preoperative imaging for tumor, node, metastasis (TNM) staging of gastric cancer? A meta-analysis. Gastric Cancer. 2012;15 Suppl 1:S3–18.
22. Fischer B, et al. Preoperative staging of lung cancer with combined PET-CT. N Engl J Med. 2009;361(1):32–9.
23. Lardinois D, et al. Staging of non-small-cell lung cancer with integrated positron-emission tomography and computed tomography. N Engl J Med. 2003;348(25):2500–7.
24. Hanna GG, et al. Conventional 3D staging PET/CT in CT simulation for lung cancer: impact of rigid and deformable target volume alignments for radiotherapy treatment planning. Br J Radiol. 2011;84(1006):919–29.

25. Antoch G, et al. Whole-body dual-modality PET/CT and whole-body MRI for tumor staging in oncology. JAMA. 2003;290(24):3199–206.
26. Antoch G, et al. Accuracy of whole-body dual-modality fluorine-18-2-fluoro-2-deoxy-D-glucose positron emission tomography and computed tomography (FDG-PET/CT) for tumor staging in solid tumors: comparison with CT and PET. J Clin Oncol. 2004;22(21):4357–68.
27. Skougaard K, et al. CT versus FDG-PET/CT response evaluation in patients with metastatic colorectal cancer treated with irinotecan and cetuximab. Cancer Med. 2014;3(5):1294–301.
28. Venook AP. Epidermal growth factor receptor-targeted treatment for advanced colorectal carcinoma. Cancer. 2005;103(12):2435–46.
29. Lenz HJ, et al. Multicenter phase II and translational study of cetuximab in metastatic colorectal carcinoma refractory to irinotecan, oxaliplatin, and fluoropyrimidines. J Clin Oncol. 2006;24(30):4914–21.
30. Contractor KB, Aboagye EO. Monitoring predominantly cytostatic treatment response with 18F-FDG PET. J Nucl Med. 2009;50 Suppl 1:97S–105.
31. Kuwatani M, et al. Modalities for evaluating chemotherapeutic efficacy and survival time in patients with advanced pancreatic cancer: comparison between FDG-PET, CT, and serum tumor markers. Intern Med. 2009;48(11):867–75.
32. Siegel R, et al. Cancer treatment and survivorship statistics, 2012. CA Cancer J Clin. 2012;62 (4):220–41.
33. Israel O, Kuten A. Early detection of cancer recurrence: 18F-FDG PET/CT can make a difference in diagnosis and patient care. J Nucl Med. 2007;48 Suppl 1:28S–35.
34. Antoniou AJ, et al. Follow-up or surveillance F-18-FDG PET/CT and survival outcome in lung cancer patients. J Nucl Med. 2014;55(7):1062–8.
35. Keidar Z, et al. PET/CT using F-18-FDG in suspected lung cancer recurrence: diagnostic value and impact on patient management. J Nucl Med. 2004;45(10):1640–6.
36. Nanni C, et al. 18F-FACBC compared with 11C-Choline PET/CT in patients with biochemical relapse after radical prostatectomy: a prospective study in 28 patients. Clin Genitourinary Cancer. 2014;12(2):106–10.
37. Cheung TT, et al. C-11-Acetate and F-18-FDG PET/CT for clinical staging and selection of patients with hepatocellular carcinoma for liver transplantation on the basis of Milan criteria: surgeon's perspective. J Nucl Med. 2013;54(2):192–200.
38. Kashyap R, et al. Role of N-13 ammonia PET/CT in diagnosing pancreatic necrosis in patients with acute pancreatitis as compared to contrast enhanced CT – results of a pilot study. Pancreatology. 2014;14(3):154–8.
39. Cherry SR, et al. MicroPET: a high resolution PET scanner for imaging small animals. IEEE Trans Nucl Sci. 1997;44(3):1161–6.
40. Tai YC, et al. Performance evaluation of the microPET focus: a third-generation microPET scanner dedicated to animal imaging. J Nucl Med. 2005;46(3):455–63.
41. Chang JM, et al. False positive and false negative FDG-PET scans in various thoracic diseases. Korean J Radiol. 2006;7(1):57–69.
42. Rosenbaum SJ, et al. False-positive FDG PET uptake – the role of PET/CT. Eur Radiol. 2006;16(5):1054–65.
43. Chung JH, et al. Overexpression of Glut1 in lymphoid follicles correlates with false-positive F-18-FDG PET results in lung cancer staging. J Nucl Med. 2004;45(6):999–1003.
44. Soderlund TA et al. Beyond 18F-FDG: characterization of PET/CT and PET/MR scanners for a comprehensive set of positron emitters of growing application – 18F, 11C, 89Zr, 124I, 68Ga and 90Y. J Nucl Med, 2015.
45. Zhou J, et al. Fluorine-18-labeled Gd3+/Yb3+/Er3+ co-doped NaYF4 nanophosphors for multimodality PET/MR/UCL imaging. Biomaterials. 2011;32(4):1148–56.

Chapter 23
Clinical Efficacy of PET/CT Using ^{68}Ga-DOTATOC for Diagnostic Imaging

Yuji Nakamoto, Takayoshi Ishimori, and Kaori Togashi

Abstract Positron emission tomography/computed tomography (PET/CT) using ^{68}Ga-labelled DOTA^0-Tyr^3 octreotide (DOTATOC) is one of the diagnostic imaging tools in somatostatin receptor scintigraphy. There have been many studies demonstrating the clinical usefulness of this diagnostic imaging method, especially for detecting neuroendocrine tumors (NETs). It often yields clinically relevant information for determining therapeutic management in NET patients. However, we have found that the usefulness of the information provided depends on the clinical situation; for example, it was considered especially helpful when recurrence/metastasis was suspected after surgery for histopathologically proven NET. In addition to NETs, DOTATOC PET/CT sometimes provides useful information in patients with tumor-induced osteomalacia (TIO), in which fibroblast growth factor 23 produced by a mesenchymal tumor causes hypophosphatemia, resulting in osteomalacia. As these mesenchymal tumors frequently express somatostatin receptors, DOTATOC PET/CT would be expected to detect causative lesions in TIO. Furthermore, many renal cell carcinomas (RCC) are not FDG avid. DOTATOC PET/CT could be helpful for detecting unexpected lesions when recurrence or metastasis is suspected after surgery for RCC. DOTATOC PET/CT is also able to reveal additional findings even in sarcoidosis, an inflammatory disease. The clinical value of DOTATOC PET/CT is discussed, based on our clinical experience.

Keywords PET/CT • DOTATOC • Neuroendocrine tumor • Tumor-induced osteomalacia

Y. Nakamoto, M.D., Ph.D. (✉) • T. Ishimori • K. Togashi
Department of Diagnostic Imaging and Nuclear Medicine, Kyoto University Graduate School of Medicine, 54 Shogoinkawahara-cho, Sakyo-Ku, Kyoto 606-8507, Japan
e-mail: ynakamo1@kuhp.kyoto-u.ac.jp

Y. Kuge et al. (eds.), *Perspectives on Nuclear Medicine for Molecular Diagnosis and Integrated Therapy*, DOI 10.1007/978-4-431-55894-1_23

23.1 Current Status of Somatostatin Receptor Scintigraphy in Japan

In diagnostic imaging of cancers, positron emission tomography (PET) using ^{18}F-labeled fluorodeoxyglucose (FDG) has been widely accepted clinically for staging and restaging, monitoring therapy response, and detecting unknown primary sites. However, there are some tumors for which FDG PET/CT does not provide relevant information owing to their insufficient FDG avidity. Such tumors include well-differentiated neuroendocrine tumors (NETs), which often cannot be identified as hypermetabolic areas on FDG PET/CT [1]. A major characteristic of NETs is that they express somatostatin receptors. For scintigraphy targeting such receptors, a radiolabeled octreotide, which has high affinity for somatostatin receptors and is very stable in vivo, has been used in Europe and the United States. Compounds labeled with ^{111}In or ^{99m}Tc are used as tracers for single photon emission computed tomography (SPECT), and tracers labeled with ^{68}Ga are used for PET.

[111]In-pentetreotide (OctreoScan) is a commercially available radiopharmaceutical. It is routinely used clinically in Europe and the United States. However, it is not currently approved for use in Japan (as of July 2015), although clinical trials were conducted about the year 2000. Patients must travel to Europe to receive this examination or personally arrange importation of this radiopharmaceutical to enable them to undergo scintigraphy in one of several academic institutions. The number of patients with gastroenteropancreatic NETs is relatively small compared with the number with other common cancers, but its incidence has been increasing [2] so that it is becoming a serious issue. In our institution, PET/CT with ^{68}Ga-DOTATOC for somatostatin receptor scintigraphy has performed since 2011. More than 300 patients have had this examination here over the last 4 years.

23.2 Usefulness in NET According to Clinical Situation

There have been many reports demonstrating the clinical usefulness of PET/CT with ^{68}Ga-DOTATOC or other ^{68}Ga-labeled PET tracers in NETs. It has been reported that it is superior to FDG PET/CT in well-differentiated NET and medullary thyroid cancer [3–5] and scintigraphy using ^{111}In-labeled compounds [6]. Its diagnostic accuracy, including sensitivity and specificity, is reasonably high (more than 90 %) according to a few meta-analyses [7, 8]. However, there are some patients with high hormone levels, indicating the presence of NETs, in whom DOTATOC PET/CT reveals no additional information.

We investigated the clinical value of DOTATOC PET/CT in relation to the clinical situation [9]. We divided patients into three groups: groups A, B, and C. In group A, PET/CT was performed after metastatic NET had been confirmed histopathologically, but the primary tumor had not been identified by other conventional imaging modalities. In group B, PET/CT was performed to evaluate suspected recurrent lesions due to high hormone levels after the patient had undergone curative surgery for histologically proven NET. Conventional imaging had been negative before DOTATOC PET/CT. In group C, NET was suspected based on laboratory data without definitive localization of the primary site by conventional imaging.

In group A, there were 14 patients who were suspected of having a primary NET because of pathologically proven liver metastasis (9 patients), nodal metastasis (3 patients), or bone metastasis (2 patients). In four of the nine patients with liver metastasis, DOTATOC PET/CT demonstrated positive findings, indicating a suspected primary tumor in the duodenum (2 patients), jejunum (1 patient), and pancreatic tail (1 patient) with the maximum standardized uptake value (SUVmax) ranging from 2.8 to 19.7. DOTATOC PET/CT showed no abnormal findings in the remaining five patients. In three patients with nodal metastasis, DOTATOC PET/CT revealed abnormal uptake in the duodenum (1 patient) and jejunum (2 patients). In two patients with bone metastasis, DOTATOC PET/CT was negative in one but showed intense focal uptake in the prostate in the other, suggesting prostate cancer. However, the uptake was found, by biopsy, to be due to benign prostatic hypertrophy. Thus, a final diagnosis of a gastroenteropancreatic NET was obtained in 7 of the 14 patients (50 %).

In group B, seven patients underwent surgery for a NET. Except for one patient with a high insulin level, DOTATOC PET/CT detected ten lesions in six patients with the SUVmax ranging from 7.9 to 70.1. Two patients had histopathological confirmation after surgery, and the remaining four patients were followed up with no surgical treatment. Thus, DOTATOC PET/CT provided additional information in six of seven patients (86 %). PET/CT imaging in a representative patient with nodal metastasis is shown in Fig. 23.1.

In group C, a total of 25 patients with suspected NET due to high hormone levels underwent DOTATOC PET/CT. A pancreatic NET with SUVmax 68.5 was clearly shown by DOTATOC PET/CT in a patient with a suspected ACTH-producing tumor, followed by surgical confirmation. In the remaining 24 patients, DOTATOC

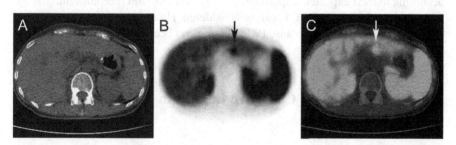

Fig. 23.1 A 51-year-old woman with suspected recurrent gastrinoma. Axial CT (**a**), DOTATOC PET (**b**), and fused (**c**) images are shown. A duodenal gastrinoma was removed by surgery, but recurrence was suspected because of rising serum gastrin levels. Intense focal uptake around the lateral segment of the liver is apparent on the DOTATOC PET and fused images (*arrows*). A lymph node metastasis was confirmed by surgery

PET/CT did not provide any additional clinically relevant information. The detection rate was significantly lower than in the other groups (Fisher's exact test, $p < 0.01$).

We concluded that DOTATOC PET/CT is useful for detecting NET, especially when recurrence or metastases are suspected because of high hormone levels after surgery for a primary NET and that it is hardly helpful in patients in whom only the hormone levels are high and the tumor has not been localized.

It is reasonable that DOTATOC PET/CT would be expected to yield relevant information when recurrence or metastasis is suspected due to high hormone levels after surgery for a functioning NET, since the pretest probability is high. In the patient shown in Fig. 23.1, a small lymph node was visualized retrospectively on contrast-enhanced CT (figure not shown), but it was difficult to distinguish from a benign inflammatory node on the basis of size. In addition, it would take time to confirm the characteristics during follow-up owing to its slow growth. The high accumulation of DOTATOC in a subcentimeter node is considered a useful finding for raising the suspicion of recurrence or metastasis after surgery for NET. Conversely, among the patients without a history of NET, only in one patient was DOTATOC PET/CT helpful, and it was negative in the remaining 24 patients. Some reasons might be considered. Primary sites may be too small to be detected by imaging modalities. If lesions are extremely small, uptake of DOTATOC could be underestimated because of the partial volume phenomenon. Also, when the primary tumor is located in the upper abdomen or alimentary tract, uptake could easily be influenced by respiratory motion or peristalsis, resulting in underestimation of uptake. In addition, high hormone levels do not always mean the presence of NET because hyperfunctioning can cause high hormone levels, e.g., nesidioblastosis in hyperinsulinemia or G-cell hyperplasia in hypergastrinemia. Furthermore, it has been reported that somatostatin receptor subtypes 2 and 5 are not well expressed in many insulinomas [10]. For these reasons, DOTATOC PET/CT may fail to show the primary tumor.

Peptide receptor radionuclide therapy (PRRT) using ^{177}Lu-labeled or ^{90}Y-labeled octreotide has been used to treat NETs in Europe. To stratify patients according to their expected response to therapy, somatostatin receptor scintigraphy, including DOTATOC PET/CT, can be considered. However, we have no sufficient data so far on this subject because PRRT has not yet been performed in our country.

23.3 Localization of Causative Lesions in Tumor-Induced Osteomalacia

It is known that DOTATOC PET/CT is useful not only in the imaging of NETs but also in other diseases. Tumor-induced osteomalacia (TIO) is considered a suitable target for somatostatin receptor scintigraphy. TIO, which is also known as oncogenic osteomalacia, is a rare paraneoplastic syndrome. Phosphaturic mesenchymal tumors secrete fibroblast growth factor 23 (FGF-23), causing hypophosphatemia due to suppression of the reabsorption of phosphorus in the proximal renal tubule and activation of vitamin D synthesis. Consequently, these tumors cause osteomalacia. Total resection of this mesenchymal tumor is essential to achieve complete cure, but localization of the causative lesions remains a challenge because they are usually small, slow growing, and are located at peculiar sites. Therefore, somatostatin receptor scintigraphy can be expected to be useful because these tumors often express somatostatin receptors [11].

There have been several studies investigating the potential usefulness of somatostatin receptor scintigraphy for detecting these mesenchymal tumors. As a preliminary evaluation in our institution, DOTATOC PET/CT has been performed for this purpose. We analyzed 14 patients (5 men and 9 women, mean age 46 years) with TIO who underwent DOTATOC PET/CT. All these patients had been suspected of having TIO due to hypophosphatemia (<2.5 mg/dl) and a high serum FGF-23 level (49–1,020 pg/ml). Overall, DOTATOC PET/CT showed 12 sites of abnormal uptake in eight patients. However, three lesions corresponding to bone were found to be fractured or pseudofractured, i.e., false-positive. Therefore, nine lesions in seven patients were finally considered to be the cause of the TIO. These lesions were located in the sphenoid bone, spine, rib, pelvic bone, tibia, and muscles. In the remaining six patients, DOTATOC PET/CT was negative. One patient is shown in Fig. 23.2. The serum FGF-23 levels in seven patients with true-positive DOTATOC PET/CT findings tended to be higher than in patients who had no causative tumor detected, but the difference was not significant. FDG PET/CT revealed only two abnormal foci in this population. Our preliminary data suggest that DOTATOC PET/CT would be a useful noninvasive technique for localizing causative tumors in patients with TIO and that fractures or pseudofractures caused by osteomalacia can be a pitfall in interpreting DOTATOC PET/CT images.

This is one of the hot topics in somatostatin receptor scintigraphy. Chong et al. found that ^{111}In-octreotide SPECT(/CT) was better than FDG PET/CT in detecting primary mesenchymal tumors causing TIO, with a sensitivity of 95 % [12]. Jing et al. showed the clinical value of ^{99m}Tc-HYNIC-TOC with a sensitivity of 86 % [13]. Other studies have demonstrated 100 % sensitivity of DOTATATE PET/CT in detecting causative lesions, although the number of cases is small [14–16]. In our experience, DOTATOC PET/CT does not always show the causative lesions, but this noninvasive technique may be considered even when TIO is suspected and the results of venous sampling are positive, because unexpected lesions can sometimes be detected by DOTATOC PET/CT.

23.4   Restaging in Renal Cell Carcinoma

Renal cell carcinoma (RCC) may be a target for somatostatin receptor scintigraphy because some recurrent or metastatic lesions from RCC are not FDG avid [17] and it has been reported that OctreoScan shows RCC metastasis [18]. At this time, experience with DOTATOC PET/CT in RCC is limited [19]. We have performed a

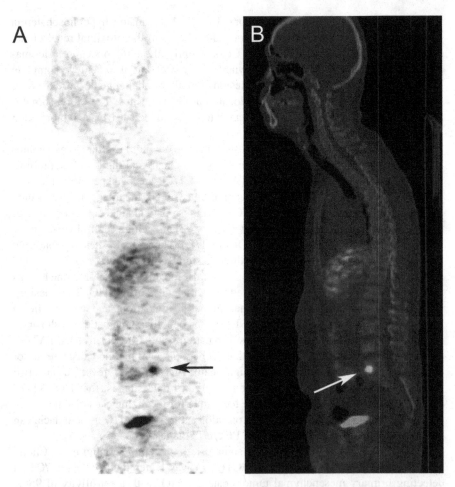

Fig. 23.2 A 54-year-old man with tumor-induced osteomalacia. Sagittal DOTATOC PET (**a**) and fused (**b**) images are shown. This patient was suspected of having tumor-induced osteomalacia due to his high FGF-23 level and hypophosphatemia. Intense focal uptake in the lumbar spine is apparent on the DOTATOC PET and fused images (*arrows*). The lesion was resected, and the patient's phosphorus level returned to normal

preliminary evaluation of the clinical efficacy of DOTATOC PET/CT in patients with suspected recurrent RCC after surgery. Seven consecutive patients who had surgery for histologically proven RCC and who were suspected of having recurrence of RCC underwent DOTATOC PET/CT for restaging. We retrospectively reviewed the PET/CT images and compared available FDG PET/CT findings. In this investigation, there were 18 recurrent or metastatic lesions in seven patients. Of the 18 lesions, 13 in six patients with clear-cell carcinoma were clearly shown on DOTATOC PET/CT, with SUVmax ranging from 2.8 to 23.3 (average 9.7). Excluding 2 of 13 lesions that were not assessed by FDG PET/CT, only three lesions were positive on FDG PET/CT. Four lesions were negative on DOTATOC PET/CT, but positive on FDG PET/CT in a patient with papillary carcinoma.

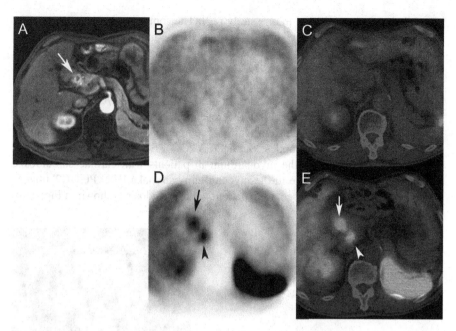

Fig. 23.3 A 76-year-old man with a hypervascular pancreatic tumor. Contrast-enhanced MR (**a**), FDG PET (**b**), FDG PET/CT (**c**), DOTATOC PET (**d**), and DOTATOC PET/CT (**e**) images are shown. The contrast-enhanced MR image (**a**) shows a well-enhanced mass in the pancreatic head (*arrow*). The FDG PET image (**b**) shows no abnormal uptake corresponding to this lesion, but the DOTATOC PET (**d**) and the DOTATOC PET/CT (**e**) images show DOTATOC accumulation in this tumor (*arrows*). A pancreatic neuroendocrine tumor and pancreatic metastasis from renal cell carcinoma was suspected. The final diagnosis was metastatic pancreatic tumor from renal cell carcinoma. Physiological uptake in a part of pancreas is also seen on the DOTATOC PET images (*arrowheads*)

Overall, the sensitivities of DOTATOC PET/CT and FDG PET/CT were 86 % and 67 %, respectively, on a patient basis and 72 % and 56 %, respectively, on a lesion basis, in our population.

A hypervascular tumor seen in the pancreas in a patient with a history of RCC may be difficult to differentiate from pancreatic NET and metastasis from RCC (Fig. 23.3). However, when inconclusive findings are obtained by conventional imaging, DOTATOC PET/CT would be useful for detecting unexpected additional metastatic lesions, just as FDG PET sometimes provides useful information if FDG-avid tumors are present.

23.5 Sarcoidosis

As somatostatin receptors are expressed on activated lymphocytes, it is expected that sarcoidosis, an inflammatory disorder, may also be visualized. The use of somatostatin receptor scintigraphy with ¹¹¹In-pentetreotide in patients with sarcoidosis was investigated in one study [20]. The somatostatin receptor imaging was able to demonstrate active granulomatous disease in the patients with sarcoidosis, and pathological uptake of radioactivity in the parotid glands during imaging was correlated with higher serum ACE concentrations. However, the efficacy of somatostatin receptor imaging in sarcoidosis has not yet been established, and there are few articles regarding the clinical utility of DOTATOC PET/CT in sarcoidosis. In our experience, DOTATOC PET/CT reveals a similar or greater number of lesions than a conventional gallium scan. As compared with FDG PET/CT, uptake may be lower in involved nodes, but DOTATOC PET/CT could be useful for evaluating involvement of the myocardium in patients with cardiac sarcoidosis, because physiological uptake in the myocardium can make FDG PET/CT images difficult to evaluate. A representative patient with sarcoidosis is shown in Fig. 23.4.

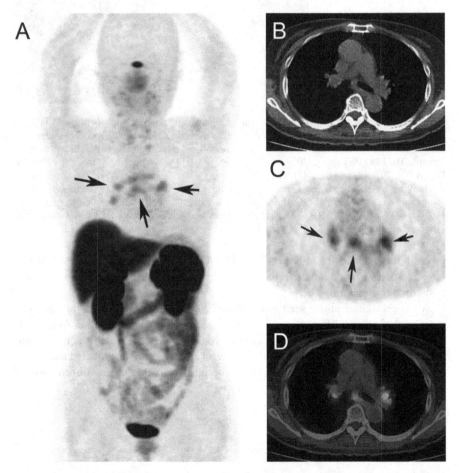

Fig. 23.4 A 65-year-old woman with suspected sarcoidosis. A maximum intensity projection image (**a**) and axial CT (**b**), DOTATOC PET (**c**), and fused (**d**) images are shown. Moderate to intense uptake of DOTATOC is observed in hilar and mediastinal lymph nodes (*arrows*)

23.6 Conclusion

DOTATOC PET/CT is a useful imaging modality for detecting NETs, as has been reported in many articles; however, its efficacy depends on the clinical situation. It may be helpful especially when recurrence or metastasis is suspected after surgery of NET, but additional information might not be obtained simply when hormone levels are high. DOTATOC PET/CT is also considered helpful for identifying causative lesions in TIO, although fracture or pseudofracture can be a pitfall. DOTATOC PET/CT could have a clinical impact in restaging of RCC or in detecting involved lesions in sarcoidosis, but further investigations with more patients are required.

Conflict of Interest None.

References

1. van Essen M, Sundin A, Krenning EP, Kwekkeboom DJ. Neuroendocrine tumours: the role of imaging for diagnosis and therapy. Nat Rev Endocrinol. 2014;10:102–14.
2. Ito T, Igarashi H, Nakamura K, Sasano H, Okusaka T, Takano K, et al. Epidemiological trends of pancreatic and gastrointestinal neuroendocrine tumors in Japan: a nationwide survey analysis. J Gastroenterol. 2015;50:58–64.
3. Kayani I, Bomanji JB, Groves A, Conway G, Gacinovic S, Win T, et al. Functional imaging of neuroendocrine tumors with combined PET/CT using 68Ga-DOTATATE (DOTA-DPhe1, Tyr3-octreotate) and 18F-FDG. Cancer. 2008;112:2447–55.
4. Kayani I, Conry BG, Groves AM, Win T, Dickson J, Caplin M, et al. A comparison of 68Ga-DOTATATE and 18F-FDG PET/CT in pulmonary neuroendocrine tumors. J Nucl Med. 2009; 50:1927–32.
5. Conry BG, Papathanasiou ND, Prakash V, Kayani I, Caplin M, Mahmood S, et al. Comparison of (68)Ga-DOTATATE and (18)F-fluorodeoxyglucose PET/CT in the detection of recurrent medullary thyroid carcinoma. Eur J Nucl Med Mol Imaging. 2010;37:49–57.
6. Buchmann I, Henze M, Engelbrecht S, et al. Comparison of 68Ga-DOTATOC PET and 111In-DTPAOC (Octreoscan) SPECT in patients with neuroendocrine tumours. Eur J Nucl Med Mol Imaging. 2007;34:1617–26.
7. Treglia G, Castaldi P, Rindi G, Eisenhut M, Runz A, Schäfer M, et al. Diagnostic performance of Gallium-68 somatostatin receptor PET and PET/CT in patients with thoracic and gastro-enteropancreatic neuroendocrine tumours: a meta-analysis. Endocrine. 2012;42:80–7.

8. Geijer H, Breimer LH. Somatostatin receptor PET/CT in neuroendocrine tumours: update on systematic review and meta-analysis. Eur J Nucl Med Mol Imaging. 2013;40:1770–80.

9. Nakamoto Y, Sano K, Ishimori T, Ueda M, Temma T, Saji H, et al. Additional information gained by positron emission tomography with (68)Ga-DOTATOC for suspected unknown primary or recurrent neuroendocrine tumors. Ann Nucl Med. 2015;29:512–8.

10. Portela-Gomes GM, Stridsberg M, Grimelius L, Rorstad O, Janson ET. Differential expression of the five somatostatin receptor subtypes in human benign and malignant insulinomas – predominance of receptor subtype 4. Endocr Pathol. 2007;18:79–85.

11. Houang M, Clarkson A, Sioson L, Elston MS, Clifton-Bligh RJ, Dray M, et al. Phosphaturic mesenchymal tumors show positive staining for somatostatin receptor 2A (SSTR2A). Hum Pathol. 2013;44:2711–8.

12. Chong WH, Andreopoulou P, Chen CC, Reynolds J, Guthrie L, Kelly M, et al. Tumor localization and biochemical response to cure in tumor-induced osteomalacia. J Bone Miner Res. 2013;28:1386–98.

13. Jing H, Li F, Zhuang H, Wang Z, Tian J, Xing X, et al. Effective detection of the tumors causing osteomalacia using [Tc-99m]-HYNIC-octreotide (99mTc-HYNIC-TOC) whole body scan. Eur J Radiol. 2013;82:2028–34.

14. Clifton-Bligh RJ, Hofman MS. Duncan E, Sim IeW, Darnell D, Clarkson A, et al. Improving diagnosis of tumor-induced osteomalacia with Gallium-68 DOTATATE PET/CT. J Clin Endocrinol Metab. 2013;98:687–94.

15. Breer S, Brunkhorst T, Beil FT, Peldschus K, Heiland M, Klutmann S, et al. 68Ga DOTA-TATE PET/CT allows tumor localization in patients with tumor-induced osteomalacia but negative 111In-octreotide SPECT/CT. Bone. 2014;64:222–7.

16. Jadhav S, Kasaliwal R, Lele V, Rangarajan V, Chandra P, Shah H, et al. Functional imaging in primary tumour-induced osteomalacia: relative performance of FDG PET/CT vs somatostatin receptor-based functional scans: a series of nine patients. Clin Endocrinol (Oxf). 2014;81:31–7.

17. Nakatani K, Nakamoto Y, Saga T, Higashi T, Togashi K. The potential clinical value of FDG-PET for recurrent renal cell carcinoma. Eur J Radiol. 2011;79:29–35.

18. Edgren M, Westlin JE, Kälkner KM, Sundin A, Nilsson S. [111In-DPTA-D-Phe1]-octreotide scintigraphy in the management of patients with advanced renal cell carcinoma. Cancer Biother Radiopharm. 1999;14:59–64.

19. Peter L, Sänger J, Hommann M, Baum RP, Kaemmerer D. Molecular imaging of late somatostatin receptor-positive metastases of renal cell carcinoma in the pancreas by 68Ga DOTATOC PET/CT: a rare differential diagnosis to multiple primary pancreatic neuroendocrine tumors. Clin Nucl Med. 2014;39:713–6.

20. Kwekkeboom DJ, Krenning EP, Kho GS, Breeman WA, Van Hagen PM. Somatostatin receptor imaging in patients with sarcoidosis. Eur J Nucl Med. 1998;25:1284–92.

Chapter 24
Correlation of 4′-[methyl-^{11}C]-Thiothymidine Uptake with Ki-67 Immunohistochemistry in Patients with Newly Diagnosed and Recurrent Gliomas

Yuka Yamamoto and Yoshihiro Nishiyama

Abstract *Purpose*: 4′-[methyl-^{11}C]-thiothymidine (4DST) has been developed as an in vivo cell proliferation marker based on the DNA incorporation method. We evaluated 4DST uptake on PET in patients with newly diagnosed and recurrent gliomas and correlated the results with proliferative activity.

Methods: 4DST PET was investigated in 32 patients, including 21 with newly diagnosed gliomas and 11 with recurrent gliomas. PET imaging was performed at 15 min after 4DST injection. The standardized uptake value (SUV) was determined by region-of-interest analysis. The maximal SUV for tumor (T) and the mean SUV for contralateral normal brain tissue (N) were calculated and T/N ratio was determined. Proliferative activity as indicated by the Ki-67 index was estimated in tissue specimens.

Results: The sensitivity of 4DST PET for the detection of newly diagnosed and recurrent gliomas was 86 % and 100 %, respectively. In newly diagnosed gliomas, there was a weak correlation between T/N ratio and Ki-67 index ($r = 0.45$; $p < 0.05$). In recurrent gliomas, there was no significant difference between T/N ratio and Ki-67 index.

Conclusion: In newly diagnosed gliomas, 4DST PET seems to be useful in the noninvasive assessment of proliferation.

Keywords ^{11}C-4DST • PET • Glioma • Proliferation

Y. Yamamoto (✉) • Y. Nishiyama
Department of Radiology, Faculty of Medicine, Kagawa University, 1750-1 Ikenobe, Miki-cho, Kita-gun, Kagawa 761-0793, Japan
e-mail: yuka@kms.ac.jp

Y. Kuge et al. (eds.), *Perspectives on Nuclear Medicine for Molecular Diagnosis and Integrated Therapy*, DOI 10.1007/978-4-431-55894-1_24

24.1 Introduction

Markers of proliferative activity are essential for individualized patient therapy and management of brain gliomas [1]. Because tissue sampling is often obtained by stereotactic biopsy and, therefore, represents only a small part of the primary tumor, there is a probability of true malignant potential being underestimated [2]. Thus, noninvasive imaging-based technology for the detection of malignant progression is required to select the best possible treatment regimen.

Positron emission tomography (PET) is now an indispensable modality for assessment of various tumors. The radiotracer 3′-deoxy-3′-[^{18}F]fluorothymidine (FLT) has been investigated as a promising PET tracer for evaluating tumor proliferating activity in brain tumors [3–5]. A theoretic limitation of FLT as a radiotracer for the salvage pathway of DNA synthesis is that it is not incorporated into DNA because of the lack of a 3′-hydroxyl [6].

Toyohara et al. developed 4′-thiothymidine labeled with ^{11}C at the methyl group (4′-[methyl-^{11}C]-thiothymidine [4DST]), as a new candidate for cell proliferation imaging that is resistant to degradation by thymidine phosphorylase and is incorporated into DNA [7, 8]. A ^{11}C-4DST PET pilot study of 6 patients with various brain tumors showed that ^{11}C-4DST PET is feasible for brain tumor imaging and can be performed with acceptable dosimetry and pharmacologic safety at a suitable dose for adequate imaging [9]. In a mixed population of patients with newly diagnosed and recurrent gliomas, Toyota et al. has recently demonstrated that 4DST PET is feasible for evaluating cell proliferation [10]. These results indicate that 4DST has great potential for imaging cell proliferation.

The purpose of this study was to evaluate 4DST uptake in patients with newly diagnosed and recurrent gliomas and to correlate the results with proliferative activity as indicated by the Ki-67 index.

24.2 Materials and Methods

24.2.1 Patients

A total of 32 patients (15 men, 17 women) with brain gliomas who underwent 4DST PET examination were selected. Of the patients, 21 had newly diagnosed gliomas and 11 presented with recurrent gliomas that had been treated with surgery, chemotherapy and radiotherapy previously.

Pathologic diagnosis had been obtained by stereotactic biopsy or open surgery. Grading of the tumor was performed according to the World Health Organization (WHO) classification for neuroepithelial tumors [11]. Distribution of tumor grades according to WHO classification was as follows: grade II ($n = 7$), grade III ($n = 9$), and grade IV ($n = 16$).

24.2.2   4DST Synthesis and PET Imaging

The radiotracer 4DST was produced using an automated synthesis system with HM-18 cyclotron (QUPID; Sumitomo Heavy Industries Ltd, Tokyo, Japan). The 4DST was synthesized using the method described by Toyohara et al. [9].

All acquisitions were performed using a Biograph mCT 64-slice PET/CT scanner (Siemens Medical Solutions USA Inc., Knoxville, TN, USA). Data acquisition began with CT at the following settings: no contrast agent, 120 kV, 192 mA, 1.0-s tube rotation time, 3-mm slice thickness, 3-mm increments, and pitch 0.55. PET emission scanning of the head region with a 15-min acquisition of one bed position was performed 15 min after intravenous injection of 4DST (6 MBq/kg). The PET data were acquired in three-dimensional mode and were reconstructed by the baseline ordered-subset expectation maximization (OSEM) bases, with incorporating correction with point spread-function and time-of-flight model (5 iterations, 21 subsets).

24.2.3   Data Analysis

Visual image analysis was performed by an experienced nuclear physician. Tumor lesions were identified as areas of focally increased uptake, exceeding that of normal brain background.

Semiquantitative analysis was performed using the standardized uptake value (SUV). The region of interest (ROI) was placed over the entire tumor using the transverse PET image. For the reference tissue, a circular ROI of 15 × 15 mm was manually placed on the uninvolved contralateral hemisphere in the same plane that showed maximum 4DST tumor uptake. Radioactivity concentration values measured in the ROI were normalized to injected dose per patient's body weight by calculation of SUV. The maximal SUV for tumor and the mean SUV for reference tissue were calculated. Tumor-to-contralateral normal brain tissue (T/N) ratio was determined by dividing the tumor SUV by that of the contralateral hemisphere.

24.2.4   Ki-67 Immunohistochemistry

Formalin-fixed, paraffin-embedded sections of resected specimens from brain tumor were made for immunohistochemical staining. The Ki-67 index was estimated as the percentage of Ki-67-positive cell nuclei per 500–1,000 cells in the region of the tumor with the greatest density of staining.

24.2.5 Statistical Analysis

All semiquantitative data were expressed as mean $\pm$ SD. The Ki-67 index and the T/N ratio were compared using linear regression analysis. Differences were considered statistically significant at $p < 0.05$.

24.3 Results

24.3.1 4DST Uptake

In newly diagnosed gliomas, 4DST PET detected 3 of 7 grade II gliomas, all 6 grade III gliomas, and all 8 grade IV gliomas. In recurrent gliomas, 4DST PET detected all 3 grade III gliomas and all 8 grade IV gliomas. Although 4DST PET in newly diagnosed gliomas showed a slightly lower detection rate than that in recurrent gliomas (86 % vs. 100 %), the difference was not statistically significant.

24.3.2 4DST Uptake and Ki-67 Immunohistochemistry

In newly diagnosed gliomas, linear regression analysis indicated a weak correlation between T/N ratio and the Ki-67 index ($r = 0.45$, $p < 0.05$; Fig. 24.1a). In recurrent gliomas, there was no significant difference between T/N ratio and the Ki-67 index ($r = 0.31$, $p = 0.36$; Fig. 24.1b).

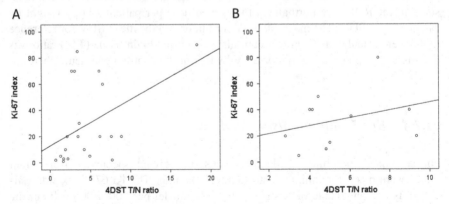

Fig. 24.1 Linear regression analysis demonstrates a weak correlation between 4DST T/N ratio and proliferative activity (Ki-67 index) in newly diagnosed gliomas ($r = 0.45$, $p < 0.05$) (A). There was no significant correlation between 4DST T/N ratio and proliferative activity (Ki-67 index) in recurrent gliomas ($r = 0.31$, $p = 0.36$) (B)

24.4   Discussion

In the present study, we evaluated 4DST uptake in patients with newly diagnosed and recurrent gliomas. 4DST PET was feasible for imaging both newly diagnosed and recurrent gliomas. 4DST PET was found to be useful in the assessment of tumor proliferation in newly diagnosed gliomas.

   Increased cell proliferation and DNA replication is a characteristic of malignant transformation [12]. The assessment of cellular proliferation rate by means of PET is useful as a noninvasive clinical approach. In a previous study, an initial clinical trial in only 6 patients with brain tumor was indicated that 4DST PET was feasible for imaging brain tumors [9]. Toyota et al. evaluated 4DST uptake and proliferative activity in 20 patients with gliomas, including 11 recurrent gliomas [10]. They showed a weak correlation between 4DST T/N ratio and Ki-67 index [10]. The present study also showed a weak correlation between 4DST T/N ratio and Ki-67 index in newly diagnosed gliomas. Minamimoto et al. evaluated 4DST uptake and Ki-67 index in patients with non-small cell lung cancer [13]. They showed a significant correlation between 4DST maximal SUV and Ki-67 index [13]. However, Ito et al. showed no significant correlation between 4DST maximal SUV and Ki-67 index in head and neck squamous cell carcinoma [14]. One possible reason for Ito et al.'s findings may be that the Ki-67 index was mainly obtained from biopsy specimens and not from resected specimens.

   The present study showed no significant correlation between 4DST T/N ratio and Ki-67 index in recurrent gliomas. Eleven patients with recurrent gliomas in the present study had received chemoradiotherapy before the PET study. Radiation and chemoradiotherapy, used as an adjuvant therapy of gliomas, can cause loosening of endothelial tight junctions, vascular leakage, or endothelial cell death and increase vascular permeability [15]. Radiation could also act to increase vascular permeability not only in the blood-brain barrier (BBB) but also in the blood-tumor barrier (BTB) [15]. We suspect that in recurrent gliomas, breakdown of BBB and BTB contributes to the degree of 4DST uptake in addition to increased proliferation. Furthermore, there is biological difference between newly diagnosed and recurrent gliomas. In recurrent gliomas, recurrent tumor and treatment-induced necrosis frequently coexist.

   Because the most proliferating part of the tumor is mainly responsible for tumor progression, 4DST analysis enables a more precise estimation of the malignancy. More important indication is the possibility that the cell proliferation imaging could be used for early evaluation of treatment effects. In the report by Toyohara et al., although ^{11}C-methionine PET detected all the contrast-enhanced lesions visualized with MRI, a clinically stable tumor with contrast enhancement was not detected with 4DST [9]. The role of 4DST in therapy monitoring has not been evaluated so far. Further prospective studies involving a larger number of patients in a variety of tumor types are required to determine the clinical usefulness of 4DST PET for early evaluation of treatment response.

24.5 Conclusion

4DST PET was feasible for imaging both newly diagnosed and recurrent gliomas.
4DST PET seems to be useful in assessment of noninvasive tumor proliferation in
newly diagnosed gliomas.

References

1. DeAngelis LM. Brain tumors. N Engl J Med. 2001;344:114–23.
2. Ceyssens S, Van Laere K, de Groot T, Goffin J, Bormans G, Mortelmans L. [^{11}C]methionine
   PET, histopathology, and survival in primary brain tumors and recurrence. AJNR Am J
   Neuroradiol. 2006;27:1432–7.
3. Hatakeyama T, Kawai N, Nishiyama Y, et al. ^{11}C-methionine (MET) and ^{18}F-fluorothymidine
   (FLT) PET in patients with newly diagnosed glioma. Eur J Nucl Med Mol Imaging.
   2008;35:2009–17.
4. Jacobs AH, Thomas A, Kracht LW, et al. ^{18}F-fluoro-$_L$-thymidine and ^{11}C-methylmethionine as
   markers of increased transport and proliferation in brain tumors. J Nucl Med. 2005;46:1948–58.
5. Ullrich R, Backes H, Li H, et al. Glioma proliferation as assessed by 3'-fluoro-3'-deoxy-l-
   thymidine positron emission tomography in patients with newly diagnosed high-grade glioma.
   Clin Cancer Res. 2008;14:2049–55.
6. Rasey JS, Grierson JR, Wiens LW, et al. Validation of FLT uptake as a measure of thymidine
   kinase-1 activity in A549 carcinoma cells. J Nucl Med. 2002;43:1210–7.
7. Toyohara J, Kumata K, Fukushi K, Irie T, Suzuki K. Evaluation of [methyl-^{14}C]4-
   '-thiothymidine for in vivo DNA synthesis imaging. J Nucl Med. 2006;47:1717–22.
8. Toyohara J, Okada M, Toramatsu C, Suzuki K, Irie T. Feasibility studies of 4'-[methyl-^{11}C]
   thiothymidine as a tumor proliferation imaging agent in mice. Nucl Med Biol. 2008;35:67–74.
9. Toyohara J, Nariai T, Sakata M, et al. Whole-body distribution and brain tumor imaging with
   ^{11}C-4DST: a pilot study. J Nucl Med. 2011;52:1322–8.
10. Toyota Y, Miyake K, Kawai N, et al. Comparison of 4'-[methyl-11C]thiothymidine
    (11C-4DST) and 3'-deoxy-3'-[18F]fluorothymidine (18F-FLT) PET/CT in human brain gli-
    oma imaging. EJNMMI Res. 2015;5:7.
11. Louis DN, Ohgaki H, Wiestler OD, et al. The 2007 WHO classification of tumours of the
    central nervous system. Acta Neuropathol. 2007;114:97–109.
12. la Fougère C, Suchorska B, Bartenstein P, Kreth FW, Tonn JC. Molecular imaging of gliomas
    with PET: opportunities and limitations. Neuro Oncol. 2011;13:806–19.
13. Minamimoto R, Toyohara J, Seike A, et al. 4'-[Methyl-11C]-thiothymidine PET/CT for
    proliferation imaging in non-small cell lung cancer. J Nucl Med. 2012;53:199–206.
14. Ito K, Yokoyama J, Miyata Y, et al. Volumetric comparison of positron emission tomography/
    computed tomography using 4'-[methyl-11C]-thiothymidine with 2-deoxy-2-18F-fluoro-D-
    glucose in patients with advanced head and neck squamous cell carcinoma. Nucl Med
    Commun. 2015;36:219–25.
15. Cao Y, Tsien CI, Shen Z, et al. Use of magnetic resonance imaging to assess blood-brain/blood-
    gliomas barrier opening during conformal radiotherapy. J Clin Oncol. 2005;23:4127–36.

Chapter 25
Impact of Respiratory-Gated FMISO-PET/CT for the Quantitative Evaluation of Hypoxia in Non-small Cell Lung Cancer

Shiro Watanabe, Kenji Hirata, Shozo Okamoto, and Nagara Tamaki

Abstract Hypoxia is present in various solid tumors, including non-small cell lung cancer (NSCLC) and is associated with treatment resistance and poor prognosis. ^{18}F-Fluoromisonidazole (FMISO) is a major PET tracer for hypoxia imaging. Previous studies have evaluated the potential role of FMISO-PET as a prognostic tool and assessed tumor reoxygenation following nonsurgical treatment in NSCLC. However, for cancers located in the thorax or abdomen, the patient's breathing causes motion artifacts and misregistration between PET and CT images. PET/CT with the respiratory-gating technique improves the measurement of lesion uptake and tumor volume. We investigated the usefulness of respiratory gating for FMISO-PET/CT-based quantification of hypoxia. Among the 14 patients examined, hypoxia was observed in three patients with non-gated acquisition and in five patients with respiratory gating. The SUVmax, tumor-to-muscle ratio, tumor-to-blood ratio, and hypoxic volume were statistically significantly higher in respiratory-gated (RG) images than in non-respiratory-gated (NG) images. RG FMISO-PET/CT may be useful for the accurate quantification of hypoxia.

Keywords Non-small cell lung cancer • Hypoxia • FMISO • Respiratory gating

25.1 Background

Lung cancer is one of the most common cancers and is the leading cause of cancer death worldwide. Although survival rates have improved in non-small cell lung cancer (NSCLC), the long-term outcome remains poor compared with other cancers. Locoregional failure is not rare, particularly after chemoradiotherapy, and may be attributed to intrinsic tumor resistance to radiotherapy and/or chemotherapy

S. Watanabe (✉) • K. Hirata • S. Okamoto
Department of Nuclear Medicine, Hokkaido University Graduate School of Medicine, North 15th, West 7th, Kitaku, Sapporo 060-8638, Japan
e-mail: shirow@med.hokudai.ac.jp

N. Tamaki
Department of Nuclear Medicine, Graduate School of Medicine, Hokkaido University, Sapporo, Japan

© The Author(s) 2016   319
Y. Kuge et al. (eds.), *Perspectives on Nuclear Medicine for Molecular Diagnosis and Integrated Therapy*, DOI 10.1007/978-4-431-55894-1_25

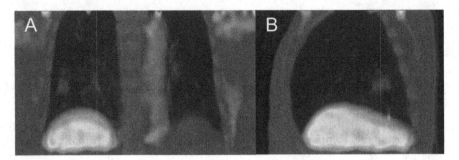

Fig. 25.1 Coronal (**a**) and sagittal (**b**) sections of thorax of a NSCLC patient in FMISO-PET/CT. The PET scan shows significant blurring and misregistration of a malignant lung lesion and the liver boundary compared with the CT scan

[1]. Intratumoral hypoxia accelerates radioresistance and chemoresistance, and thus hypoxic tumors require a 2.5–3 times radiotherapy dose to achieve the same cytotoxic effect [2]. Hypoxia may also promote metastatic spread [3].

[18]F-Fluoromisonidazole (FMISO) is a major PET tracer for hypoxia imaging. The combination of positron emission tomography (PET) and computed tomography (CT) is valuable in cancer diagnosis, follow-up, and treatment management. Previous studies have evaluated the potential role of FMISO-PET as a prognostic tool and in the assessment of the presence of tumor reoxygenation following nonsurgical treatment of NSCLC [1, 4].

However, if the tumor is located in the thorax or abdomen, the patient's breathing causes motion artifacts, resulting in misregistration between PET and CT images (Fig. 25.1) [5]. Because CT is used for attenuation correction of PET images, such misregistration affects image reconstruction. The patient's breathing leads to marked displacement of most of the internal organs, from the apical region of the lungs down to the abdominal organs. Internal organ movement has a degrading effect on image quality and quantitative values in terms of spatial resolution and contrast [6]. Respiratory gating is a technique for improving the measurement of lesion uptake and tumor volume in PET/CT [7]. Motion management is becoming an important issue in both diagnostic and therapeutic applications. A series of studies in ^{18}F-fluorodeoxyglucose PET/CT have shown that respiratory-gated (RG) 4D-PET/CT and breath-holding protocols allow compensation for image degradation and artifacts induced by respiratory movements [6]. In contrast, there has been no study in which RG FMISO-PET/CT was evaluated. We investigated the usefulness of respiratory gating in FMISO-PET/CT-based quantification of hypoxia.

25.2 Materials and Methods

25.2.1 Subjects

We examined 14 patients [8 men, 6 women; median age (range) 78 (50–90) year] with pretreatment stages I–III NSCLC (Table 25.1). None of the patients had ever

Table 25.1 Patient characteristics

Characteristic	Number/value
Male (Female)	8 (6)
Median age (range) [year]	78 (50–90)
Administered FMISO activity [MBq]	397.6 ± 15.7
T stage	
I	8
II	5
III	1
Tumor length (range) [mm]	29.3 (12.0–53.8)

received radiotherapy. The respiratory status of the patients was not considered as an exclusion criterion. All these patients gave their written informed consent to participate in this study. This study was approved by the Institutional Review Board of Hokkaido University.

25.2.2 FMISO-PET/CT Studies

PET images were acquired using a whole-body time-of-flight PET/CT scanner (GEMINI-TF; Philips). We administered 400 MBq of ^{18}F-FMISO intravenously. Four hours after injection, static emission scans with the field of view covering the entire thorax were obtained in the 3D mode. Our protocol included a 4D CT scan and a 30-min list-mode PET acquisition in one bed position centered on the primary tumor. Respiratory signals were detected using a respiratory monitor system (Philips Bellows) with a length sensor in a belt strapped around the patient's upper abdomen.

The PET scanning protocol is shown in Fig. 25.2. To reconstruct RG images, the respiratory cycle was divided into five phases of the same duration. The third phase, which corresponds to expiration, was used for reconstruction. Non-respiratory-gated (NG) images were reconstructed with 6 min of acquisition of PET data (i.e., sub-dataset of 12–18 min were extracted from the complete dataset of 30 min). For all PET image reconstructions, photon attenuation was corrected using 4D CT images. Reconstructions were performed using 3D-RAMLA (ordered subset expectation maximization).

25.2.3 Image Analysis

FMISO uptake 4 h after injection was quantified using (1) standardized uptake values (SUV = 1 g/mL X measured radioactivity X body weight/injected radioactivity), (2) tumor-to-muscle ratio (TMR), and (3) tumor-to-blood ratio (TBR). Paraspinal muscles were used as the reference muscle. Venous blood was sampled immediately before the PET/CT scanning and counted for radioactivity

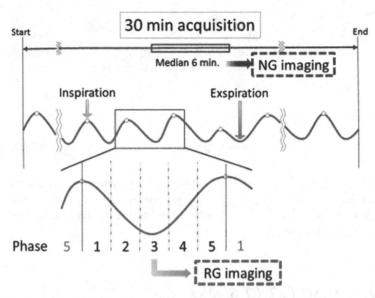

Fig. 25.2 Summary of the PET scan protocol. All the acquisitions lasted 30 min. For respiratory-gated imaging, the third phase, which corresponds to expiration, was used for reconstruction. Non-respiratory-gated images were reconstructed with 6 min of acquired PET data (i.e., 12–18 min)

using a cross-calibrated well counter. We also calculated hypoxic volume (HV) as an area TBR higher than 1.5 [8]. Patients having nonzero HV were considered as having hypoxic tumor. Differences in SUVmax, TMR, TBR, and HV between RG and NG images were statistically analyzed for significance.

25.2.4 Statistical Analysis

All results are expressed here as mean ± standard deviation (SD). A statistical paired t-test was employed to evaluate the statistical significance of the differences in SUVmax, TMR, and TBR between RG and NG. HV was compared between RG and NG images using the Wilcoxon signed-rank test because of the non-normal distribution of HV. P values smaller than 0.05 were considered statistically significant.

25.3 Results and Discussion

In all the 14 patients, the tumor was visually identifiable from its higher signal intensities than the surrounding lung tissues (Figs. 25.3 and 25.4). Quantitatively, SUVmax, TMR, and TBR were all significantly higher on RG images (1.93 ± 1.11,

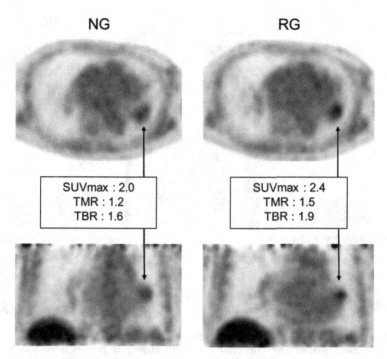

Fig. 25.3 Axial and coronal sections of NG and RG PET images of a patient with a NSCLC lesion in the left lower lobe. In addition to the difference in morphological appearances of the lesion between the NG and RG images, there are considerable increases in SUVmax, TMR, and TBR

1.46 ± 0.78, and 1.42 ± 0.87, respectively) than on NG images (2.09 ± 1.11, 1.61 ± 0.78, and 1.53 ± 0.87, respectively) (Table 25.2, Fig. 25.5).

Whereas the NG images showed tumor hypoxia in three patients, the RG images identified tumor hypoxia in two more patients (i.e., a total of 5 patients). In patients with hypoxia, HV on NG images was 12.8 ± 22.6, whereas that on RG images was 13.2 ± 22.7, which was significantly higher (Table 25.3).

The results of this study showed significant differences in various quantitative values between RG and NG. Theoretically, RG is less affected by motion artifacts, and thus the images acquired with RG are considered to be more accurate than those with NG. Our data suggest the risk of using non-respiratory gating for FMISO PET in NSCLC, because non-respiratory gating could significantly underestimate tumor hypoxia. Instead, the use of respiratory gating is recommended as a standard technique for treatments targeting a hypoxic region.

The ability to determine the degree and extent of hypoxia in NSCLC is not only important prognostically but also in the selection of candidate patients for hypoxia-modifying treatments. [9] Among different treatments, radiotherapy would most benefit from hypoxia imaging techniques. Radiobiological modeling suggests that hypoxia would have a greater impact on the efficacy of a single-large-fraction treatment than on that of fractionated treatment because of the lack of

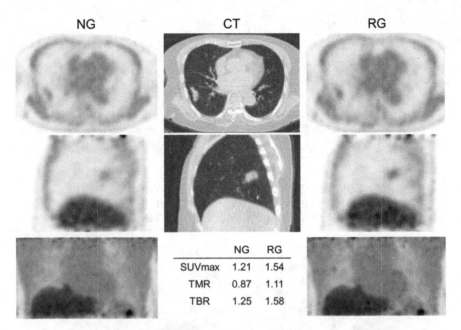

Fig. 25.4 Images of an 87-year-old female with stage II NSCLC in the right lower lobe. In non-respiratory-gated maximum intensity projection (MIP) imaging, no primary lesion was detected. However, in respiratory-gated MIP imaging, the lesion was visually detected

Table 25.2 SUVmax, TMR, and TBR of lesions on RG and NG images

	SUVmax		TMR		TBR	
	NG	RG	NG	RG	NG	RG
Mean	1.93	2.09	1.46	1.61	1.42	1.53
SD	1.11	1.11	0.78	0.78	0.87	0.86

Abbreviations: *NG* non-gating, *RG* respiratory gating, *SD* standard deviation, *SUVmax* maximum standardized uptake value, *TBR* tumor-to-blood ratio, *TMR* tumor-to-muscle ratio

reoxygenation in the former [9]. Information on tumor hypoxia may be used to modify the radiation planning, especially the treatment fraction, to maximize cytotoxic effects.

However, as mentioned above, respiratory motion during PET image quantification can introduce image misregistration errors, and if uncorrected images are acquired, such errors may eventually hinder adequate patient management [10]. As a combined treatment strategy with functional information provided by PET imaging, correction of PET images for respiratory motion artifacts may increase the efficacy of individually tailored therapy. If FMISO-PET imaging predicts local failure, then it can be used for guiding the selection of patients who would benefit from dose escalation, modification of fractionation, or additional treatment with a hypoxic cell radiosensitizer.

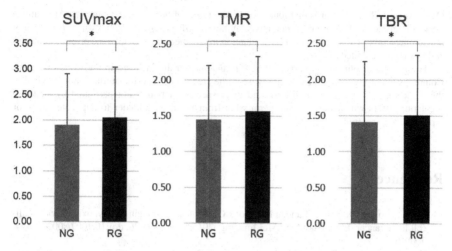

Fig. 25.5 SUVmax, TMR, and TBR were significantly higher on RG images than on NG images (*$p < 0.05$, paired *t*-test)

Table 25.3 Increase in HV with RG

Age	Sex	HV in NG	HV in RG
72	Male	0	0.19
50	Male	9.15	9.92
62	Female	52.54	53.12
85	Male	2.05	2.69
81	Male	0.00	0.13
Mean		12.8	13.2
SD		22.6	22.7

Abbreviations: *HV* hypoxic volume, *NG* non-gating, *RG* respiratory gating, *SD* standard deviation

One of the limitations of our study was the relatively small number of patients examined. Further clinical study will be required to clarify the diagnostic value of the quantitative evaluation of hypoxia with RG in association with local recurrence and prognosis.

25.4 Conclusion

Respiratory gating in FMISO-PET/CT could provide higher sensitivity of hypoxic evaluation and accurate quantification of hypoxia.

References

1. Yip C, Blower PJ, Goh V, Landau DB, Cook GJ. Molecular imaging of hypoxia in non-small-cell lung cancer. Eur J Nucl Med Mol Imaging. 2015;42(6):956–76. doi:10.1007/s00259-015-3009-6.
2. Gray LH, Conger AD, Ebert M, Hornsey S, Scott OC. The concentration of oxygen dissolved in tissues at the time of irradiation as a factor in radiotherapy. Br J Radiol. 1953;26 (312):638–48. doi:10.1259/0007-1285-26-312-638.
3. Gilkes DM, Semenza GL, Wirtz D. Hypoxia and the extracellular matrix: drivers of tumour metastasis. Nat Rev Cancer. 2014;14(6):430–9. doi:10.1038/nrc3726.
4. Cherk MH, Foo SS, Poon AM, Knight SR, Murone C, Papenfuss AT, et al. Lack of correlation of hypoxic cell fraction and angiogenesis with glucose metabolic rate in non-small cell lung cancer assessed by 18F-Fluoromisonidazole and 18F-FDG PET. J Nucl Med Off Publ Soc Nucl Med. 2006;47(12):1921–6.
5. Callahan J, Kron T, Schneider-Kolsky M, Hicks RJ. The clinical significance and management of lesion motion due to respiration during PET/CT scanning. Cancer Imaging Off Publ Int Cancer Imaging Soc. 2011;11:224–36. doi:10.1102/1470-7330.2011.0031.
6. Bettinardi V, Picchio M, Di Muzio N, Gilardi MC. Motion management in positron emission tomography/computed tomography for radiation treatment planning. Semin Nucl Med. 2012;42(5):289–307. doi:10.1053/j.semnuclmed.2012.04.001.
7. Jani SS, Robinson CG, Dahlbom M, White BM, Thomas DH, Gaudio S, et al. A comparison of amplitude-based and phase-based positron emission tomography gating algorithms for segmentation of internal target volumes of tumors subject to respiratory motion. Int J Radiat Oncol Biol Phys. 2013;87(3):562–9. doi:10.1016/j.ijrobp.2013.06.2042.
8. Okamoto S, Shiga T, Yasuda K, Ito YM, Magota K, Kasai K, et al. High reproducibility of tumor hypoxia evaluated by 18F-fluoromisonidazole PET for head and neck cancer. J Nucl Med Off Publ Soc Nucl Med. 2013;54(2):201–7. doi:10.2967/jnumed.112.109330.
9. Meng X, Kong FM, Yu J. Implementation of hypoxia measurement into lung cancer therapy. Lung Cancer (Amsterdam, Netherlands). 2012;75(2):146–50. doi:10.1016/j.lungcan.2011.09.009.
10. Grootjans W, de Geus-Oei LF, Meeuwis AP, van der Vos CS, Gotthardt M, Oyen WJ, et al. Amplitude-based optimal respiratory gating in positron emission tomography in patients with primary lung cancer. Eur Radiol. 2014;24(12):3242–50. doi:10.1007/s00330-014-3362-z.

Printed in the United States
By Bookmasters